Fundamentals of Epidemiology and Biostatistics: Combining the Basics

Ray M. Merrill, PhD, MPH, MS
Brigham Young University
Provo, Utah

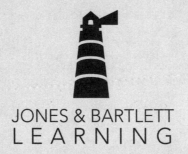

JONES & BARTLETT
LEARNING

World Headquarters
Jones & Bartlett Learning
5 Wall Street
Burlington, MA 01803
978-443-5000
info@jblearning.com
www.jblearning.com

Jones & Bartlett Learning books and products are available through most bookstores and online booksellers. To contact Jones & Bartlett Learning directly, call 800-832-0034, fax 978-443-8000, or visit our website, www.jblearning.com.

Production Credits

Publisher: Michael Brown
Managing Editor: Maro Gartside
Editorial Assistant: Chloe Falivene
Editorial Assistant: Kayla Dos Santos
Associate Production Editor: Rebekah Linga
Senior Marketing Manager: Sophie Fleck Teague
Manufacturing and Inventory Control Supervisor: Amy Bacus

Composition: Circle Graphics, Inc.
Cover Design: Michael O'Donnell
Cover Image: © Terry Chan/ShutterStock, Inc.
Printing and Binding: Edwards Brothers Malloy
Cover Printing: Edwards Brothers Malloy

To order this product, use ISBN: 978-1-4496-6753-5

Library of Congress Cataloging-in-Publication Data
Merrill, Ray M.
  Fundamentals of epidemiology and biostatistics : combining the basics / Ray M. Merrill.
      p. ; cm.
  Includes bibliographical references and index.
  ISBN 978-1-4496-4772-8 (pbk.) — ISBN 1-4496-4772-3 (pbk.)
  I. Title.
  [DNLM: 1. Epidemiologic Methods. WA 950]
  614.4—dc23
                              2011047992

6048

Printed in the United States of America
16 15 14 13 12   10 9 8 7 6 5 4 3 2

DEDICATION

To Amy Valette

CONTENTS

PREFACE

Fundamentals of Epidemiology and Biostatistics: Combining the Basics is an introductory text for students in epidemiology, clinical medicine, health policy and management, nursing, and various allied health fields. Students and professionals in all these settings should have knowledge of the basic principles of epidemiology and biostatistics. There are many subfields of public health and medical research, but epidemiology and biostatistics are fundamental to all these areas of study.

This book is intended to be used in a single course offered during a block or semester. Its primary purpose is to present the distinct and complementary roles of epidemiology and biostatistics to public health and clinical medicine in the context of substantive, interesting, and current applications. *Fundamentals of Epidemiology and Biostatistics: Combining the Basics* presents the material in a clear, concise, and accurate manner. Readers of this book will gain an appreciation of the fact that identifying, understanding, and solving public and clinical health problems often require thinking in terms of principles and practices in the areas of epidemiology and biostatistics.

Some of the special features of this book include the following:

Topics: This text includes fundamental concepts and methods that are required for a basic understanding and interpretation of epidemiology and biostatistics for public health and clinical medicine. The outline follows a logical sequence.

Substantive examples: Practical and relevant public health and clinical examples are used in each chapter.

Actual data: Many of the examples presented are based on actual data involving health-related states or events.

Assignment problems: Each chapter has a set of questions to determine students' mastery of the material.

Graphical excellence: Introductory statistical graphics that can be produced with spreadsheet or charting software are presented in order to effectively present data.

Computer applications: Computer applications using SAS are used to demonstrate data analysis throughout the book; procedure code is provided in Appendix A.

Statistical inference: Concepts of sampling, hypothesis testing, P values, and confidence intervals are presented.

Causal inference: Ways to support conclusions about cause-and-effect relationships are presented.

Structure: The book sets off definitions, historical information, and certain formulas in boxes, and key words are in italic type in order to enhance readability and strengthen prominent points.

This book has four major biostatistics themes: descriptive statistical procedures (Chapters 2–5), probability (Chapters 6 and 7), statistical inference (Chapter 8), and statistical techniques for determining appropriate sample size and assessing data (Chapters 9, 11, and 13).

In the chapters covering descriptive statistics, we define terms important in the application of epidemiology and biostatistics, present scales of measurement and ways to summarize and present nominal and ordinal data, describe two methods to standardize rates, introduce life tables, present the method for calculating years of potential life lost, and describe standard ways to summarize and present numerical data. We also introduce statistical notation and present several types of graphs that are useful for describing the distribution of health-related states and events.

In the two chapters covering probability, we introduce probability concepts, probability distributions, probability distribution for sample statistics (called sampling distributions), Bayes' Theorem, and selected sampling methods. Statistical inference is introduced in a single chapter that addresses methods for estimating population parameters and how to examine and test hypotheses. Finally, the statistical techniques part of the book includes various methods for calculating sample size for different types of research questions and selected approaches for analyzing research questions about relationships among variables and about patient survival across time.

These four major biostatistics themes play a fundamental role in conducting observational and experimental epidemiologic studies, which investigate the distribution and determinants of health-related states or events in human populations. The primary purpose of this study is to prevent and control health problems. The study design is central to epidemiology. Several study designs employed in epidemiology are introduced and described, along with the quantitative elements of these designs. Chapter 1 provides a description of the distinct yet complementary roles of epidemiology and biostatistics in public health and clinical medicine and the basic study designs used in epidemiologic research. Chapter 10 focuses on selected observational study designs, while Chapter 12 focuses on experimental study designs. Finally, because drawing conclusions about causality is critical in epidemiology for developing appropriate disease and health-related prevention and control measures, this topic concludes the book (Chapter 14). Criteria for establishing cause-and-effect relationships are discussed, and selected causal models are presented.

After completing this book, the student should be able to:

- Describe the distinct but complementary roles of epidemiology and biostatistics in public health and clinical medicine.
- Apply descriptive epidemiology and biostatistics procedures to understand and describe the distribution of health-related states or events.
- Apply probability concepts and probability distribution theory to understanding and describing health problems, identifying the efficacy of medical screening and testing procedures, and sampling in order to obtain a representative group of study participants.
- Derive estimators from a sample that is used to estimate an unknown population parameter and measure the precision in the estimators using confidence intervals.
- Apply the steps of hypothesis testing to answer research questions about means and proportions in single groups, in two independent groups in one group, in two dependent groups, in more than two independent groups, or in more than two dependent groups.
- Determine appropriate sample size and assess various types of research questions.
- Identify and apply appropriate observational or experimental study designs to answer specific public health or medical research questions.
- Estimate survival curves using the life table (actuarial) method or the product-limit (Kaplan-Meier) method and evaluate statistical significance of differences between curves using the log-rank test.
- Apply causal theory and causal criteria to identify determinants of health-related states or events.
- Apply the study of the distribution and determinants of health-related states or events to prevent and control health problems.
- Apply SAS in studying the distributions and determinants of health-related states or events in human populations.

ABOUT THE AUTHOR

Ray M. Merrill, PhD, MPH, MS, is a professor of epidemiology and biostatistics at Brigham Young University. He is also an adjunct professor in the Department of Family and Preventive Medicine and the Department of Health Promotion and Education at the University of Utah. He is a former cancer prevention fellow at the U.S. National Cancer Institute and a visiting scientist in the Unit of Epidemiology for Cancer Prevention at the International Agency for Research on Cancer, Lyon, France. He has won several awards for his research in epidemiology and is currently a fellow of the American College of Epidemiology and of the American Academy of Health Behavior. He teaches classes in epidemiology and biostatistics and is the author of over 200 peer-reviewed publications and 5 books.

CHAPTER 1

Introduction

This chapter introduces health professionals in community medicine, health policy and management, nursing, and various health fields allied to epidemiology and biostatistics. We begin by defining *health* and presenting analytic competencies fundamental to public health. We then define *epidemiology*, along with study designs and the scientific method, which are integral parts of epidemiology. *Biostatistics* is also defined, and its supportive role in epidemiology is described. The role epidemiology and biostatistics play in providing health professionals with the skills necessary to meet the analytic competencies of public health is emphasized.

HEALTH

The World Health Organization (WHO) defines *health* as a state of complete physical, mental, and social well-being and not merely the absence of disease or infirmity.[1] *Physical health* is the ability of the human body to function properly and includes physical fitness and activities of daily living; *mental health* is the ability to think clearly, reason objectively, and act properly; and *social health* is the ability to have satisfying relationships and interaction within social institutions and societal mores. In more recent years, three additional dimensions of health have been added: *emotional health* (one's ability to cope, adjust, and adapt), *spiritual health* (one's personal beliefs and choices), and *environmental health* (one's surroundings, such as habitat or occupation). The field of medicine concerned with safeguarding and improving the health of a community as a whole is *public health*.[2] Safeguarding and improving the public's health is accomplished by efforts in preventive medicine, health education, control of communicable diseases, application of sanitary measures, and monitoring environmental hazards.[3]

To meet the goals of public health, core functions have been set forth that involve assessment, policy development, and assurance.[4] Ten essential public health services have also been given.[5] The 3 core functions of public health and the 10 essential public health services categorized under the appropriate core functions are presented in **Table 1.1**. Analytic competencies for each of the 10 services are also shown in the table. Because the focus of this text is on analytic competencies in public health, other

TABLE 1.1   Competencies for the 10 Essential Public Health Services

I. Assessment

- Monitor health status to identify and solve community health problems.
- Diagnose and investigate health problems and health hazards in the community.

Analytic competencies[6]

- Define the problem.
- Determine appropriate use of data and statistical methods for problem identification and resolution, as well as program planning, implementation, and evaluation.
- Select and define variables relevant to defined public health problems.
- Evaluate the integrity and comparability of data and identify gaps in data sources.
- Understand how the data illuminate ethical, political, scientific, economic, and overall public health issues.
- Understand basic research designs used in public health.
- Make relevant inferences from data.

II. Policy development

- Inform, educate, and empower people about health issues.
- Mobilize community partnerships and action to identify and solve health problems.
- Develop policies and plans that support individual and community health efforts.

III. Assurance

- Enforce laws and regulations that protect health and ensure safety.
- Link people to needed personal health services and assure the provision of health care when otherwise unavailable.

- Define a problem.
- Make relevant inferences from data.

- Assure competent public and personal healthcare workforce.

- Determine appropriate use of data and statistical methods for problem identification and resolution, and program planning, implementation, and evaluation.

TABLE 1.1 Competencies for the 10 Essential Public Health Services (*continued*)

III. Assurance	Analytic competencies[6]
• Evaluate effectiveness, accessibility, and quality of personal and population-based health services.	• Evaluate the integrity and comparability of data and identify gaps in data sources. • Understand how the data illuminate ethical, political, scientific, economic, and overall public health issues. • Understand basic research methodologies used in public health and health services research. • Make relevant inferences from data.
• Research for new insights and innovative solutions to health problems.	• Define a problem. • Determine appropriate use of data and statistical methods for problem identification and resolution, and program planning, implementation, and evaluation. • Select and define variables relevant to defined public health problems. • Evaluate the integrity and comparability of data and identify gaps in data sources. • Understand how the data illuminate ethical, political, scientific, economic, and overall public health issues. • Understand basic research designs used in public health. • Make relevant inferences from data.

Data from: U.S. Department of Health and Human Services. The public health workforce: An agenda for the 21st century. A report of the Public Health Functions Project. http://www.health.gov/phfunctions/pubhlth.pdf. Accessed June 14, 2011.

competencies such as communication skills, policy and development/program planning skills, cultural skills, financial planning and management skills, and other basic public health skills are not listed.

Many disciplines are involved in public health research, but it rests upon a scientific core of epidemiology. Monitoring, diagnosing, and investigating disease and health-related events are primary functions of epidemiology that assist in decisions about appropriate action and identify whether progress is being made in prevention and control efforts. Biostatistical methods also play a critical

Definitions

Research is a scientific or scholarly investigation that aims to advance human knowledge.

Epidemiology is the study of the distribution and determinants of health-related states or events in specified human populations, and the application of this study to prevent and control health problems.[11]

Definitions

Surveillance is the process of observing or monitoring.

Monitoring is a process in which changes in health status over time or among populations are identified in order to recognize health problems and to assess progress toward health goals or objectives.

Diagnosing is the act or process of identifying or determining the nature of a case of a disease or distinguishing one disease from another.

Investigating is the act or process of inquiry or systematic study to discover and examine the facts so as to establish the truth.

Biostatistics is the science of statistics applied to biologic or medical data; it is a contraction of biology and statistics.

role in public health and, in particular, are fundamental to carrying out descriptive and analytic epidemiologic studies. Because epidemiology draws heavily on biostatistics, the distinction between the two is often unclear. However, there are some important differences that will be discussed in this chapter.

EPIDEMIOLOGY

The first known epidemiologist, also known as the father of medicine, is the Greek physician Hippocrates (460–377 BCE). Hippocrates addressed how selected diseases were related to time and seasons, place, environmental conditions, and especially in relation to water and the seasons. He also taught about causal factors, how diseases affect people, and how diseases spread. He classified illness as acute, chronic, endemic, and epidemic.[7–10]

The public health problem is established through observed or measured phenomena in the population of interest. Characterizing acute, chronic, endemic, and epidemic disease states and conditions according to person, place, and time factors remains an important way epidemiologists are able to identify unique features that may provide clues or evidence regarding the source of the agent and the nature of the exposure leading to given health problems.

The word *epidemiology* is based on three Greek words: *epi*, the prefix, meaning "on, upon, or befall"; *demos*, the root, meaning "the people"; and *logos*, the suffix, meaning "the study of." In accordance with medical terminology, the suffix is read first and then the prefix and the root, such that the word *epidemiology* literally means "the study of that which befalls the people." Today, *epidemiology* involves the study of the distribution and determinants of diseases and health-related events (e.g., body weight and diet). To better understand the word *epidemiology*, descriptions of the various parts of the definition are presented in **Table 1.2**.

Disease processes are complex and require that we understand biology, anatomy, physiology, histology, biochemistry, microbiology, and related medical sciences. A *disease* is any impairment of normal physiological function affecting all or part of an organism, especially a specific pathological change, which may be caused by pathogens (viruses, bacteria, fungi, or parasites capable of producing disease); chemicals

TABLE 1.2   Defining Epidemiology

Term	Description
Study	A careful examination of a phenomenon; implies sound methods of scientific investigation. Contributing factors to epidemiology include advances in biology, medicine, statistics, and social and behavioral sciences.
Distribution	Distribution refers to the frequency and pattern of a health-related state or event. Frequency is the number of occurrences of a health-related state or event; pattern involves presenting the distribution by person, place, and time characteristics.
Determinants	Determinants are factors that produce an effect, result, or consequence in another factor. A determinant is a cause. Determinants may be: • Physical stresses—excessive heat, cold, and noise; radiation (electromagnetic, ultrasound, microwave, or x-irradiation); climate change; ozone depletion; housing; and so on • Chemicals—drugs, acids, alkali, heavy metals (lead and mercury), poisons (arsenic), and some enzymes • Biological—disease-causing infectious agents or pathogens (viruses, bacteria, fungi, and parasites) • Psychosocial milieu—families and households, socioeconomic status, social networks and social support, neighborhoods and communities, access to health care, formal institutions, and public policy
Health-related states or events	*Health-related states or events* refers to the fact that epidemiology involves more than just the study of disease states; it also includes the study of events, behaviors, and conditions associated with health: • A *disease* is an interruption, cessation, or disorder of body functions, systems, or organs (e.g., cholera, angina, breast cancer, and influenza). • An *event* is something that takes place (e.g., vehicular collisions, workplace injuries, drug overdose, and suicide). • A *behavior* is a manner of conducting oneself (e.g., physical activity, diet, and safety precautions). • A *condition* is an existing circumstance (e.g., an unhealthy state, a state of fitness, something that is essential to the occurrence of something else).
Application	Application refers to the fact that the information obtained through epidemiology is applied to better prevent and control health problems.

Definitions

Epidemic refers to the occurrence of cases of an illness, specific health-related behavior, or other health-related events clearly in excess of normal expectancy in a community or region.

Endemic refers to the constant presence or usual frequency of a specific disease in a particular population; a disease is said to be endemic when it continually prevails in a region.

Pandemic is an epidemic that is extensive, involving large regions, countries, or continents.

Acute diseases or conditions are characterized by the rapid onset of symptoms that are usually severe with short duration.

Chronic diseases or conditions are long-lasting or recurrent, lasting three months or more.

(e.g., drugs, acids, heavy metals); inherent weaknesses (e.g., suppressed immune system, susceptibility gene); lifestyle (e.g., lack of physical activity, smoking, obesity); and physical stresses (e.g., radiation, extreme temperatures, workplace injuries), and is characterized by an identifiable group of signs or symptoms. The ability of a pathogen to get into a susceptible host and cause a disease is called *invasiveness*. The disease-evoking power of a pathogen is called *virulence*.

In general, diseases may be classified as congenital and hereditary diseases, allergies and inflammatory diseases, degenerative diseases, metabolic diseases, or cancer. *Congenital and hereditary diseases* are often caused by genetic and familial tendencies toward certain inborn abnormalities; injury to the embryo or fetus by environmental factors, chemicals, or agents such as drugs, alcohol, or smoking; or innate developmental problems possibly caused by chemicals or agents. They can also be a fluke of nature. Examples are Down syndrome, hemophilia, and heart disease present at birth.[12] *Allergies* and *inflammatory diseases* are caused by the body reacting to an invasion of or injury by a foreign object or substance. Allergies, viruses, bacteria, or other microscopic and microbiological agents can cause an inflammatory reaction in the body. Some inflammatory reactions may result in the body forming antibodies. Antibodies are formed as a first line of defense. They are protein substances or globulins derived from B and T lymphocytes that originate in the bone marrow.[12] *Degenerative diseases* cause a lower level of mental, physical, or moral state than is normal or acceptable. Degenerative diseases are often associated with the aging process but in some cases may not be age related. Arteriosclerosis, arthritis, and gout are examples of degenerative chronic diseases.[12] *Metabolic diseases* cause the dysfunction, poor function, or malfunction of certain organs or physiologic processes in the body, leading to disease states. Glands or organs that fail to secrete certain biochemicals to keep the metabolic process functioning in the body cause metabolic disorders. For example, adrenal glands may stop functioning properly, causing Addison's disease; the cells may no longer use glucose normally, causing diabetes; or the thyroid gland may fail, resulting in a goiter, hyperthyroidism, or cretinism (hypothyroidism).[12] *Cancer* is a collective name that refers to a group of many diseases with one common characteristic: uncontrolled cell growth or the loss of the cell's ability to perform apoptosis (cell suicide). The gradual increase in the number of uncontrolled dividing cells creates a mass of tissue called a tumor (neoplasm). When a tumor is malignant, meaning it is capable of spreading to surrounding tissue or remote places in the body, it is called cancer.[13]

Infectious diseases are caused when pathogens enter, survive, and multiply in the host. An infectious disease may or may not be contagious. Infectious disease is contagious if it is capable of being communicated or transmitted. Infectious diseases may be either acute or chronic. Noninfectious diseases are noncommunicable, but may be either acute or chronic. Health-related events are noninfectious and may be acute or chronic (**Table 1.3**).

Cancer is a disease that may be infectious or noninfectious. Although cancer is generally thought of as being lifestyle related (e.g., tobacco, diet), 10–20% of all cancer has been related to parasites, bacteria, and viruses.[14,15] For example, Epstein-Barr virus is associated with Burkitt's lymphoma, human papillomavirus is associated with cervical

TABLE 1.3 Classification of Selected Diseases

	Communicable		Noncommunicable	
	Acute	**Chronic**	**Acute**	**Chronic**
Infectious	Influenza/pneumonia	Cancer	Anthrax	
	Cholera	Leprosy	Legionnaires' disease	
	Lyme disease	Polio	Tetanus	
	Mumps	Syphilis		
	Measles	Tuberculosis		
Noninfectious			Accidents	Alcoholism
			Drug abuse	Arthritis
			Epilepsy	Cancer
			Heart attack	Cardiovascular disease
			Homicide	
			Seizures	Diabetes mellitus
			Stroke	Oral health problems
			Suicide	
				Paralysis

cancer, hepatitis B virus is associated with liver cancer, human T-cell lymphotrophic virus is associated with adult T-cell leukemia, Kaposi's sarcoma–associated herpesvirus is associated with Kaposi's sarcoma, and bacterium *H. pylori* is associated with stomach cancer. Some known inherited conditions that increase the risk of cancer include hereditary retinoblastoma linked to retinoblastoma; xeroderma pigmentosum linked to skin cancer; Wilms' tumor linked to kidney cancer; Li-Fraumeni syndrome linked to sarcomas, leukemia, and cancers involving the brain and breast; familial adenomatous polyposis linked to colorectal cancer; Paget's disease of the bone linked to bone cancer; and Fanconi's aplastic anemia linked to leukemia, and liver and skin cancers.

Each disease has a natural history of progression if no medical intervention is taken and the disease runs its full course. There is a stage of susceptibility, a stage of presymptomatic disease, a stage of clinical disease, and a stage of outcome (recovery, disability, or death). The stage of susceptibility precedes the disease and reflects the likelihood a host has of becoming ill from a given source. The stage of presymptomatic disease involves the time from exposure and subsequent pathologic changes up to the time of clinical symptoms. This time is called the incubation period. In the context of chronic disease, it is called the latency period. The stage of clinical disease is when signs and symptoms are manifest. The final stage reflects the patient's prognosis. Factors that influence these stages include primary prevention, secondary prevention, and tertiary prevention.

Understanding and influencing health-related behaviors is also complex and involves psychology, sociology, and economics. Many behavior change models are based on the idea that health education itself is not sufficient to promote behavior change. The Health Belief Model is a widely used conceptual framework for understanding health behavior.[17] In this model, behavior change requires a rational decision-making process that considers perceived susceptibility to illness, perceived consequences or seriousness of the illness, belief that recommended action is appropriate or efficacious to reduce risk, and belief that the benefits of action outweigh the costs.[18–20] Two exten-

Definitions

Primary prevention is preventing a disease or disorder before it happens through activities such as lifestyle changes; community health education; school health education; good prenatal care; good behavior choices; proper nutrition; and safe and healthful conditions at home, school, and the workplace.

Secondary prevention is aimed at the health screening and detection activities used to identify disease. It also aims to block the progression of disease or prevent an injury from developing into an impairment or disability.

Tertiary prevention consists of limiting any disability by providing rehabilitation (attempt to restore an afflicted person to a useful, productive, and satisfying quality of life) where a disease, injury, or disorder has already occurred and caused damage. Prompt diagnosis and treatment, followed by proper rehabilitation and posttreatment recovery, proper patient education, behavior changes, and lifestyle changes are all necessary to improve the patient's prognosis.[16]

TABLE 1.4 Concepts, Definitions, and Applications of the Health Belief Model		
Concept	**Definition**	**Application**
Perceived susceptibility	One's opinion of chances of getting a condition	Define population(s) at risk, risk levels; personalize risk based on a person's features or behavior; heighten perceived susceptibility if too low
Perceived severity	One's opinion of how serious a condition and its consequences are	Specify consequences of the risk and the condition
Perceived benefits	One's belief in the efficacy of the advised action to reduce risk or seriousness of impact	Define action to take; how, where, when; clarify the positive effects to be expected
Perceived barriers	One's opinion of the tangible and psychological costs of the advised action	Identify and reduce barriers through reassurance, incentives, assistance
Cues to action	Strategies to activate "readiness"	Provide how-to information, promote awareness, reminders
Self-efficacy	Confidence in one's ability to take action	Provide training, guidance in performing action

Data from: Glanz K, Marcus Lewis F, Rimer BK. *Theory at a Glance: A Guide for Health Promotion Practice.* Bethesda, MD: National Institutes of Health; 1997.

sions of these concepts in more recent years include cues to action and self-efficacy (**Table 1.4**).[21]

TRANSMISSION OF DISEASE

The ability of a disease to be transmitted from one person to another or to spread throughout the population is called *communicability.* The communicability of a disease is determined by how likely a pathogen or agent will be transmitted from a diseased or infected person to another susceptible person. Infectious communicable diseases may be transmitted vertically or horizontally. *Vertical transmission* refers to the transmission from an individual to its offspring through the placenta, milk, or vagina. *Horizontal transmission* refers to the transmission of an infectious agent from an infected individual to a susceptive contemporary.

Definitions

Fomites are objects such as clothing, towels, and utensils that can harbor a disease agent and are capable of transmitting it.

A **vector** is an invertebrate animal (e.g., tick, mite, mosquito, blood-sucking fly) that is capable of transmitting an infectious agent among vertebrates.

A **reservoir** is the habitat (living or nonliving) in or on which an infectious agent lives, grows, and multiplies and on which it depends for its survival in nature.

Zoonoses are those diseases and infections that are transmitted between vertebrate animals and humans.

A **vehicle** is a nonliving intermediary such as a fomite, food, or water that conveys the infectious agent from its reservoir to a susceptible host.

A **carrier** contains, spreads, or harbors an infectious organism.

Horizontal transmission may involve direct transmission, a common vehicle, an airborne pathogen, or a vector-borne pathogen. Examples of direct transmission include chlamydia, cytomegalovirus, genital warts, gonorrhea, herpes, intestinal parasites, scabies, and syphilis, which are caused by infectious agents passed from one person to another during sexual contact. Examples of a common vehicle include water-borne diseases caused by pathogenic microorganisms that are directly transmitted by consuming contaminated water, food-borne illness (commonly called food poisoning) caused by the consumption of a number of food-borne bacteria and viruses (e.g., *E. coli* O157:H7, salmonella), or blood-borne diseases caused mainly by parasites and viruses (e.g., malaria is one of the most common blood-borne diseases on earth, affecting nearly a half-billion people). Examples of airborne pathogens include pathogenic microorganism spread by droplet nuclei through the air by coughing, sneezing, singing, or talking (e.g., haemophilus influenza, measles, meningitis, mumps, pertussis, tuberculosis, diphtheria, plague, and varicella). Examples of vector-borne pathogens are pathogens transmitted by blood-feeding arthropods. Some vector-borne diseases include malaria, dengue, yellow fever, louse-borne typhus, plague, leishmaniasis, sleeping sickness, West Nile encephalitis, Lyme disease, Japanese encephalitis, Rift Valley fever, and Crimean-Congo hemorrhagic fever.

DESCRIPTIVE EPIDEMIOLOGY

The definition of epidemiology indicates both descriptive and analytic features. Various methods in descriptive epidemiology, which are related to "distribution" (see the definition of epidemiology), are used to monitor the health of a population, identify a public health problem and its extent, and identify unique characteristics associated with those experiencing the health problem. Thus, clues may be obtained as to the determinants of the health problem. However, it is analytic epidemiology that provides methods to test hypotheses about causal associations.

The application of epidemiologic methods to assess the distribution of health problems in human populations is the essence of descriptive epidemiology. Descrip-

History

An Irish cook, Mary Mallon (1869–1938), also called Typhoid Mary, was believed to be responsible for 53 cases of typhoid fever in a 15-year period. She was a cook who served in many homes that were stricken with typhoid. The disease followed, but never preceded, her employment. Bacteriologic examination of Mary Mallon's feces showed that she was a chronic carrier of typhoid. Mary seemed to sense that she was giving people sickness, because when typhoid appeared, she would leave with no forwarding address. Mary Mallon illustrated the importance of concern over the chronic typhoid carrier causing and spreading typhoid fever. Like 20% of all typhoid carriers, Mary suffered no illness from the disease. Epidemiologic investigations have shown that carriers might be overlooked if epidemiologic searches are limited to the water, food, and those with a history of the disease.[22,23]

tive epidemiology is used to describe the health of communities and to identify health problems and priorities according to person (who?), place (where?), and time (when?) factors (**Table 1.5**). Descriptive epidemiology also involves characterizing the nature of the health problem (what?).

Characteristics of disease cases themselves, in terms of a variety of person characteristics, may portray the uniqueness of the patient population. If a given attribute emerges as being common, at-risk groups may be identified and the idea of a specific exposure may be presented. Birthplace, workplace, community, and so on may identify differences in environmental factors that provide evidence of potential risk behaviors or factors for disease. Place characteristics may also play a role in disseminating environmental pathogens or chemical agents that may influence disease. Time plays various roles in descriptive epidemiology. Monitoring health status over time is useful for identifying and solving community health problems. Time trends can identify health problems that are endemic or epidemic. An epidemic may arise from a specific source or from infections transmitted from one infected person to another.[24] The time from the point of exposure until clinical symptoms arise is the incubation period. Knowing the incubation period of the disease can help narrow the likely cause and lead to a solution to the problem. Some examples of incubation periods are 12–36 hours for botulism, 2–3 weeks for chicken pox, 12–72 hours (usually about 24 hours) for the common cold, 1–3 days for influenza, 2 weeks or longer for rabies, 1–3 days for scarlet fever, 4–12 weeks for tuberculosis, and 7–21 days for whooping cough.[16] For chronic disease, the time from exposure to clinical symptoms is called the latency period. The latency period for several cancer types can be several years (e.g., about 20 to 25 years for smoking and lung cancer, and 40 or more years for a blistering sunburn during childhood or adolescence and melanoma of the skin). Comparing time trends of chronic disease

TABLE 1.5	Defining Descriptive Epidemiology		
Characteristic	**Question**	**Attributes**	**Examples**
Person	Who is affected?	Inherent	Age, gender, race/ethnicity, blood type, genetics, family structure
		Acquired	Immunity, marital status, education, beliefs, traditions
		Activities	Occupation, leisure, medication use, religious practices
		Conditions	Air quality, water quality, food quality, housing conditions, living conditions, safety of the environment, areas for walking and exercising, health services
Place	Where are they affected?		Birthplace, workplace, classroom, school, cafeteria, jail, country, state, county, census tract; water supplies, sewage disposal outflows, ecological habitats, air-flow patterns in buildings, prevailing wind currents, milk distribution routes
Time	When are they affected?		Epidemic curve
			Incubation period
			Secular or seasonal trend
			Latency period
			Duration of the course of the health-related state or event
			Life expectancy of the host or pathogen
Health-related state or event	What observed features distinguish the health-related state or event?		An instance of something; an occurrence
			Clinical signs and symptoms

and conditions in relation to suspected risk factors may also provide clues as to the cause of the disease.

If the duration time of the epidemic is reflected on a graph, with the vertical axis representing frequency and the horizontal axis representing time, the shape of the graph is called the epidemic curve. The time begins at the point of exposure and extends over the course of the epidemic, and may reflect hours, days, weeks, or longer. The shape of the epidemic curve reflects whether the exposure occurred at a point in time or was continuous.

A *case definition* consists of a set of criteria that identifies what is involved.[25] A standard case definition ensures that cases are consistently diagnosed, regardless of where or when they are diagnosed or by whom. If case definitions are inconsistently applied, classifying the health problem becomes problematic. A case definition may be limited according to person, place, and time criteria. Person criteria typically include clinical symptoms (e.g., diarrhea, stomach cramps, and sometimes vomiting or fever for *Salmonella* food poisoning) or clinical tests (e.g., pneumonia on chest X-ray). Place criteria may require the case be employed at a certain location, and time criteria may require that a case be diagnosed during a certain time period. For certain rare but lethal communicable diseases (e.g., plague) where a quick response is needed, a loose case definition may be appropriate. For certain other situations where a quick response is less critical and identifying causal associations is important (e.g., cancer), a stricter set of criteria for establishing the presence of the disease is warranted. The identifying features (e.g., signs, symptoms, disease progression, place and type of exposure, lab findings) will depend on the condition and disease under investigation.

> **Definition**
>
> A **case definition** in epidemiology is a set of standard criteria for diagnosing a particular disease or health-related condition, by specifying clinical criteria and limitations on person, place, and time factors.

ANALYTIC EPIDEMIOLOGY

Analytic epidemiology is the application of epidemiologic methods to study the determinants of health-related states or events in human populations. Analytic epidemiology answers questions about why and how a health-related state or event occurred. Analytic methods involve formulating and testing hypotheses about associations between exposure and outcome variables. Statistical measures of association are used, and causal theory is often employed. Analytic studies provide greater evidence than do descriptive studies to support a hypothesis of causal association.

Analytic epidemiologic study designs employ a comparison group in order to evaluate associations between exposure and outcome variables. For example, selected future health outcomes are compared between those exposed and those not exposed (cohort study), or previous exposure status is compared between cases and noncases (case-control study). Use of a comparison group is also important in evaluating the efficacy and effectiveness of prevention and control programs.[26] For

Definitions

Efficacy refers to the ability of a program to produce a desired effect among those who participate in the program compared with those who do not.

Effectiveness refers to the ability of a program to produce benefits among those who are offered the program.

A **case report** is an in-depth investigation of a problem or situation of a single individual; it includes qualitative descriptive research of the facts in chronological order.

A **case series** is a small group of patients with a similar diagnosis.

A **cross-sectional study** is a collection of data at a single point in time for each participant or system being studied. It is assumed that the phenomena of interest remain static through the period of study.

An **ecologic study** refers to aggregate data involved instead of individual-level data, such as comparing injury rates from one occupation to another.

In an **experimental study**, participants are deliberately manipulated for the purpose of studying an intervention effect. An intervention is assigned to selected participants to determine its effect on a given outcome.

example, researchers may be interested in whether the recovery time is quicker among heart attack patients who adhere to a given dietary program compared with those who do not. If those who comply with the program have much quicker recovery than those who do not comply, the dietary program is efficacious, but if the program is so strict that very few are able to adhere to it, it is not efficient.

STUDY DESIGNS

A study design is a detailed plan or approach for systematically collecting, analyzing, and interpreting data; it is a formal approach of scientific or scholarly investigation. Study designs in epidemiology are classified as descriptive or analytic. A descriptive study design is used to assess and monitor the health of communities and identify health problems and priorities according to who is affected, where they are affected, and when they were most likely affected. It also involves describing what the health problem is. These study designs include case studies, cross-sectional studies, and ecologic studies. Descriptive epidemiologic studies also lend support to more definitive evaluation using analytic methods.

Although these study designs are generally classified as descriptive, in some cases when a specific research hypothesis is formulated and cross-sectional or ecologic data is used to assess the hypothesis, we may refer to it as an analytic study.

Analytic study designs are used to test one or more predetermined hypotheses about associations between exposure and outcome variables. Analytic epidemiology provides information on how and why a health-related state or event occurred. There are both observational (i.e., the observed variables are not controlled by the investigator) and experimental (i.e., the exposure status is controlled by the investigator) study designs. For exposures that cannot be ethically assigned in an experimental study (e.g., requiring participants to smoke or not smoke cigarettes), exposure–disease relationships are better assessed in observational study designs. Analytic observational study designs include case control, cohort, case crossover, and nested case control.

Experimental (or intervention) study designs may involve a between-group design, a within-group design, or a combination of both types of designs. The strongest methodological design is a between-group design in which the outcome of interest is compared between one group receiving the intervention of interest and another group receiving no active treatment (preferably a placebo) or a currently accepted treatment. A within-group design (also called a time-series design) may also be used, but the outcome of interest is compared before and after an intervention. The between-group design is more prone to individual type confounding factors (e.g., gender, race, genetic susceptibility). The within-group design is more susceptible to confounding from time-related factors (e.g., learning effects where participants do better on follow-up cognitive tests because they learned from the baseline test, influences from the media, or other external factors).

SCIENTIFIC METHOD

Epidemiology employs the scientific method to identify and solve public health problems. The scientific method involves using appropriate study designs and statistical methods for investigating an observable occurrence and acquiring new knowledge. Descriptive epidemiologic methods are used to identify the presence of a health problem. Once the research problem is established, hypotheses are formulated to evaluate possible explanations for the health problem. Hypothesis testing is central to the scientific method. After the researcher has formulated a research hypothesis, data are collected and assessed to either support or fail to support the hypothesis. If the hypothesis is rejected, alternatives are considered. If the data are consistent with the purported hypothesis, the hypothesis is retained. Information is

---

Definitions

A **case-control study** involves grouping people as cases (persons experiencing a health-related state or event) and controls, and investigating whether the cases are more or less likely than the controls to have had past experiences, lifestyle behaviors, or exposures.

A **cohort** is a group or body of people, often defined by experiencing a common event (e.g., birth, training, or enrollment) in a given time period.

A **cohort study** involves grouping people into exposure categories (e.g., smokers versus nonsmokers) and investigating whether exposure classifications are associated with one or more health outcomes in the future.

A **case-crossover study** compares the exposure status of a case immediately before its occurrence with that of the same case at a prior time.

A **nested case-control study** is a case-control study nested within a cohort study (also called a case-cohort study).

analyzed in epidemiology in much the same way as it is analyzed in prospective laboratory experiments, but because the investigator often does not have control over the exposure and outcome measures, extra care must be taken to find convincing evidence that the hypothesized chain of events is not due to bias.

BIOSTATISTICS

Biostatistics can be thought of as having two parts, *bio*, meaning biology (the science concerned with the phenomena of life and living organisms, and in public health specifically referring to human life), and *statistics*. The word *statistics* has multiple meanings, such as data or numbers, the process of collecting and analyzing data for patterns and relationships, and the description of a field of study. Working with numbers may involve using statistical methods that summarize and describe person, place, and time factors, and applying statistical methods to draw certain conclusions that can be applied to public health. The application of statistics is broad, but when applied to biology or medicine, it is termed *biostatistics*.[24]

> **Definition**
>
> **Statistics** is the science of data and involves collecting, classifying, summarizing, organizing, analyzing, and interpreting data.

Several important individuals helped develop the use of statistics in the context of biology, including Sir Ronald A. Fisher (1890–1962), Sewall G. Wright (1889–1988), and J. B. S. Haldane (1892–1964). In 1930, Fisher published *The Genetical Theory of Natural Selection*, wherein he developed a number of basic statistical methods; Wright and Haldane used statistics in developing modern population genetics. These

> **History**
>
> Florence Nightingale (1820–1910), a British nurse, possessed one of the greatest analytical minds of her time. In 1854, Nightingale was appointed head of a contingent of nurses sent to care for soldiers in the Crimean War, where she effected changes in hospital sanitation that significantly reduced soldiers' mortality rates from illness. In 1856, Nightingale returned to England and spent the rest of her life enacting reform of army sanitation, hospitals, and a number of other public health efforts. Much of her work was accomplished through gathering and sharing statistics and writing reports and letters. She used data as a tool for improving city and military hospitals; monitored disease mortality rates, which showed that with improved sanitary methods in hospitals, the rates of death decreased; and developed applied statistical methods to display her data, showing that statistics provided an organized way of learning and improving medical and surgical practices.[33–35]

and other biostatisticians played a critical role in adding quantitative discipline to the study of biology.[27–32]

Biostatistics may be divided into four general areas: descriptive, probability, inferential, and statistical techniques. Descriptive biostatistics involves methods of organizing, summarizing, and describing numerical data relating to living organisms. A second area of biostatistics study is probability as it relates to living organisms. Probability covers random variables and probability distributions; sampling methods, sampling distributions and the central limit theorem. A third area of biostatistics involves inference about a population's characteristics from information in the sample. Finally, there are several statistical methods that are used for investigating a range of problems involving biologic data, which we refer to as statistical techniques.

Biostatistics can involve the application of statistics to any living system, whether human, animal, plant, fungus, or microorganism. On the other hand, epidemiology focuses on human populations. Hence, biostatistics within epidemiology involves the study of the frequency, patterns, and relationships of health-related states or events in human populations. However, unlike epidemiology, biostatistics does not focus on the study of determinants of health-related states or events in human populations; that is, although understanding causal processes is a primary focus in epidemiology, it is not a focus of biostatistics.

EVALUATING THE LITERATURE

The ability to access the scientific literature is vital for health professionals in order to stay current in their knowledge about disease management and prevention. Medical practitioners should read the literature to stay abreast of the most effective screening and diagnostic procedures and treatments and the most effective approach for implementing the treatments. In addition, knowledge of likely health outcomes according to specific prognostic indicators is important for counseling patients. From a disease prevention point of view, the literature indicates risk factors associated with a given health-related state or event and describes health promotion and disease prevention programs. Public health officials are often required to draw upon the literature in their health planning and decision making for establishing health programs with appropriate priorities. The literature also may guide public health professionals in carrying out health programs. Publishers ask the health professionals themselves to critically assess the articles submitted for possible inclusion in their journals. In order for an article to properly inform our health efforts and not be misleading, it must provide valid information about medicine and public health. Finally, participating in or directing research requires that we understand what is currently known about a topic before we can advance knowledge on that topic.

A review involving 585 articles in the medical literature indicated that physicians with prior training in epidemiology and biostatistics are better prepared for reading medical literature.[36] Several studies have assessed the extensive use of study designs and statistical methods in medical and health-related journals. These studies have involved biomedical journals,[37] general medical journals,[38–40] rheumatology and internal medicine journals,[41] psychiatric journals,[42] family practice journals,[43] ophthalmic journals,[44] rehabilitation literature,[45] radiology journals,[46] public health journals,[47] surgical journals,[48] and health education journals.[49] A high percentage of articles in these journals involve study designs and statistical methods. For example, Merrill and colleagues assessed the use and types of study designs and the statistical methods employed in three representative health education journals from 1994 through 2003.[49] Editorials, commentaries, program/practice notes, and perspectives represented 17.6% of the journals' content. More commonly, the articles used cross-sectional designs (27.5%), reviews (23.2%), and analytic designs (i.e., case-control, cohort, and experimental studies) (18.4%). In addition, over the study period, the use of cross-sectional study designs increased 3.3% annually and the use of analytic study designs increased 5.5% annually, whereas the use of review articles decreased by 9.3% annually. The use of statistics in the articles surveyed also showed an increasing trend (e.g., 2.4% for descriptive statistics, 4.4% for parametric test statistics, 3.5% for nonparametric test statistics, 6.8% for generalized linear models, and 6.7% for validation statistics).

Although peer-reviewed journals are often rigorously reviewed prior to acceptance and publication, almost all reported studies have limitations. In 1992, a comprehensive report involving 28 papers that examined the scientific adequacy of study design, data collection, and statistical methods of 4,235 published medical studies found that only 20% met the researcher's criteria for validity.[50] They also found that poorly designed studies were more likely to report positive findings (i.e., 80% versus 25%). In 2002, a review of 34 commonly reviewed journals found that many journals failed to report how or whether their studies dealt with confounding factors.[51] Many studies have also been shown to suffer from various statistical problems in medical research.[52–56] As health professionals, it is ultimately our responsibility to conclude whether the results of a published paper are valid.

A basic knowledge of epidemiology and biostatistics makes the medical and health-related literature accessible, such that current knowledge can be gained and applied. The content of this text will provide health practitioners with the skills they need to meet the analytic competencies listed in the outset of this chapter.

EXERCISES

1. *Health* has been defined as consisting of six interactive dimensions. Are there any of these six dimensions that are not important to your own health?
2. The 3 core public health functions involve assessment, policy development, and assurance. Relate these functions to the 10 essential public health services.
3. Define the terms *monitoring* and *diagnosing* and indicate how they are distinct and why they are important in public health.
4. It has been said that public health intervention focuses on prevention rather than treatment. What are some ways in which disease prevention may be achieved?
5. What are two ways in which epidemiology is distinct from biostatistics?
6. What is meant by the phrase "application of this study" in the definition of epidemiology?
7. Epidemiology is commonly referred to as the foundation of public health. Why?
8. With respect to treating a health problem, how would an epidemiology approach differ from a clinical approach?
9. Epidemiology involves more than just the study of disease. Explain.
10. Classify each of the following as (A) primary prevention, (B) secondary prevention, or (C) tertiary prevention.

    ____ vitamin-fortified foods
    ____ fluoridation of public water supplies
    ____ wearing protective devices
    ____ health promotion
    ____ cancer screening
    ____ lifestyle changes
    ____ physical therapy for stroke victims
    ____ halfway houses for recovering alcoholics
    ____ shelter homes for the developmentally challenged
    ____ fitness programs for heart attack patients
    ____ community health education
    ____ ensuring healthful conditions at home, school, and workplace

11. Self-efficacy is a concept of the Health Belief Model. Define this term and state where it fits in the six dimensions of health.

12. Classify the following as involving (A) direct transmission or (B) indirect transmission.

    ____ mosquito conveys the infectious agent
    ____ mucous membrane to mucous membrane (STDs)
    ____ herpes type 1 acquired from contact with an infected animal

13. In what way can a pathogen be indirectly transmitted from an infected person or animal?

14. List three common types of indirect transmission.

15. Zoonoses are diseases and infections transmitted between vertebrate animals and humans. Provide examples of direct and indirect transmission of a pathogen involving a vertebrate animal.

16. Which question does a case definition answer in descriptive epidemiology?

17. Classify each of the following as (A) descriptive epidemiology or (B) analytic epidemiology.

    ____ Identify the extent of a public health problem.
    ____ Identify the efficacy of a new drug.
    ____ Monitor the change in obesity for a given community over time.
    ____ Identify primary risk factors for disease.

18. Which descriptive study designs are observational?

19. Which analytic study design is *not* observational?

20. List the four general areas of biostatistics introduced in this chapter.

21. A primary purpose for taking a class that covers principles of epidemiology and biostatistics is to provide you with skills for reading the health literature. What are some of the ways this may be so?

REFERENCES

1. World Health Organization. Definition of health. World Health Organization. https://apps.who.int/aboutwho/en/definition.html. Accessed June 16, 2011.

2. *Dorland's Medical Dictionary for Health Consumers*. Philadelphia, PA: Saunders; 2007.

3. *The American Heritage Medical Dictionary*. Boston, MA: Houghton Mifflin Company; 2007.

4. Institute of Medicine. *The Future of Public Health*. Washington, DC: National Academy Press; 1988.

5. Centers for Disease Control and Prevention. 10 essential public health services. National Public Health Performance Standards Program (NPHPSP). http://www.cdc.gov/nphpsp/essential Services.html. Published December 9, 2010. Accessed June 16, 2011.

6. U.S. Department of Health and Human Services Public Health Service. The public health workforce: an agenda for the 21st century. A report of the Public Health Functions Project. http://www.health.gov/phfunctions/pubhlth.pdf. Published 1998. Accessed June 14, 2011.

7. Hippocrates. Airs, waters, places. In Buck C, Llopis A, Najera E, Terris M, eds. *The Challenge of Epidemiology: Issues and Selected Readings*. Washington, DC: World Health Organization; 1988:18–19.

8. *Dorland's Illustrated Medical Dictionary*. 25th ed. Philadelphia, PA: Saunders; 1974.

9. Cumston CG. *An Introduction to the History of Medicine*. New York, NY: Alfred A. Knopf; 1926.

10. Garrison FH. *History of Medicine*. Philadelphia, PA: Saunders; 1926.

11. Last JM, ed. *A Dictionary of Epidemiology*. 3rd ed. New York, NY: Oxford University Press; 1995.

12. Crowley LV. *Introduction to Human Disease*. 2nd ed. Boston, MA: Jones and Bartlett; 1988.

13. U.S. National Institutes of Health. Understanding cancer. National Cancer Institute. http://www .cancer.gov/cancertopics/understandingcancer/cancer. Published 2010. Accessed June 28, 2011.

14. Doll R, Peto R. The causes of cancer: quantitative estimates of avoidable risks of cancer in the United States today. *J Natl Cancer Inst*. 1981;66:1191–1308.

15. Doll R. Epidemiological evidence of the effects of behavior and the environment on the risk of human cancer. *Recent Results Cancer Res*. 1998;154:3–21.

16. Merrill RM. *Introduction to Epidemiology*. 5th ed. Sudbury, MA: Jones and Bartlett Publishers; 2010.

17. Prochaska JO, DiClemente CC. Stages of change in the modification of problem behaviors. *Prog Behav Modif*. 1992;28:184–218.

18. Rosenstock IM. Why people use health services. *Milbank Mem Fund Q*. 1966;44:94–127.

19. Rosenstock IM. Historical origins of the health belief model. *Health Educ Q*. 1974;2:328–335.

20. Janz NK, Becker MH. The health belief model: a decade later. *Health Educ Q*. 1984;11:1–47.

21. Glanz K, Marcus Lewis F, Rimer BK. *Theory at a Glance: A Guide for Health Promotion Practice*. Bethesda, MD: National Institutes of Health; 1997.

22. Nester EW, McCarthy BJ, Roberts CE, Pearsall NN. *Microbiology: Molecules, Microbes and Man*. New York, NY: Holt, Rinehart and Winston; 1973.

23. Health News. *Medical Milestone: Mary Mallon, Typhoid Mary*. New York, NY: New York Department of Health; November 1968.

24. *Stedman's Medical Dictionary for the Health Professions and Nursing: Illustrated 5th Edition*. New York, NY: Lippincott Williams & Wilkins; 2005.

25. *McGraw-Hill Concise Dictionary of Modern Medicine*. New York, NY: McGraw-Hill Companies, Inc.; 2002.

26. Oleckno WA. *Essential Epidemiology: Principles and Application*. Long Grove, IL: Waveland Press; 2002.

27. Hald A. *A History of Mathematical Statistics*. New York, NY: Wiley; 1998.

28. Wright S. *Evolution and the Genetics of Populations: Genetics and Biometric Foundations*. Vol. 1. New ed. Chicago, IL: University of Chicago Press; 1984.

29. Wright S. *Evolution and the Genetics of Populations: Genetics and Biometric Foundations*. Vol. 2. New ed. Chicago, IL: University of Chicago Press; 1984.

30. Wright S. *Evolution and the Genetics of Populations: Genetics and Biometric Foundations.* Vol. 3. New ed. Chicago, IL: University of Chicago Press; 1984.

31. Wright S. *Evolution and the Genetics of Populations: Genetics and Biometric Foundations.* Vol. 4. New ed. Chicago, IL: University of Chicago Press; 1984.

32. Majumder PP. Haldane's contributions to biological research in India. *Resonance.* 1998;3:32–35.

33. Cook ET. *The Life of Florence Nightingale.* Vols. 1–2. London: Macmillan; 1913.

34. Bostridge M. *Florence Nightingale: The Making of an Icon.* New York, NY: Farrar, Straus and Giroux; 2008.

35. McDonald L, ed. *Florence Nightingale: An Introduction to Her Life and Family.* Collected Works of Florence Nightingale, vol. 1. Waterloo, Ontario: Wilfrid Laurier University Press; 2001.

36. Weiss ST, Samet JM. An assessment of physician knowledge of epidemiology and biostatistics. *J Med Educ.* 1980;55(8):692–697.

37. Pilcik T. Statistics in three biomedical journals. *Physiol Res.* 2003;51:39–43.

38. Wang Q, Zhang B. Research design and statistical methods in Chinese medical journals. *JAMA.* 1998;280:283–285.

39. Colditz GA, Emerson JD. The statistical content of published medical research: some implications for biomedical education. *Med Educ.* 1985;19:248–255.

40. Emerson JD, Coldtiz GA. Use of statistical analysis in the *New England Journal of Medicine.* *N Engl J Med.* 1983;309:709–713.

41. Cardiel MH, Goldsmith CH. Type of statistical techniques in rheumatology and internal medicine journals. *Revista de Investigación Clínica.* 1995;47:197–201.

42. Miettunen J, Nieminen P, Isohanni M. Statistical methodology in general psychiatric journals. *Nordic J Psychiatry.* 2002;56:223–228.

43. Fromm BS, Snyder VL. Research design and statistical procedures used in the *Journal of Family Practice.* *J Fam Pract.* 1986;23:565–566.

44. Juzych MS, Shin DH, Seyedsadr M, Siengner SW, Juzych LA. Statistical techniques in ophthalmic journals. *Arch Opthalmol.* 1992;110:1225–1229.

45. Schwartz SJ, Sturr M, Goldberg G. Statistical methods in rehabilitation literature: a survey of recent publications. *Arch Phys Med Rehab.* 1996;77:497–500.

46. Elster AD. Use of statistical analysis in the *AJR* and *Radiology*: frequency, methods, and subspecialty differences. *AJR Am Journal Roentgenol.* 1994;163:711–715.

47. Levy PS, Stolte K. Statistical methods in public health and epidemiology: a look at the recent past and projections for the next decade. *Stat Meth Med Res.* 2000;9:41–55.

48. Reznick RK, Dawson-Saunders E, Folse JR. A rationale for the teaching of statistics to surgical residents. *Surgery.* 1987;101:611–617.

49. Merrill RM, Lindsay CA, Shields EC, Stoddard J. Have the focus and sophistication of research in health education changed? *Health Educ Behav.* 2007;34(1):10–25.

50. Williamson JW, Goldschmidt PG, Colton T. The quality of medical literature: an analysis of validation assessments. In Bailar JC, Mosteller F, eds. *Medical Uses of Statistics.* Boston, MA: Massachusetts Medical Society; 1992.

51. Mullner M, Matthews H, Altman DG. Reporting on statistical methods to adjust for confounding: a cross-sectional survey. *Ann Intern Med.* 2002;136:122–126.

52. Williams JL, Hathaway CA, Koster KL, Layne BH. Low power, type II errors, and other statistical problems in recent cardiovascular research. *Am J Physiol.* 1997;273:H487–H493.

53. Hyran M. Appropriate analysis and presentation of data is a must for good clinical practice. *Acta Neurochir Suppl.* 2002;83:121–125

54. Skovlund E. A critical review of papers from clinical cancer research. *Acta Oncol.* 1998;36:339–345.

55. Vrbos LA, Lorenz MA, Peabody EH, McGregor M. Clinical methodologies and incidence of appropriate statistical testing in orthopaedic spine literature. Are statistics misleading? *Spine.* 1993;18(8):1021–1029.

56. McCance I. Assessment of statistical procedures used in papers in the *Aust Vet J.* 1995; 72(9):322–328.

Data and Descriptive Measures

The definition of epidemiology includes the study of the distribution of health-related states or events in human populations. The word *distribution* refers to frequency and pattern. Describing and presenting the frequency and pattern of health-related states or events provides insights into the presence of a new disease or adverse health effect, the extent of the public health problem, and who is at greatest risk. In addition, an understanding of the frequency and pattern of health-related states or events is useful for informing health planning and resource allocation and identifying avenues for future research that may provide clues about causal relationships. The study of the distribution of health-related states or events in human populations is the essence of descriptive epidemiology and heavily relies on biostatistics.

Biostatistics is the science of statistics applied to biologic or medical data, wherein statistics is the science of data and involves collecting, classifying, summarizing, organizing, analyzing, and interpreting data. Epidemiology draws upon biostatistics as it applies to human populations. In this chapter, we formally define terms that are important in the application of epidemiology and biostatistics, and we present scales of measurement and ways to summarize and present nominal, ordinal, and numerical data.

DATA AND RELATED CONCEPTS

To begin, data are obtained by observing or measuring some characteristic or property of the population of interest. An object (person or thing) upon which we collect data is an experimental unit. The properties being observed or measured are called variables.

All data and the variables we measure are either quantitative or qualitative. Quantitative data are observations measured on a numerical scale and can be measured as how many, how long, how much, and so on. Examples

Definitions

Data are pieces of information and may be thought of as observations or measurements of a phenomenon of interest.

An **experimental unit** is a person or thing upon which we collect data.

A **variable** is a characteristic that varies from one observation to the next and can be measured or categorized.

Definitions

Quantitative data are observations or measurements that are numerical.

Qualitative data are observations that can only be classified into one of a group of nonnumerical categories; a general description of properties that cannot be described numerically.

of quantitative data include biometric measures such as blood pressure, cholesterol, and glucose; the number of patients a crisis center will serve during a given week; and the dose of radiation. On the other hand, qualitative data are nonnumerical and can only be classified into one of a group of categories. Examples of qualitative data include marital status, racial/ethnic classification, and place of residence.

We can also think of qualitative data as a way to describe qualities, such as hot, yellow, and longer. Qualitative research is based on an individual's, typically subjective, analysis. Among epidemiologic study designs, only the case study design is a qualitative description of the facts in chronological order. A case study design may be a case report or a case series. A *case report* involves a description of a single individual whereas a *case series* involves a description of a small number of cases with a similar diagnosis. The case study design may be thought of as a snapshot description of a problem or situation for an individual or group. The case study is useful for providing in-depth descriptions of the disease state, providing clues about a new disease or adverse health effect resulting from an exposure or experience, and identifying potential areas of new research. However, conclusions stemming from a case study are limited to the individual, group, and/or context under study and cannot be used to establish a causal relationship.

History

A case report involved a description of a 74-year-old woman who experienced airway obstruction when a piece of meat became lodged in her trachea.[1] The patient became unconscious as a bystander unsuccessfully applied the Heimlich maneuver. However, the Heimlich maneuver was again attempted while the woman was in a supine position, this time successfully. The woman was then taken to the emergency room, where it was discovered that a 2-cm rupture occurred in the lesser curvature of her stomach. Contusions were also identified over the fundus and posterior stomach. Surgery corrected the problem, and she was discharged six days after later, with no complications from the surgery. The value of this case study was to emphasize that gastric perforation and other complications may result from the Heimlich maneuver, and that patients treated with the Heimlich maneuver should be evaluated for such problems.

A case series occurred from October 4, 2001, to November 2, 2001, when 10 cases of inhalational anthrax were identified in the United States. These cases were intentionally caused by the release of *Bacillus anthracis*. Epidemiologic investigation identified that the outbreak involved cases in the District of Columbia, Florida, New Jersey, and New York. The *B. anthracis* spores were delivered through the mail in letters and packages. The ages of the cases ranged from 43 to 73 years, with 70% being male, and all but one were confirmed to have handled a letter or package containing *B. anthracis* spores. The incubation period ranged from 4 to 6 days. Symptoms at the onset included fever or chills, sweat, fatigue or malaise, minimal or nonproductive cough, dyspnea, and nausea or vomiting. Blood tests and chest radiographs were also used to further characterize symptoms.[2] An understanding of the symptoms that characterize inhalational anthrax cases may result in earlier diagnosis of future cases.

Case series may also identify the emergence of a new disease or epidemic if the disease exceeds what is expected. For instance, on June 4, 1981, the Centers for Disease Control (CDC) published a report that described five young men, all active homosexuals, who were treated for biopsy-confirmed *Pneumocystis carinii* pneumonia at three different hospitals in Los Angeles, California, during the period from October 1980 to May 1981. This was the first report of a disease that a year later would be called acquired immune deficiency syndrome (AIDS).[3] Descriptive epidemiologic studies to follow indicated that the agent causing AIDS was transmitted through homosexual behavior,[4,5] heterosexual behavior,[6,7] and blood (needle sharing among drug users and blood transfusions),[8–10] and from mothers with AIDS to their infants.[11]

POPULATIONS, SAMPLES, AND RANDOM SAMPLING

When we examine epidemiologic data, we do so because the data characterize some phenomenon of interest. The data set that represents the target of interest is called a population. Since epidemiology focuses on human populations, the population refers to a group of people where the individuals share one or more observable personal or observational characteristics from which data may be collected and evaluated. Social, economic, family (marriage and divorce), work and labor force, and geographic factors are examples of what may characterize populations. In biostatistics, the population is not limited to people, and in statistics, the population is not limited to living organisms; however, when epidemiology applies biostatistics, it involves human populations.

Many populations are too large to observe or measure because of time and cost. Thus, we are often required to select a subset of values from the population. Inferences about the population are then made, based on information contained in the sample. A sample is always smaller than the population. Some advantages of studying samples instead of populations are that they can be studied

> **Definitions**
>
> A **population** is a set or collection of items of interest in a study. In public health, where the focus is on human populations, a population refers to a collection of individuals who share one or more observable personal or observational characteristics from which data may be collected and evaluated.
>
> A **sample** is a subset of items that have been selected from the population.

more quickly and at lower cost, it may be impossible to access the entire population, and sample results may be more accurate than results based on a population.

The most common type of sampling procedure is a random sample. Random sampling is used to obtain a representative subgroup of the population. The method of random sampling is relatively easy to implement if the population is small, but it becomes more difficult with larger populations. With larger populations, we can only approximate random sampling. Most epidemiologic studies involving random selection rely on statistical software packages (e.g., Excel, SAS, SPSS, Minitab) with random number generators to automatically obtain the random sample.

> **Definition**
>
> A **random sample** is a sample in which every element in the population has an equal chance of being selected.

SCALES OF MEASUREMENT

The scale in which a characteristic is measured has implications for the way the information is summarized and displayed. The scale of measurement involves the precision with which a characteristic is measured, which also determines the methods for summarizing, organizing, and analyzing the data. There are three scales of measurement used in epidemiology: nominal, ordinal, and numerical. A list of these measurement scales, along with selected statistics and graphs used to evaluate this data, are presented in **Table 2.1**. A description of the different statistics and graphs will be presented later in this chapter.

The nominal scale is sometimes called qualitative observations because it describes a quality of a person or thing being studied. It may also be called a categorical observation because the levels of the variable fit into categories. A nominal scale variable is dichotomous (binary) if it has two levels, or multichotomous if it has more than two levels. If there was an outbreak of cholera, you could determine case status (nominal data) and identify the number of cases in the defined area (discrete data). If you were interested in assessing the risk of death from leukemia according to the level of radiation exposure, death from leukemia (yes, no) is nominal data, and dose of radiation exposure is continuous data. We could group the exposure level into exposed or unexposed to radiation (nominal data) or no exposure, low exposure, medium exposure, and high exposure (ordinal data).

SUMMARIZING AND PRESENTING NOMINAL AND ORDINAL DATA

Data must be summarized before they can be used as a basis for making inferences about some phenomenon under investigation. Tabular and graphic formats are generally known as empirical frequency distributions. Tabular and graphic empirical frequency distributions are useful for describing data or extracting information from a set of data.

TABLE 2.1 Scales of Measurement				
Scale	**Description**	**Example**	**Statistics**	**Graphs**
Nominal	Qualitative observations or categorical observations	Sex, race, marital status, education status, exposed (yes, no), disease (yes, no)	Frequency Relative frequency	Contingency tables Bar chart Spot map Area map
Ordinal	Qualitative observations or categorical observations	Preference rating (e.g., agree, neutral, disagree) Rank-order scale	Frequency Relative frequency	Bar chart
Numerical	Quantitative observations. There are two types: continuous (interval), which has values on a continuum, and discrete scales, which has values equal to integers.	Dose of ionizing radiation Number of fractures	Geometric mean Arithmetic mean Median Mode Range Variance Standard deviation Coefficient of variation	Bar chart (for discrete data) Histogram or frequency polygon Box plot Stem-and-leaf plot

It is often of interest for a set of data to identify the pattern or grouping into which the data fall. A *frequency table* or distribution is the number of observations (e.g., cases) falling into each of several values or ranges of values (e.g., time periods). Frequency distributions are portrayed as a frequency table or graph. The strength of a frequency distribution table is that it allows us to readily see the overall pattern of the data, and it easily communicates information.

For nominal or ordinal data, we present the number of values in the data set that fall in each level of the variable. Along with frequencies reported for each level of the variable, relative frequencies are often presented in the table. *Relative frequency* is the proportion of cases that fall into each level of the variable.

Definitions

A **frequency distribution** is a tabular summary of a set of data that shows the frequency or number of data items that fall in each of several distinct classes. A frequency distribution is also known as a frequency table.

The **relative frequency** of a category is the frequency of that category divided by the total number of observations, where n is the total number of observations (i.e., the sample size).

$$Relative\ frequency = \frac{Frequency}{n}$$

A **proportion** is the number of observations with the characteristic of interest divided by the total number of observations. It is used to summarize counts.

A **rate** is a number of cases of a particular outcome divided by the size of the population in that time period, multiplied by a base (e.g., 100, 1,000, 10,000, or 100,000).

EXAMPLE 2.1

In a study involving attitudes about smoking prevention and control responsibilities and behaviors among physicians in Jordan, the level of agreement with several statements was of interest (**Table 2.2**).[12]

Combining the frequency of cases (nominal scale variable) for a selected time interval with the corresponding at-risk population produces a rate. A *rate* is calculated by summing the frequency of cases during a specified time period and then dividing the total number of cases by the population at risk of becoming a case. Deriving rates for different subgroups of the population (e.g., age, sex, geographic area, and exposure history) can assist us in identifying high-risk groups and provide clues about causality. Such information is a prerequisite to the development and targeting of appropriate prevention and control measures.

The purpose of the *rate base* (which is a multiple of the rate by 10 to the nth power) is to help us better understand, interpret, and communicate the result of our calculations.

EXAMPLE 2.2

Suppose the proportion of people with access to health care in a given population is 0.75. If we multiply this value by 100, we can say that 75 out of every 100 people (i.e., 75%) have access to health care.

EXAMPLE 2.3

In 2008, the rate of malignant female breast cancer in 17 cancer registries in the United States was 0.00134.[13] By multiplying the rate by 100,000, we can say that 134 per 100,000 women were diagnosed with breast cancer in the United States. You may agree that expressing the rate per 100 (previous example) or 100,000 (this example) is a preferred way to communicate the information.

TABLE 2.2	Level of Agreement with Selected Statements Related to Smoking and Health and Physician Responsibilities as Role Models for Their Patients among 251 Physicians in Amman, Jordan, 2006		
	Number	**Relative frequency**	**Percentage of all participants**
Smoking in enclosed public places should be prohibited			
Strongly agree	185	0.74	74
Agree	63	0.25	25
Disagree	3	0.01	1
Physicians should routinely advise their smoking patients to quit smoking			
Strongly agree	137	0.55	55
Agree	103	0.41	41
Disagree	11	0.04	4
Patient's chances of quitting smoking are increased if a health professional advises him or her to quit			
Strongly agree	65	0.26	26
Agree	88	0.35	35
Disagree	98	0.39	39

Data from: Merrill RM, Madanat H, Layton JB, Hanson CL, Madsen CC. Smoking prevalence, attitudes, and perceived smoking prevention and control responsibilities and behaviors among physicians in Jordan. *Int Q Community Health Educ.* 2006–2007;26(4):397–413.

In addition to a rate, which is a proportion relative to time, we summarize and describe case data using a *ratio*, which is a relationship between two quantities, expressed as the quotient of one divided by the other. The ratio is particularly useful in epidemiology as we compare the risk of disease according to selected groups.

EXAMPLE 2.4

In 17 cancer registries in the United States in 2008, there were 41,154 cases of malignant prostate cancer in whites and 6,635 cases in blacks. These frequencies become much more meaningful when we compare them with the respective white and black male populations. The population for white males was 30,349,061, and the population for black males was 4,335,504.[13] The incidence rates of prostate cancer for white and black males are:

$$Rate_W = \frac{41,154}{30,349,061} = 0.00136$$

$$Rate_B = \frac{6,635}{4,335,504} = 0.00153$$

Definitions

A **ratio** is a part divided by another part. It is the number of observations with the characteristic of interest divided by the number without the characteristic of interest.

Vital statistics are quantitative data concerning the important events in human life or the conditions and aspects affecting it, such as births, deaths, marriages, migrations, health, and disease.

In order to make these incidence rates more interpretable, we can multiply them by a rate base. In this situation, 100,000 appears to be an appropriate value. Hence, the malignant prostate cancer incidence rate in whites was 136 per 100,000, and for blacks it was 153 per 100,000. The ratio of the incidence rate in blacks to the incidence rate in whites is 1.125; that is, the rate is 1.125 times (12.5%) greater in blacks than whites.

Quantitative data concerning a population—such as the number of births, marriages, and deaths; health; and disease—are referred to as vital statistics. There are several statistical measures involving births, deaths (mortality), and illness (morbidity). Originally, mortality and birth data were more readily available, but over the past century, diagnosis and reporting have improved such that morbidity statistics are becoming more and more common. In this section, selected morbidity, mortality, and birth measures are presented according to their numerator, denominator, and rate base (**Table 2.3**). Each of these measures involves the same general formula, where x refers to cases, y refers to the sample or population, and n is a whole number of 0 or greater:

$$\frac{x}{y} \times 10^n$$

EXAMPLE 2.5

In the 17 cancer registries in the United States in 2008, there were 43,318 cases of malignant breast cancer in white females and 5,074 in black females. The population for white females was 30,416,622, and the population for black females was

TABLE 2.3	Measures of Morbidity		
Measure	**Numerator (*x*)**	**Denominator (*y*)**	**Expressed per number at risk (rate base)**
Incidence rate	Number of new cases of a specified disease reported during a given time interval.	Estimated population at midinterval	Varies
Attack rate (also called cumulative incidence rate)	Number of new cases of a specified disease reported during an epidemic period.	Population at start of the epidemic period	Usually 100
Secondary attack rate	Number of new cases of a specified disease among contacts of known cases.	Size of contact population at risk	Usually 100
Person-time rate (also called incidence density rate)	Number of new cases reported during a given time interval.		
Prevalence proportion	Number of current cases, new and old, of a specified disease at a given point in time; a measure that reflects incidence, death (or survival), and cure; indicates the burden of a health problem.	Estimated population at the same point in time	Usually 100

4,672,358.[13] The population values were mid-year estimates on July 1, 2008. The incidence rates of breast cancer for white and black females are:

$$Rate_W = \frac{43,318}{30,416,622} \times 100,000 = 142 \; per \; 100,000$$

$$Rate_B = \frac{5,074}{4,672,358} \times 100,000 = 109 \; per \; 100,000$$

The ratio of the incidence rate in whites to the incidence rate in blacks is 1.303. In other words, the malignant breast cancer incidence rate in whites is 1.303 times (30.3%) greater than that in blacks.

The incidence rate is commonly used to describe the risk of chronic health-related states or events, whereas the attack rate is used to reflect the risk of acute health-related states or events. In epidemiology, an attack rate is the cumulative incidence of illness in a group of people observed over a short period of time, usually in relation to an infectious agent. The cumulative incidence of illness in a group of clinically exposed people during a short period of time may be referred to as a clinical attack rate (i.e., percent of people clinically exposed who get sick).

EXAMPLE 2.6

Suppose in a small community of 460 residents, 87 attended a social event that included a meal prepared by several individuals. Within three days, 39 of those who attended the event became ill with a condition diagnosed as *Salmonella enterocolitis*. The *attack rate* among attendees was:

$$\frac{39}{87} \times 100 = 44.8 \; per \; 100$$

A secondary attack rate is useful for identifying the contagious nature of a disease.

EXAMPLE 2.7

Suppose in a community of 4,320, public health authorities found 120 persons with condition X in 80 households. A total of 480 persons lived in the 80 affected households. Assuming that each household had only one primary case, the *secondary attack rate* is:

$$\frac{120 - 80}{480 - 80} \times 100 = \frac{40}{400} \times 100 = 10 \; per \; 100$$

In some situations, it is more accurate to add up the time people are at risk instead of the number of people. Workers at a factory may work full time, part time, or overtime. Since we only want to include the time people are at risk in the denominator of a rate calculation, we might want to consider the time people worked per week.

EXAMPLE 2.8

Suppose 300 workers were employed at a given company. In this company, 75% of the employees worked 40 hours per week and 25% worked 20 hours per week. During a given week, 105 of the employees complained of respiratory problems. What is the *person-time rate* of respiratory problems?

$$\frac{105}{300(40 \times 0.75 + 20 \times 0.25)} \times 100 = \frac{105}{10500} \times 100 = 1 \; per \; 100 \; hours \; worked$$

Prevalence is a statistic that is useful for describing the magnitude of a public health problem at a point in time. The measure of burden is also more commonly used than the incidence rate for assessing diseases where it is difficult to identify when they became a case (e.g., arthritis or diabetes). Prevalence is a dynamic measure reflecting the influences of incidence, mortality, and cure; that is, new cases add to the prevalent pool of cases until they either die or recover. For some diseases where it is difficult to say that someone has recovered, they may be considered a prevalent case until death. This is the approach taken by the United States National Cancer Institute.[14]

EXAMPLE 2.9

In 2009 in Texas, 385,900 out of 1,754,091 adults self-reported having been told by a doctor that they had arthritis.[15] The *prevalence proportion* is:

$$\frac{385,900}{1,754,091} \times 100 = 22 \ per \ 100$$

The prevalence proportion for men was 18% ($n = 1,488,000$), and the prevalence proportion for women was 27% ($n = 2,371,000$). The prevalence of arthritis for women was 1.5 times (or 50%) greater than the prevalence for men.

Many mortality measures are used in epidemiology (**Table 2.4**). The first and most basic measure of death is the crude mortality rate. The word *crude* is used because it is not adjusted for age or other factors.

EXAMPLE 2.10

In 2007, the number of deaths in the United States was 1,203,812 for males and 1,219,699 for females. The corresponding mid-year population estimates were 148,466,361 and 152,823,971, respectively.[13] The male and female *mortality rates* are:

$$Rate_M = \frac{1,203,812}{148,466,361} \times 100,000 = 811 \ per \ 100,000$$

$$Rate_F = \frac{1,219,699}{152,823,971} \times 100,000 = 798 \ per \ 100,000$$

Cause-specific death rates are also of primary interest.

TABLE 2.4   Measures of Mortality

Measure	Numerator (x)	Denominator (y)	Expressed per number at risk (rate base)
Mortality rate	Total number of deaths reported during a given time interval	Estimated midinterval population	1,000 or 100,000
Cause-specific death rate	Number of deaths assigned to a specific cause during a given time interval	Estimated midinterval population	100,000
Proportional mortality ratio	Number of deaths assigned to a specific cause during a given time interval	Total number of deaths from all causes during the same time interval	100
Death-to-case ratio	Number of deaths assigned to a specific disease during a given time interval	Number of new cases of that disease reported during the same time interval	100
Infant mortality rate	Number of deaths under 1 year of age during a given time interval	Number of live births reported during the same time interval	1,000
Maternal mortality rate	Number of deaths assigned to pregnancy-related causes during a given time interval	Number of live births reported during the same time interval	100,000
Maternal mortality ratio	Number of deaths of women during or shortly after a pregnancy	100,000 live births	
Abortion rate	Number of abortions done during a given time interval	Number of women ages 15–44 during the same time interval	1,000

EXAMPLE 2.11

In 2007 in the United States, the *mortality rate* from suicide and self-inflicted injuries was:

$$Rate_M = \frac{27,264}{148,466,361} \times 100,000 = 18.4 \ per \ 100,000$$

$$Rate_F = \frac{7,328}{152,823,971} \times 100,000 = 4.8 \ per \ 100,000$$

Thus, the rate was 3.8 times (280%) greater for males than for females.[13]

EXAMPLE 2.12

In 2007, the *mortality rate* from homicide and legal intervention was:

$$Rate_M = \frac{14,919}{148,466,361} \times 100,000 = 10.0 \ per \ 100,000$$

$$Rate_F = \frac{3,829}{152,823,971} \times 100,000 = 2.5 \ per \ 100,000$$

Thus, the rate was 4.0 times (300%) greater for males than for females.[13]

EXAMPLE 2.13

The *proportional mortality ratio* in 2007 in the United States for diabetes mellitus was:

$$\frac{71,380}{2,423,511} \times 100 = 2.9 \ per \ 100$$

Thus, the percentage of deaths attributed to diabetes mellitus out of all deaths occurring in the U.S. population in 2007 is 2.9.[13]

The death-to-case ratio has historically been used to measure acute infectious diseases. However, it can also be used in poisonings, chemical exposures, or other short-term deaths not caused by disease. It has limited usefulness in the study of chronic disease because the time of onset may be hard to determine and the time of diagnosis to death is longer. Thus, the number of deaths in a current time period may have little relationship to the number of new cases that occur. An exception might include very lethal diseases such as pancreatic cancer.

EXAMPLE 2.14

In Hawaii, the *death-to-case ratio* for pancreatic cancer in 2007 was:

$$\frac{155}{195} \times 100 = 79.5 \ per \ 100$$

Thus, the death-to-case ratio for pancreatic cancer in Hawaii is about 80%.[13]

The infant mortality rate is a commonly used health status indicator of populations and a key measure of the health status of a community or population. This measure represents prenatal and postnatal nutritional care or the lack thereof. Declining infant mortality in developing countries has been linked primarily with affordable health services, improvements in the status of women, nutrition standards, universal immunization, and the expansion of prenatal obstetric services.[16]

EXAMPLE 2.15

In the United States in 2010, the *infant mortality rate* was[17]:

$$\frac{253,380}{4,223,000} \times 100 = 6 \; per \; 100$$

The maternal mortality rate is a general indicator of the overall health of a population. It further represents the status of women in society and the functioning of the healthcare system. This indicator is influenced by general socioeconomic conditions; unsatisfactory health conditions related to sanitation, nutrition, and care preceding the pregnancy; incidence of the various complications of pregnancy and childbirth, and availability and utilization of healthcare facilities, including prenatal and obstetric care.

Complications during pregnancy and childbirth are a leading cause of death and disability among women of reproductive age in developing countries. The maternal mortality ratio is a related measure that represents the risk associated with each pregnancy (i.e., the obstetric risk). It is a useful measure for evaluating the quality of the healthcare system.

EXAMPLE 2.16

The world estimated maternal mortality ratio in 2008 by region was[18]:

$$Rate_{Developed \; Regions} = \frac{1,700}{12,142,857} \times 100,000 = 14 \; per \; 100,000 \; live \; births$$

$$Rate_{Developing \; Regions} = \frac{355,000}{122,413,793} \times 100,000 = 290 \; per \; 100,000 \; live \; births$$

The deliberate termination of a pregnancy before the fetus is capable of living outside the womb is an induced abortion.

History

Edgar Sydenstricker (1881–1936) was an epidemiologist who helped advance the study of disease statistics. The development of a morbidity statistics system in the United States was quite slow. One problem was that morbidity statistics cannot be assessed and analyzed in the same manner that mortality (death) statistics can. Sydenstricker struggled with the mere definition of sickness and recognized that to all persons, disease is an undeniable and frequent experience. Birth and death come to a person only once, but illness comes often. This was especially true in Sydenstricker's era, when sanitation, public health, microbiology, and disease control and prevention measures were still being developed.[19]

In the early 1900s, morbidity statistics of any given kind were not regularly collected on a large scale. Interest in disease statistics came only when the demand for them arose from special populations and when the statistics would prove useful socially and economically. Additionally, Sydenstricker noted that there were barriers to collecting homogeneous morbidity data in large amounts. These obstacles included differences in data collection methods and definitions, time elements, and the existence of peculiar factors that affect the accuracy of all records.[19]

Sydenstricker suggested that morbidity statistics should be classified into five general groups in order to be of value: reports of communicable disease; hospital and clinical records; insurance, industrial establishment, and school illness records; illness surveys; and records of the incidence of illness in a population continuously or frequently observed.[19]

Under the direction of the United States Public Health Service, Sydenstricker and his colleagues conducted a morbidity study in the years 1921 to 1924. The study involved 1,079 individuals who were observed for 28 months. The study found that only 5% of illnesses were of short duration of 1 day or less, and that 40% were not only disabling but caused bed confinement as well. It was also discovered that the illness rate was 100 times the annual death rate. In addition, morbidity was shown to vary by age. Incidence of 4 or more attacks of illness in a given year was highest in children aged 2–9 years (45%) and lowest in those aged 20–24 years (11%). By age 35, the rate rose again, to 21%. When severity of illness was looked at, it was found that the greatest resistance to disease was in children between 5 and 14 years. The lowest resistance to disease was in early childhood, 0–4 years, and toward the end of life.[19,20]

EXAMPLE 2.17

The *abortion rate* in the United States in 2008 was[21]:

$$\frac{1,212,350}{61,935,767} \times 1,000 = 19.6 \; per \; 1,000 \; women \; aged \; 15–44 \; years$$

Selected measures of natality are presented in **Table 2.5**. The birth rate is the nativity or childbirths per 1,000 people per year. In general, the birth rate is based on birth counts from a universal system of registration of births, deaths, and marriages, and population estimates from a census. The birth rate is commonly combined with death rates and migration rates to estimate population growth. Birth rates of 10 to 20 per 1,000 are considered low, whereas birth rates from 40 to 50 per 1,000 are considered high. A low birth rate may cause stress on a society because there are fewer people of working age to

TABLE 2.5	Measures of Natality		
Measure	**Numerator (x)**	**Denominator (y)**	**Expressed per number at risk (rate base)**
Birth rate	Number of live births reported during a given time interval	Estimated total population at midinterval	1,000
Fertility rate	Number of live births reported during a given time interval	Estimated number of women ages 15–44 (or sometimes 15–49) years at midinterval	1,000
Rate of natural increase	Number of live births minus the number of deaths during a given time interval	Estimated total population at midinterval	1,000

support the aging population. On the other hand, a high birth rate can cause stress on a society as an increasing number of children require education and jobs as they enter the workforce. There are also environmental challenges that a large population can produce.

The numerator and denominator for calculating the crude birth rate is given in Table 2.5.

EXAMPLE 2.18

In 2009, the United States' *birth rate* was[22]:

$$\frac{4,131,019}{306,001,407} \times 1,000 = 13.5 \ per \ 1,000$$

The birth rate varied considerably by race/ethnicity. For example, the rate per 1,000 was 11.0 for non-Hispanic whites, 15.8 for non-Hispanic blacks, 13.9 for American Indian or Alaska Natives, 16.2 for Asians or Pacific Islanders, and 20.6 for Hispanics.[22]

The fertility rate represents the number of live births per 1,000 women of child-bearing age.

EXAMPLE 2.19

In the United States, the 2009 *fertility rate* was[22]:

$$\frac{4,131,019}{61,934,318} \times 1,000 = 66.7 \ per \ 1,000$$

The fertility rate per 1,000 women was 58.5 for non-Hispanic whites, 68.9 for non-Hispanic blacks, 62.8 for American Indian or Alaska Natives, 68.7 for Asians or Pacific Islanders, and 93.3 for Hispanics.[22]

The rate of natural increase is the crude birth rate minus the crude death rate of a population. If we ignore migration, a positive rate of natural increase means the population increased, and a negative number means the population decreased.

EXAMPLE 2.20

The *rate of natural increase* in the United Kingdom in 2011 was[17]:

$12 - 9 = 3$ *per* 1,000

On the other hand, the rate of natural increase in Russia in 2011 was:

$11 - 16 = -5$ *per* 1,000

The 2011 estimated world birth rate was 19 per 1,000, and the estimated death rate was 8 per 1,000. Hence, the natural increase was 11 per 1,000.[23]

SUMMARIZING AND PRESENTING NUMERICAL DATA

Frequency distribution tables presented earlier in this chapter also apply to numerical data. For example, a frequency distribution table is presented for a discrete variable in **Table 2.6**. The number of children that make up the classes and frequencies associated with each class are shown. Also presented in the table are relative frequencies (the proportion of cases in each class divided by the total frequencies). Cumulative values of the frequencies and relative frequencies are also informative.

TABLE 2.6 Frequency Distribution of the Number of Children among 20 Women			
Number of children	Frequency	Relative frequency	Percentage of all women
0	4	0.2	20
1	8	0.4	40
2	4	0.2	20
3	2	0.1	10
4 or more	2	0.1	10
Total		1.0	100

To construct a frequency distribution for continuous data, we select the number of classes, the class interval or width of the classes, and the class boundaries or the values that form the interval for each class. Then we count the number of values in the data set that fall in each class.

Steps for Constructing a Frequency Distribution

1. Determine the *number of classes* as the integer that exceeds the value for the approximate number of classes. To approximate the number of classes:

$$[2 \times (\textit{Size of the data set})]^{0.3333}$$

2. Determine the *class interval or width* as the larger value than the approximate width that is determined as:

$$\frac{\text{Highest value} - \text{Lowest value}}{\text{Number of classes}}$$

3. Determine the *class boundaries*. The lower boundary for the first class is an arbitrary value below the lowest data value. Then find the upper boundary for the first class by adding the class width. Find the boundaries for each remaining class by successively incrementing by the class width. The classes should cover all of the actual data values so that each data point falls into a distinct class.

4. Present the *frequency* for each class in the table.

EXAMPLE 2.21

Suppose we wanted to construct a frequency distribution of ages for 50 students 18 to 33 years. Step 1 gives 5; step 2 gives 3; and steps 3 and 4 give **Table 2.7.**

TABLE 2.7   Frequency Distribution for 50 Students According to Age Group

Class limits	Class boundaries	Class frequency	Relative frequency	Percentage of all students
18–20	17.5–20.5	18	0.36	36
21–23	20.5–23.5	12	0.24	24
24–26	23.5–26.5	11	0.22	22
27–29	26.5–29.5	8	0.16	16
30–33	29.5–33.5	1	0.02	2
Total		50	1.00	100

TABLE 2.8 Measures of Central Location	
Measure	Description
Arithmetic mean	Arithmetic average of a distribution of data
Geometric mean	The *n*th root of the product of *n* observations
Median	The middle value in an ordered array of data; if an ordered array has an even number of observations, average the two middle values
Mode	Number or value that occurs most frequently in a distribution of data

To summarize and describe numerical scale data, we use measures of central location and dispersion. A measure of central location is a single value that best represents a group of persons who are described in a frequency distribution. Common measures of central location are presented in **Table 2.8**.

The value of the geometric mean will always be less than or equal to the arithmetic mean. The *geometric mean* is more appropriate than the arithmetic mean for describing proportional growth, both exponential (constant proportional growth) and varying growth. If the frequency distribution of data is normally distributed, then the *arithmetic mean* is the preferred measure of central tendency. If the data distribution is skewed to the right or left, then the median or the mode is preferred.

A *measure of dispersion* is the spread or variability in a distribution of data. It is used to describe how much the individuals in a frequency distribution vary from each other and from the measure of central location. Biological measurements are particularly susceptible to variation from one person to another, from one observer to another, or within an individual from one point in time to another. As with measures of central location, there are several measures of dispersion that are useful in studying biological data (**Table 2.9**).

Before presenting the formulas for the measures presented in Tables 2.8 and 2.9, consider that a *parameter* is a measurement on the population level, but a *statistic* is a measurement on the sample level. Measures on the population level are fixed and invariant characteristics of the population. However, in samples, the observed measure is an estimate of the population measure. We customarily use Greek letters for population parameters and Roman letters for sample statistics. For example,

Definition

A **normal probability distribution** plots all of its values in a symmetrical fashion, and most of the results are situated around the probability's mean. Values are equally likely to plot either above or below the mean. Grouping takes place at values that are close to the mean and then tails off symmetrically away from the mean.

TABLE 2.9 Measures of Dispersion

Measure	Description
Range	Difference between the largest (maximum) and smallest (minimum) values of a frequency distribution
Interquartile range	The central portion of the distribution, calculated as the difference between the third quartile and the first quartile
Variance	Mean of the squared differences of the observations from the mean
Standard deviation	The square root of the variance
Standard error	The standard deviation divided by the square root of n
Coefficient of variation	A measure of relative spread in the data; a normalized measure of dispersion of a probability distribution that adjusts the scales of variables so that meaningful comparisons can be made

the population mean is denoted by μ and the sample mean is denoted by $\overline{X}$. Basic statistical notations in presented as follows:

Statistical Notation
Variables are denoted by capital letters (e.g., X, Y, and Z)
n = the number of observations in a *sample*
N = the number of observations in a *population*
X_i = the ith observation
X_l = the lowest observation
X_n = the highest observation in a sample
X_N = the highest observation in a population
f_i = frequency of X_i
f = total number of observations in an interval
Σ = sum

Population and statistical forms of the various measures are presented as follows.

Arithmetic Mean

$$\mu = \sum_{i=1}^{N} \frac{X_i}{N} \qquad \overline{X} = \sum_{i=1}^{n} \frac{X_i}{n} \qquad \overline{X} = \sum_{i=1}^{n} f_i \frac{X_i}{n}$$

EXAMPLE 2.22

Calculate the mean for the following sample of ages: 21, 18, 25, 31, 30, 30, and 29.

$$\overline{X} = \sum_{i=1}^{7} \frac{X_i}{n} = (21+18+25+31+30+30+29)/7 = 26.3$$

EXAMPLE 2.23

For the following data, calculate the mean.

$$\overline{X} = \sum_{i=1}^{17} f_i \frac{X_i}{n} = (3 \times 24 + 7 \times 25 + 5 \times 26 + 2 \times 27)/17 = 25.4$$

X_i	f_i
24	3
25	7
26	5
27	2

Geometric Mean

$$GM = \sqrt[n]{(X_1)(X_2)\dots(X_n)}$$

EXAMPLE 2.24

Suppose you were monitoring the level of *Enterococci* bacteria per 100 mL of sample over time and obtained the following data: 5 ent./100 mL, 25 ent./100 mL, 50 ent./100 mL, 1,000 ent./100 mL. Calculate the geometric mean for this data.

$$GM = \sqrt[4]{5 \times 25 \times 50 \times 1,000} = 50$$

Median

1. Arrange the observations in increasing or decreasing order.
2. Find the position of the 2nd quartile (i.e., 50th percentile).

$$Position\ Q_2 = \frac{(n+1)}{2}$$

3. Identify the X_i value that corresponds with the 2nd quartile. If a quartile lies on an observation, the value of the quartile is the value of that observation. If a quartile lies between observations, the value of the quartile is the value of the lower observation plus the upper observation divided by 2.

$$Midrange\ (most\ types\ of\ data) = \frac{(X_1 + X_n)}{2}$$

EXAMPLE 2.25

Suppose we are interested in the median for the data in Example 2.22. Ordering these data give the following: 18, 21, 25, 29, 30, 30, and 31. Because there are 7 observations, the position for the 2nd quartile is 4:

$$\text{Position } Q_2 = \frac{(7+1)}{2} = 4$$

Then, the 2nd quartile position corresponds with the value 29; that is,

18, 21, 25, 29, 30, 30, 31

If the number 32 were added to this data set, then the middle position would be:

$$\text{Position } Q_2 = \frac{(8+1)}{2} = 4.5$$

This corresponds with the value 29.5; that is,

$$\frac{29+30}{2} = 29.5$$

In epidemiology, we often deal with data in five-year age groups (0–4, 5–9, 10–14, etc.). To calculate the median age for a given interval of ages, apply the following formula:

$$\frac{(Beginning\ age\ in\ interval + Ending\ age\ in\ interval + 1)}{2}$$

This will be important to know when we calculate, later in this chapter, years of potential life lost for data where age is grouped into five-year intervals instead of presented by single year.

EXAMPLE 2.26

Calculate the median age for those in the age group 0–4.

$$\frac{(0+4+1)}{2} = 2.5$$

The number 1 is added to include those who are between ages 4 and 5.

Mode

To find the mode, arrange the data into a frequency distribution, showing the values of the variable (X_i) and the frequency (f_i) with which each occurs.

EXAMPLE 2.27

In the table shown in Example 2.23, 25 is the mode because its corresponding frequency of 7 is greater than any other frequency.

Range

$$X_N - X_1 \text{ or } X_n - X_1$$

EXAMPLE 2.28

For the data set 18, 21, 25, 29, 30, 30, 31, the range is $31 - 18 = 13$. In reporting the range, it is informative to also identify the minimum and maximum values used to compute the range; that is, the range is 13 (18 to 31).

Interquartile Range

1. Arrange the observations in increasing or decreasing order.
2. Find the positions of the 1st quartile (i.e., the 25th percentile) and the 3rd quartile (i.e., the 75th percentile).

   $$Position\ Q_1 = \frac{(n+1)}{4}$$

   $$Position\ Q_3 = \frac{3(n+1)}{4}$$

3. Identify the X_i values that correspond with the 1st and 3rd quartiles. If a quartile lies on an observation, the value of the quartile is the value of that observation. If a quartile lies between observations, the value of the quartile is the value of the lower observation plus the specified fraction of the difference between the observations.

EXAMPLE 2.29

For the ages 18, 21, 25, 29, 30, 30, and 31:

$$Position\ Q_1 = \frac{(7+1)}{4} = 2$$

$$Position\ Q_3 = \frac{3(7+1)}{4} = 6$$

The positions 2 and 6 correspond with the values 21 and 30:

18, 21, 25, 29, 30, 30, 31

So the interquartile range is 9 (21 to 30).

Variance

$$\sigma^2 = \frac{1}{N}\sum_{i=1}^{N}(X_i - \mu)^2$$

$$s^2 = \frac{1}{n-1}\sum_{i=1}^{n}(X_i - \overline{X})^2$$

$$s^2 = \frac{1}{\left(\sum_{i=1}^{n}f_i - 1\right)}\sum_{i=1}^{n}f_i(X_i - \overline{X})^2$$

Note that an intuitive reason for dividing the sample sum of squares by $n-1$ instead of N is because the range over which the sample values are spread is smaller than that for which the population is spread. Dividing by $n-1$ gives a better estimate of the population variance than $n-2$ or $n-3$ or some other divisor.

EXAMPLE 2.30

For our sample of ages 18, 21, 25, 29, 30, 30, and 31, the sample variance is:

$$s^2 = \frac{1}{7-1}([18-26.3]^2 + [21-26.3]^2 + [25-26.3]^2 + [29-26.3]^2$$

$$+ [30-26.3]^2 + [30-26.3]^2 + [31-26.3]^2) = 25.9$$

EXAMPLE 2.31

For the data in Example 2.23, the sample variance is computed as:

$$s^2 = \frac{1}{([3+7+5+2]-1)}(3[24-25.4]^2 + 7[25-25.4]^2 + 5[26-25.4]^2$$

$$+ 2[27-25.4]^2) = 0.87$$

The variance is a measure of variability that is used to calculate the standard deviation. The standard deviation is used in statistical tests and confidence intervals.

Standard Deviation

$$\sigma = \sqrt{\sigma^2} = \sqrt{\frac{1}{N} \sum_{i=1}^{N} (X_i - \mu)^2}$$

$$s = \sqrt{s^2} = \sqrt{\frac{1}{n-1} \sum_{i=1}^{n} (X_i - \overline{X})^2}$$

$$s = \sqrt{s^2} = \sqrt{\frac{1}{\left(\sum_{i=1}^{n} f_1 - 1\right)} \sum_{i=1}^{n} f_i (X_i - \overline{X})^2}$$

EXAMPLE 2.32

For the variance computed in Example 2.30, the standard deviation is simply:

$$s = \sqrt{25.9} = 5.1$$

Standard Error (SE) of the Mean

$$SE = \frac{\sigma}{\sqrt{N}}$$

$$SE = \frac{s}{\sqrt{n}}$$

The standard error is a statistic that applies to sampling distributions.

EXAMPLE 2.33

Continuing with Example 2.32,

$$SE = \frac{5.1}{\sqrt{7}} = 1.9$$

Coefficient of Variation

$$CV = \frac{\sigma}{\mu} \times 100$$

$$CV = \frac{s}{\overline{X}} \times 100$$

EXAMPLE 2.34

For the sample of data in Example 2.22, the coefficient of variation is:

$$CV = \frac{5.1}{26.3} \times 100 = 19.4$$

For the sample of data in Example 2.23, the coefficient of variation is:

$$CV = \frac{0.93}{25.4} \times 100 = 3.7$$

A comparison indicates that the relative variation in the first age group is much greater than that in the second age group.

EXERCISES

1. Epidemiology has a population focus. What is the meaning of *population?*
2. Classify the following as (A) nominal data, (B) ordinal data, (C) discrete data, or (D) continuous data.

    ____ integers of counts that differ by fixed amounts, with no intermediate values possible

    ____ measurable quantities not restricted to taking on integer values

    ____ ordered categories or classes

    ____ unordered categories or classes

3. Classify the following as either (A) quantitative or (B) qualitative data.

    ____ age

    ____ hometown

    ____ cholesterol level

    ____ eye color

    ____ number of siblings

4. Which type of study design is qualitative?
5. List some possible advantages of collecting and studying a sample as opposed to a population.
6. Complete the following frequency distribution table, which involves the number of children for 20 women.

Number of children	Frequency	Relative frequency	Cumulative frequency	Cumulative relative frequency
0	4			
1	8			
2	4			
3	2			
4+	2			

7. The following fraction is a(n):
   A. ratio
   B. proportion
   C. attack rate
   D. mortality rate

   $$\frac{\text{\# Women in the United States who died from breast cancer in 2012}}{\text{\# Women in the United States who died from ovarian cancer in 2012}}$$

8. The following fraction is a(n):
   A. ratio
   B. proportion
   C. attack rate
   D. mortality rate

   $$\frac{\text{\# Men in the United States who died from cancer in 2012}}{\text{\# Men in the United States who died in 2012}}$$

9. The following fraction is a(n):
   A. ratio
   B. proportion
   C. incidence rate
   D. mortality rate

   $$\frac{\text{\# Women in the United States who died from myocardial infarction in 2012}}{\text{\# Women in the United States population, midyear in 2012}}$$

10. In a recent survey, investigators found that the prevalence of disease A was higher than that of disease B. The seasonal pattern of both diseases is similar. Which factors may explain the higher prevalence of disease A?

11. In a community of 460 residents, 63 individuals attended a church social event that included a meal prepared by some of the members. Within 3 days, 34 of those attending the social became ill with a condition diagnosed as salmonellosis. Calculate the attack rate.

12. Which of the following is not true of a rate in epidemiology?

    A. The cases in the numerator are included in the denominator.

    B. The cases in the denominator must be at risk of being in the numerator.

    C. Subjects in the numerator and denominator must cover the same time period.

    D. The numerator must consist of disease cases.

13. Classify each of the following as (A) prevalence, (B) cumulative incidence rate, or (C) incidence density rate.

    ____ person-time rate

    ____ attack rate

    ____ reflects incidence, survival, cure

    ____ measure of burden

14. In a study concerned with the possible effects of air pollution on the development of chronic bronchitis, the following data were obtained. A population of 9,000 men aged 45 years was examined in January 2007. Of these, 6,000 lived in areas that exposed them to air pollution and 3,000 did not. At this examination, 90 cases of chronic bronchitis were discovered, with 60 among those exposed to air pollution. All the men initially examined who did not have chronic bronchitis were available for subsequent repeated examinations during the next 5 years. These examinations revealed 268 new cases of chronic bronchitis in the total group, with 61 among those unexposed to air pollution. Calculate (A) the prevalence proportion of chronic bronchitis as of January 2007, (B) the incidence rate (per 1,000) of chronic bronchitis for the 5 years among those exposed to air pollution, (C) the incidence rate (per 1,000) of chronic bronchitis for the 5 years among those unexposed to air pollution, and (D) the incidence rate (per 1,000) of chronic bronchitis for the 5 years among those in the total population.

15. Referring to the previous problem, how much greater is the rate among those who were exposed compared with those not exposed?

16. The Centers for Disease Control and Prevention (CDC) estimates that over 700,000 persons in the United States acquire gonorrheal infections each year, with roughly half being reported to the CDC. In 2006, 358,366 new cases of gonorrhea were reported to the CDC. The 2006 midyear U.S. civilian population was estimated to be 298,754,819.[24] For this data, we will use a value of 10^5 for 10^n. Calculate the 2006 gonorrhea incidence rate for the United States and interpret your findings.

17. Seven cases of hepatitis A occurred among 70 children attending a child-care center. Each infected child came from a different family. The total number of persons in the 7 affected families was 32. One incubation period later, 5 family members of the 7 infected children also developed hepatitis A. Calculate the attack rate in the child-care center and the secondary attack rate among family contacts of those cases and interpret your findings.

18. Of 6,000 employees at a given company, 350 experienced an injury while on the job in a given week. Of the 6,000 employees, 470 were on vacation that week, 5,000 worked 40 hours, 78 worked 50 hours per week, and the rest worked 20 hours per week. What is the person-time rate of injuries? Interpret your findings.

19. How many classes should the frequency distribution have if it contained 250 data items?

20. Suppose your data set contains BMI values that range from 18.5 to 41.9. What is the width of each class and the class boundaries, assuming you want the class interval to be an integer value?

21. The following represent the percentages of adults at least 20 years of age in 10 counties in New Jersey, in 2008, who are estimated to be physically inactive, based on survey data from the Behavior Risk Factor Surveillance System[25]: 28.2, 29.1, 26.1, 22, 22.8, 24.5, 26.7, 24.9, 22.3, and 28.7. Calculate the arithmetic mean, median, mode, variance, standard deviation, standard error, range, interquartile range, and coefficient of variation for this sample.

22. The computational formula for the standard deviation is:

$$SD = \sqrt{\dfrac{\sum X^2 - \dfrac{\left(\sum X\right)^2}{n}}{n-1}}$$

Show that the value you get applying this formula is the same as the formula introduced in the chapter for deriving the standard deviation, based on the data in the previous problem.

REFERENCES

1. Fearing NM, Harrison PB. Complications of the Heimlich maneuver: case report and literature review. *J Trauma.* 2002;53:978–979.

2. Jernigan JA, Stephens DS, Ashford DA, et al. Bioterrorism-related inhalational anthrax: the first 10 cases reported in the United States. *Emerg Infect Dis.* 2001;7(6):933–944.

3. Centers for Disease Control and Prevention. Pneumocystis pneumonia—Los Angeles. *MMWR.* 1981;30:250.

4. Centers for Disease Control and Prevention. A cluster of Kaposi's sarcoma and *Pneumocystis carinii* pneumonia among homosexual male residents of Los Angeles and Orange counties, California. *MMWR.* 1982;31:305–307.

5. Jaffe HW, Choi K, Thomas PA, et al. National case-control study of Kaposi's sarcoma and *Pneumocystis carinii* pneumonia in homosexual men: part 1, epidemiologic results. *Ann Intern Med.* 1983;99:145–151.

6. Centers for Disease Control and Prevention. Immunodeficiency among female sexual partners of males with acquired immune deficiency syndrome (AIDS)—New York. *MMWR.* 1983;31:697–698.

7. Harris C, Small CB, Klein RS, et al. Immunodeficiency in female sexual partners of men with the acquired immunodeficiency syndrome. *N Engl J Med.* 1983;308:1181–1184.

8. Centers for Disease Control and Prevention. *Pneumocystis carinii* pneumonia among persons with hemophilia A. *MMWR.* 1982;31:365–367.

9. Centers for Disease Control and Prevention. Possible transfusion-associated acquired immune deficiency syndrome (AIDS)—California. *MMWR.* 1982;31:652–654.

10. Centers for Disease Control. Acquired immune deficiency syndrome (AIDS): precautions for clinical and laboratory staffs. *MMWR.* 1982;31:577–580.

11. Centers for Disease Control and Prevention. Unexplained immunodeficiency and opportunistic infections in infants—New York, New Jersey, and California. *MMWR.* 1982;31:665–667.

12. Merrill RM, Madanat H, Layton JB, Hanson CL, Madsen CC. Smoking prevalence, attitudes, and perceived smoking prevention and control responsibilities and behaviors among physicians in Jordan. *Int Q Community Health Educ.* 2006–2007;26(4):397–413.

13. Surveillance, Epidemiology, and End Results (SEER) Program (www.seer.cancer.gov). SEER*Stat Database: Mortality—All COD, Aggregated with State, Total U.S. (1969–2007) <Katrina/Rita Population Adjustment>, National Cancer Institute, DCCPS, Surveillance Research Program, Cancer Statistics Branch. Underlying mortality data provided by NCHS. www.cdc.gov/nchs. Published June 2010. Accessed July 10, 2011.

14. Surveillance, Epidemiology, and End Results (SEER) Program. Cancer prevalence. http://seer.cancer.gov/statistics/types/prevalence.html. Published April 11, 2011. Accessed August 4, 2011.

15. Centers for Disease Control and Prevention. Arthritis. http://www.cdc.gov/arthritis/data_statistics/state_data_list.htm#texas. Published August 24, 2011. Accessed August 4, 2011.

16. Golding J, Emmett PM, Rogers IS. Breast feeding and infant mortality. *Early Hum Dev.* 1997;49 (Suppl):S143–S155.

17. U.S. Census Bureau. International programs. http://www.census.gov/population/international/data/idb/country.php. Accessed August 4, 2011.

18. WHO, UNICEF, UNFPA, and the World Bank. Trends in maternal mortality: 1990 to 2008. http://whqlibdoc.who.int/publications/2010/9789241500265_eng.pdf. Published 2010. Accessed August 4, 2011.

19. Sydenstricker E. A study of illness in a general population. *Public Health Rep.* 1926;61:12.

20. Sydenstricker E. Sex difference in the incidence of certain diseases at different ages. *Public Health Rep.* 1928;63:1269–1270.

21. Johnston, R. Historical abortion statistics, United States. http://www.johnstonsarchive.net/policy/abortion/ab-unitedstates.html. Published January 17, 2011. Accessed August 4, 2011.

22. Hamilton BE, Martin JA, Ventura SJ. Births: preliminary data for 2009. National vital statistics reports. Vol. 59, no. 3. National Center for Health Statistics. http://www.cdc.gov/nchs/data/nvsr/nvsr59/nvsr59_03.pdf. Published December 21, 2010. Accessed July 24, 2011.

23. Ross, S. The harvest fields statistics 2011. http://www.wholesomewords.org/missions/greatc.html#birdatrate. Accessed August 4, 2011.

24. Centers for Disease Control and Prevention. Gonorrhea. http://www.cdc.gov/std/stats06/gonorrhea.htm. Published November 13, 2007. Accessed December 20, 2011.

25. Centers for Disease Control and Prevention. County-level estimates of leisure-time physical inactivity. http://www.cdc.gov/diabetes/pubs/inactivity.htm. Published May 20, 2011. Accessed December 20, 2011.

CHAPTER 3

Standardizing Rates

A *rate* is the number of cases of a given outcome of interest that occurs over a specified period of time divided by the population at risk of becoming a case during that same time period. It is typically multiplied by a base 10^n (where $n = 1, 10, 100, 1,000$, etc.) in order to make the rate easier to interpret and communicate. A rate is more informative than just the number of cases because it takes into account the size of the population from which the cases derive.

A *crude rate* is a single number computed as a summary measure for an entire population. Rates that are derived in relatively small, well-defined subgroups are called *specific rates*. A problem that can occur when crude rates for different groups are compared is when the populations vary substantially with respect to characteristics such as age and gender. For example, if two populations have vastly different age distributions, we would not be sure whether differences in incidence and mortality rates are due to location or the effect of age. In this situation, age is referred to as a *confounder*; that is, because it is related to both location and the rates, it obscures the true relationship between these factors.

Anytime a health outcome of interest is related to age, if the age distribution differs between or among the groups being compared, the rates should be standardized to avoid bias from confounding. Similarly, within a group where disease rates are monitored over time, if the disease is associated with age and the age distribution changes over time, the rates should be standardized. When there is no difference in the age distribution among groups being compared or within a group being monitored over time, even though the health outcome of interest may be associated with age, age standardizing the rates for the groups is not necessary.

The purpose of this chapter is to present two methods for standardizing rates: the direct and indirect methods.

AGE-SPECIFIC RATES

Age-group specific death rates of diabetes mellitus in the United States in 2007, for males according to racial classification, are shown in **Table 3.1**.[1] Death rates are strongly associated with age, and the age distribution differs among racial groups. For example, 62% of whites, 73% of blacks, and 71% of other racial groups are aged 0–44 years. In this situation, it is more accurate to compare age-group specific death rates among the racial groups rather than their overall crude rates. The age-group specific rates are much higher for blacks than for whites or other racial groups. For example, in the age group 55–64 years, the death rates for diabetes mellitus are 128% higher in blacks compared with whites and 155% higher in blacks compared with other racial groups. In the age group 65 years and older, blacks have a 66% higher death rate than whites and 97% higher death rate than other racial groups.

Although subgroup-specific rates provide a more accurate comparison among populations than do the crude rates when confounding is an issue, many subgroup comparisons can quickly become overwhelming. Thus, it would be convenient to summarize the subgroup-specific rates into a single value that adjusts for the differences in the potential confounder. In the next section, we introduce the direct method of standardization.

DIRECT METHOD OF STANDARDIZATION

An *age-standardized rate*, also called an *age-adjusted rate*, is a weighted average of the age-group specific rates where the weights are the proportions of persons in the corresponding age groups of a standard population. The first step in applying this technique is to choose the standard population. The standard population is the population that provides the reference age distribution. For the diabetes mellitus data, we will use the white population. This choice is somewhat arbitrary; however, it is a good idea to select the larger population as the standard. We then calculate the number of cases that would have occurred among blacks and other racial groups, assuming that each had this standard population distribution while retaining its own individual age-specific diabetes mellitus death rates (**Table 3.2**). The expected numbers of cases for each group are obtained by multiplying the population by the rate and dividing by 100,000.

The age-adjusted diabetes mellitus death rate for each racial group is then calculated by dividing its total expected number of cases by the total of the standard population.

TABLE 3.1 Death Rates for Diabetes Mellitus among Males in the United States According to Racial Groups, 2007

Age	White			Black			Other		
	Population	Cases	Rate*	Population	Cases	Rate*	Population	Cases	Rate*
0–44	75,003,454	1,174	1.57	13,825,421	452	3.27	6,262,955	60	0.96
45–54	17,974,205	2,591	14.42	2,452,158	795	32.42	1,166,936	127	10.88
55–64	13,507,752	5,091	37.69	1,503,828	1,293	85.98	770,535	260	33.74
65+	14,072,083	19,877	141.25	1,260,925	2,949	233.88	666,109	789	118.45
Total	120,557,494	28,733	23.83	19,042,332	5,489	28.83	8,866,535	1,236	13.94

*Expressed per 100,000

Data from: Surveillance, Epidemiology, and End Results (SEER) Program (www.seer.cancer.gov). SEER*Stat Database: Mortality–All COD, Aggregated with State, Total U.S. (1969–2007) <Katrina/Rita Population Adjustment>, National Cancer Institute, DCCPS, Surveillance Research Program, Cancer Statistics Branch, released June 2010. Underlying mortality data provided by NCHS (www.cdc.gov/nchs). Accessed August 2, 2011.

TABLE 3.2	Expected Cases of Diabetes Mellitus Using the Direct Method				
	White	**Black**		**Other**	
Age	**Population**	**Rate***	**Expected Cases**	**Rate***	**Expected Cases**
0–44	75,003,454	3.27	2,453	0.96	720
45–54	17,974,205	32.42	5,827	10.88	1,956
55–64	13,507,752	85.98	11,614	33.74	4,558
65+	14,072,083	233.88	32,912	118.45	16,668
Total	120,557,494		52,806		23,902

*Expressed per 100,000

Data from: Surveillance, Epidemiology, and End Results (SEER) Program (www.seer.cancer.gov). SEER*Stat Database: Mortality–All COD, Aggregated With State, Total U.S. (1969–2007) <Katrina/Rita Population Adjustment>, National Cancer Institute, DCCPS, Surveillance Research Program, Cancer Statistics Branch, released June 2010. Underlying mortality data provided by NCHS (www.cdc.gov/nchs). Accessed August 2, 2011.

$$Rate_B = \frac{52,806}{120,557,494} \times 100,000 = 43.80 \; per \; 100,000$$

$$Rate_O = \frac{23,902}{120,557,494} \times 100,000 = 19.83 \; per \; 100,000$$

These age-adjusted rates are the diabetes mellitus death rates for men that would apply if all racial groups had the same age distribution as the white population. After controlling for the effect of age in this manner, we see that the higher death rates of diabetes mellitus for blacks compared with whites are much more pronounced, and that the rates are more similar between whites and other racial groups.

Had we selected the black population or the other racial group population as the standard, we would have obtained different death rates for diabetes mellitus. However, this is not important because the adjusted rate is a hypothetical construct with no meaning by itself. It is simply a construct that is based on a hypothetical standard distribution. It does not reflect the true death rate of any population, whereas the crude death rate does. These rates are only meaningful when we are comparing two or more groups. Notice, however, that we chose one of the three populations as the standard. In general, the selected standard population should not deviate much from the groups being compared. In situations in which annual rates are age adjusted over several years, it is best to apply a population as the standard that lies within the years being considered. The actual standard year does not matter as much because the standard will affect the level of the trend, but not the trend itself.[2]

INDIRECT METHOD OF STANDARDIZATION

This approach is taken when age-group specific rates are unstable because of small numbers or when there are missing numbers. The indirect method of age-adjustment involves selecting a standard population, calculating the age-specific rates for the standard population, multiplying the age-specific rates by the age-specific population values in the comparison populations to obtain the expected number of health-related states or events in each age group, and then dividing the total number of health-related states or events observed in the comparison population by the total number of expected health-related states or events. This ratio is referred to as the *standardized morbidity ratio* (SMR) (or *standardized mortality ratio*, when deaths are being considered).

$$SMR = \frac{Observed}{Expected}$$

Interpreting SMR

SMR = 1   *The health-related states or events observed were the same as expected from the age-specific rates in the standard population.*

SMR > 1   *More health-related states or events were observed than expected from the age-specific rates in the standard population.*

SMR < 1   *Fewer health-related states or events were observed than expected from the age-specific rates in the standard population.*

To illustrate, we again use the diabetes mellitus data.[1] However, this time we calculate the number of deaths that would have occurred in the black and other races population subgroups if each had taken on the age-specific death rates of the white population (**Table 3.3**). The expected numbers of cases among blacks and other racial groups are calculated by multiplying the age-specific rates for whites by the populations for the corresponding subgroups and dividing by 100,000.

The next step is to divide the observed number of deaths from diabetes mellitus in the black and other racial groups by the total expected number of impairments. The resulting value is the SMR.

TABLE 3.3	Expected Cases of Diabetes Mellitus Using the Indirect Method				
	Whites	**Black**		**Other**	
	Rate*	**Population**	**Expected Cases**	**Population**	**Expected Cases**
0–44	1.57	13,825,421	217	6,262,955	98
45–54	14.42	2,452,158	354	1,166,936	168
55–64	37.69	1,503,828	567	770,535	290
65+	141.25	1,260,925	1,781	666,109	941
Total	23.83	19,042,332	2,919	8,866,535	1,497

*Expressed per 100,000

Data from: Surveillance, Epidemiology, and End Results (SEER) Program (www.seer.cancer.gov). SEER*Stat Database: Mortality–All COD, Aggregated with State, Total U.S. (1969–2007) <Katrina/Rita Population Adjustment>, National Cancer Institute, DCCPS, Surveillance Research Program, Cancer Statistics Branch, released June 2010. Underlying mortality data provided by NCHS (www.cdc.gov/nchs). Accessed August 2, 2011.

$$SMR_B = \frac{5,489}{2,919} = 1.88$$

$$SMR_O = \frac{1,236}{1,497} = 0.83$$

These SMRs indicate that blacks have an 88% greater diabetes mellitus death rate than the white population, whereas the other racial group has a death rate that is 17% lower than that of the white population.

USES OF STANDARDIZED RATES

Standardized rates, particularly age-adjusted rates, are commonly used for monitoring trends in vital statistics and chronic diseases and conditions. The crude death rate in the United States has decreased approximately 15.8% from 1969 to 2007 (**Figure 3.1**). However, the age distribution has varied considerably during this time period. For instance, in 1969, 24.3% of the population was aged 50 years or older, whereas in 2007, this value was 30.4%. Applying the direct method of age adjustment, using the 2000 U.S. population as the standard, gives the second trend line on the graph. This trend line represents a 40.8% decrease in rates from 1969 to 2007. In other words, the

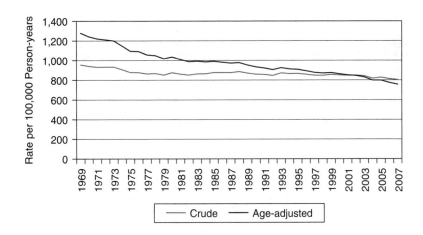

FIGURE 3.1 Trend in all cause death rates in the United States, 1969–2007. Footnote: Rates age-adjusted to the 2000 U.S. population (19 age groups—Census P25-1130).
Data from: Surveillance, Epidemiology, and End Results (SEER) Program (www.seer.cancer.gov). SEER*Stat Database: Mortality—All COD, Aggregated with State, Total U.S. (1969–2007) <Katrina/Rita Population Adjustment>, National Cancer Institute, DCCPS, Surveillance Research Program, Cancer Statistics Branch, released June 2010. Underlying mortality data provided by NCHS (www.cdc.gov/nchs). Accessed August 2, 2011.

decrease in death rates is much more pronounced when we account for changes in the age distribution over these years. Hence, to remove the confounding effect of a changing age distribution over time, we can age-adjust the rates.

The influence of cancer (**Figure 3.2**) on the decreasing death rates is much smaller than that of heart disease (**Figure 3.3**). For cancer, the age-adjusted death rate increased, peaked in about 1991, and then decreased. The age-adjusted cancer death rate decreased 10.3% from 1969 through 2007, whereas the crude rate increased by 16.8% during this time period. The age-adjusted heart disease death rate decreased 63.5% during these years, and the crude heart disease death rate decreased by 44.3% over the study period.

Applying the direct method of age adjustment to rates over time assumes that the age-group specific rates have a similar trend over time. If they are not approximately parallel, then an age-adjusted rate can mask important information (**Figure 3.4**). In the situation of nonparallel trends in age-specific rates, reporting age-group specific rates is more appropriate.

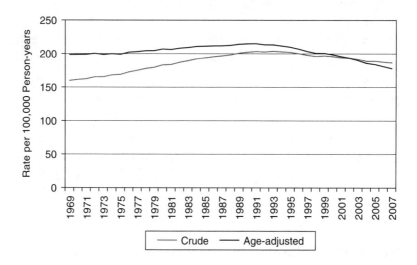

FIGURE 3.2 Trend in cancer death rates in the United States, 1969–2007. Footnote: Rates age-adjusted to the 2000 U.S. population (19 age groups—Census P25-1130).
Data from: Surveillance, Epidemiology, and End Results (SEER) Program (www.seer.cancer.gov). SEER*Stat Database: Mortality—All COD, Aggregated with State, Total U.S. (1969–2007) <Katrina/Rita Population Adjustment>, National Cancer Institute, DCCPS, Surveillance Research Program, Cancer Statistics Branch, released June 2010. Underlying mortality data provided by NCHS (www.cdc.gov/nchs). Accessed August 2, 2011.

In practice, the direct method of standardizing rates is more common than the indirect method. With computer software such as Excel, it is fairly easy to compute age-adjusted rates using either the direct or indirect methods. A rule of thumb is to use the direct method when subgroup-specific rates are available for all the groups being compared. If not, or if the subgroup rates are based on small numbers and therefore are unstable, the indirect method should be used. In addition, we should only adjust the rates if there is a confounding factor such as age or gender, or if we are not interested in comparing rates among groups or within a group over time. It is important to remember that the adjusted rates are hypothetical constructs and do not represent the actual frequency in the population of interest. For this reason, the choice of the standard population is arbitrary, although it should reflect the time period and the populations being studied.

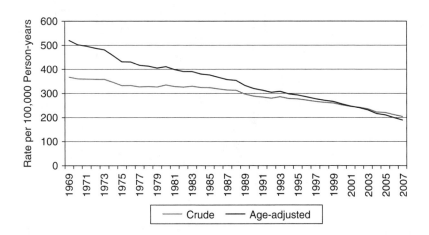

FIGURE 3.3 Trend in heart disease death rates in the United States, 1969–2007. Footnote: Rates age-adjusted to the 2000 U.S. population (19 age groups—Census P25-1130).

Data from: Surveillance, Epidemiology, and End Results (SEER) Program (www.seer.cancer.gov). SEER*Stat Database: Mortality—All COD, Aggregated with State, Total U.S. (1969–2007) <Katrina/Rita Population Adjustment>, National Cancer Institute, DCCPS, Surveillance Research Program, Cancer Statistics Branch, released June 2010. Underlying mortality data provided by NCHS (www.cdc.gov/nchs). Accessed August 2, 2011.

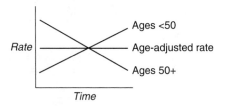

FIGURE 3.4 Trends in rates for two age groups.

EXERCISES

Age-Group Specific Deaths and Population Sizes in Florida and Utah in 2007[1]

Ages (years)	Florida		Utah	
	All Deaths	Population	All Deaths	Population
0–19	3,181	4,466,929	531	912,374
20–39	6,481	4,640,902	892	843,838
40–59	24,039	5,009,290	2,116	583,098
60–79	57,652	3,085,897	4,390	263,995
80+	76,733	996,508	6,213	65,620
Total	168,086	18,199,526	14,142	2,668,925

1. Calculate the crude mortality rates for Florida and Utah. What is your conclusion about the burden of death in the two populations?
2. Calculate the age-specific rates for Florida and Utah.
3. Compare the age-specific rates between Florida and Utah and interpret your results.
4. Using the direct method, calculate the age-adjusted rate for Utah using Florida as the standard.
5. Now compare the age-adjusted rate in Utah to the Florida rate and interpret your results.

Age-Group Specific Deaths from Pneumonia and Influenza and Population Values in Tennessee, 2007, for Whites and Blacks[1]

Ages (years)	Whites		Blacks	
	Deaths from Pneumonia and Influenza	Population	Deaths from Pneumonia and Influenza	Population
0–39	20	2,558,725	0	664,888
40–59	101	1,441,488	18	269,503
60–79	349	796,804	44	94,626
80+	815	190,332	67	21,862
Total	1,285	4,987,349	129	1,050,879

6. What is the age-specific expected number of cases in blacks, assuming they had the same rates as whites?

7. Apply the indirect method of standardization to this data, with blacks taking on the age-specific death rates of the white population. Interpret your results.

8. Is there ever a time that you would not want to age-adjust rates when comparing rates between or among groups?

9. What is an important assumption behind age-adjusted rates that are calculated for the same population over time?

10. Age-adjusted rates have been referred to as hypothetical constructs, with critics considering the actual age-adjusted rates meaningless. Explain.

11. Is the choice of the standard really arbitrary?

REFERENCES

1. Surveillance, Epidemiology, and End Results (SEER) Program (www.seer.cancer.gov). SEER* Stat Database: Mortality—All COD, Aggregated with State, Total U.S. (1969–2007) <Katrina/Rita Population Adjustment>, National Cancer Institute, DCCPS, Surveillance Research Program, Cancer Statistics Branch. Underlying mortality data provided by NCHS. www.cdc.gov/nchs. Published June 2010. Accessed August 2, 2011.

2. Merrill, RM, Hankey, BF. Monitoring progress against cancer with age-adjusted rates and trends: what role does the standard population play? *J Cancer Educ.* 2000;15:99–107.

CHAPTER 4

Describing Data with Graphs

An important way to summarize and display data is with the use of graphs. Graphs are used to convey the general patterns in a set of observations at a single glance. However, because of their simplicity, they often contain less detail than tables. Nevertheless, a loss of detail may be worth a greater level of understanding of the data. Graphs are most informative if they are relatively simple and self-explanatory. As in the case of tables, graphs should contain descriptive titles, be clearly labeled, and indicate the units of measurement. The purpose of this chapter is to present several types of graphs used in epidemiology and clinical medicine.

There are several graphical methods available for displaying data. Some selected types of graphs are presented in **Table 4.1**. In general, graphs can help clarify a public health problem. Graphs are helpful in finding patterns, trends, aberrations, similarities, and differences in data. They are useful for effectively describing and communicating health-related states or events according to person, place, and time. The building blocks of graphs are numbers, ratios, proportions, and rates.

Definition

A **graph** is a two-dimensional drawing showing a relationship between two sets of information or numbers using a line, curve, series of bars, or other symbols in a simple, compact format.

TABLE 4.1 Graphs for Describing Data

Type of Graph	When to Use
Arithmetic-scale line graph	Line graphs are used mostly for data plotted against time. An arithmetic graph has equal quantities along the y-axis and shows actual changes in magnitude of the number or rate of a health-related state or event across time.
Logarithmic-scale line graph	The y-axis is changed to a logarithmic scale. In other words, the axis is divided into cycles, with each being 10 times greater than the previous cycle. Focus is on the rate of change. A straight line reflects a constant rate of change.
Simple bar chart	A visual display of the magnitude of the different categories of a single variable, with each category or value of the variable represented by a bar.

(continues)

TABLE 4.1   Graphs for Describing Data (*continued*)

Type of Graph	When to Use
Grouped bar chart	Multiple sets of data are displayed as side-by-side bars.
Stacked bar chart	Similar to a grouped bar chart, except that each of the segments in which the bar or column is divided belongs to a different data series. It shows how a total entity is subdivided into parts.
Deviation bar chart	Illustrates differences, both positive and negative, from the baseline.
100% component bar chart	The bar is divided into proportions that are the same as the proportions of each category of the variable; it compares how components contribute to the whole in different groups.
Pie chart	Shows components of a whole.
Histogram	A graphic representation of the frequency distribution of a variable. Rectangles are drawn in such a way that their bases lie on a linear scale representing different intervals, and their heights are proportional to the frequencies of the values within each of the intervals.
Frequency polygon	A graphical display of a frequency table. The intervals are shown on the x-axis, and the frequency in each interval is represented by the height of a point located above the middle of the interval. The points are connected so that together with the x-axis they form a polygon.
Cumulative frequency	A running total of frequencies. A cumulative frequency polygon is used to graphically represent the total.
Spot map	A map that indicates the location of each case of a rare health-related state or event by a place that is potentially relevant to the health event being investigated, such as where each case lived or worked.
Area map	A map that indicates the number or rate of a health-related state or event by place, using different colors or shadings to represent the various levels of the disease, event, behavior, or condition.
Stem-and-leaf plot	A method of organizing numerical data in order of place value. The stem of the number includes all but the last digit. The leaf of the number will always be one digit.
Box plot	Also called a box-and-whisker plot, it is a graphical depiction of numerical data through six-number summaries: the mean, the smallest observation, the first quartile, the median, the third quartile, and the largest observation. The box portion of the graph represents the middle 50% of the data. The plot is useful for describing the distribution of the data, whether it is skewed, and if outliers are present.

TABLE 4.1	Graphs for Describing Data *(continued)*
Type of Graph	**When to Use**
Scatter plot	This graph is a useful summary of the association between two numerical variables. It is usually drawn before calculating a linear correlation coefficient or fitting a regression line, because these statistics assume a linear relationship in the data. It provides a good visual picture of the relationship between the two variables and aids in the interpretation of the correlation coefficient or regression model.
Population pyramid	This is a graphical illustration that shows the distribution of age groups in a population for males and females.

ARITHMETIC-SCALE AND LOGARITHMIC-SCALE LINE GRAPHS

Arithmetic-scale line graphs are useful for plotting counts, ratios, proportions, and rates. If the focus is on the rate of change, the data could be expressed on a logarithmic scale. A straight line reflects a constant rate of change.

EXAMPLE 4.1

The world population is plotted against time in **Figure 4.1**. In 1950, the average annual growth rate was 4.7%; in 1970, it was 2.07%; in 1990, it was 1.56%; and in 2010, it was 1.10%. In 2050, it is estimated to be about 0.45%.[1] By modifying the figure so that data are presented on a logarithmic scale (**Figure 4.2**), we see a decreasing rate of change.

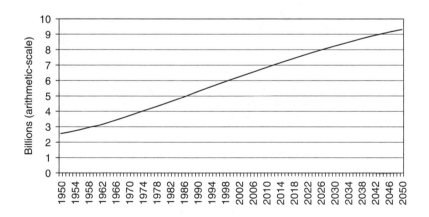

FIGURE 4.1 World population estimates, 1950–2050.
Data from: U.S. Census Bureau. http://www.census.gov/. Accessed October 25, 2011.

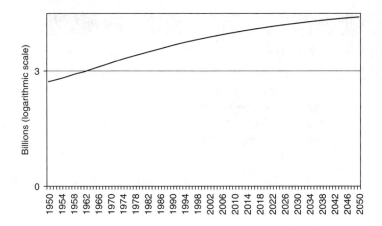

FIGURE 4.2 World population estimated rate of change, 1950–2050.
Data from: U.S. Census Bureau. http://www.census.gov/. Accessed October 25, 2011.

EXAMPLE 4.2

In the United States, the ratio (multiplied by 100) of male to female babies born according to race and calendar year is presented in **Figure 4.3**.[2] In other words, this

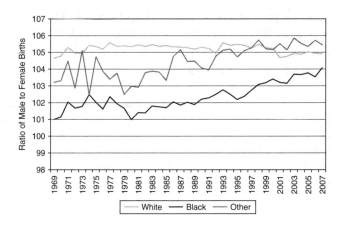

FIGURE 4.3 Number of male births for every 100 female births in the United States by racial group.
Data from: Surveillance, Epidemiology, and End Results (SEER) Program (www.seer.cancer.gov). SEER*Stat Database: Incidence—SEER 9 Regs Research Data, Nov 2010 Sub (1973–2008) <Katrina/ Rita Population Adjustment> Linked to County Attributes—Total U.S., 1969–2009 Counties, National Cancer Institute, DCCPS, Surveillance Research Program, Cancer Statistics Branch, released April 2011, based on the November 2010 submission.

graph shows the number of male births to every 100 female births in the United States. Since 1969, about 105 white males have been born to every 100 white females born. The number of males to females for blacks and other racial groups was lower than for whites in 1969, but has been steadily increasing through 2007.

BAR CHART

To display a frequency, proportion, or rate by the variable class, options include the bar chart, grouped bar chart, stacked bar chart, and 100% component bar chart. A deviation bar chart shows differences, both positive and negative, from the baseline.

EXAMPLE 4.3

In 2007, death rates due to suicide and self-inflicted injuries varied considerably between males and females and across racial groups in the United States.[2] Grouped bar charts (**Figure 4.4**), stacked bar charts (**Figure 4.5**), and 100% component bar charts (**Figure 4.6**) are useful for illustrating this variability.

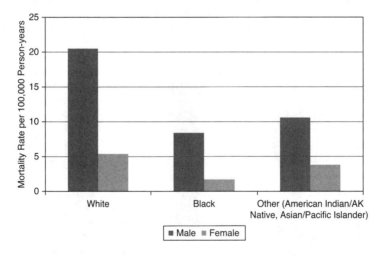

FIGURE 4.4 Suicide and self-inflicted injury, 2007. Grouped bar chart.
Data from: Surveillance, Epidemiology, and End Results (SEER) Program (www.seer.cancer.gov). SEER*Stat Database: Mortality–All COD, Aggregated with State, Total U.S. (1969–2008) <Katrina/Rita Population Adjustment>, National Cancer Institute, DCCPS, Surveillance Research Program, Cancer Statistics Branch, released September 2011. Underlying mortality data provided by NCHS (www.cdc.gov/nchs).

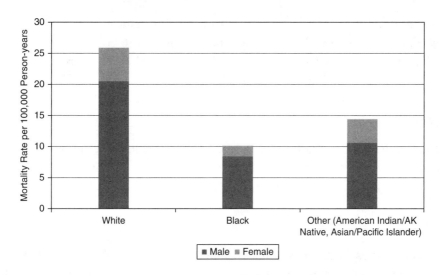

FIGURE 4.5 Suicide and self-inflicted injury, 2007. Stacked bar chart.
Data from: Surveillance, Epidemiology, and End Results (SEER) Program (www.seer.cancer.gov).
SEER*Stat Database: Mortality—All COD, Aggregated with State, Total U.S. (1969–2008) <Katrina/
Rita Population Adjustment>, National Cancer Institute, DCCPS, Surveillance Research Program, Can-
cer Statistics Branch, released September 2011. Underlying mortality data provided by NCHS (www.
cdc.gov/nchs).

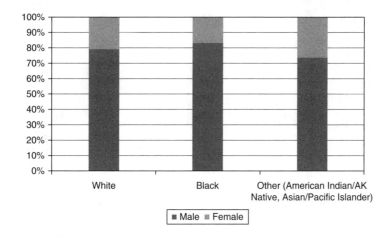

FIGURE 4.6 Suicide and self-inflicted injury, 2007. 100% component bar chart.
Data from: Surveillance, Epidemiology, and End Results (SEER) Program (www.seer.cancer.gov).
SEER*Stat Database: Mortality—All COD, Aggregated with State, Total U.S. (1969–2008) <Katrina/Rita
Population Adjustment>, National Cancer Institute, DCCPS, Surveillance Research Program, Cancer
Statistics Branch, released September 2011. Underlying mortality data provided by NCHS (www.cdc.
gov/nchs).

EXAMPLE 4.4

In the United States in 2007, the ratio of females to males varied considerably across the age span.[2] A deviation bar chart is one way to illustrate this. **Figure 4.7** shows that there are more females in the population in the age groups 40 and older, but more males in the population in the younger age groups.

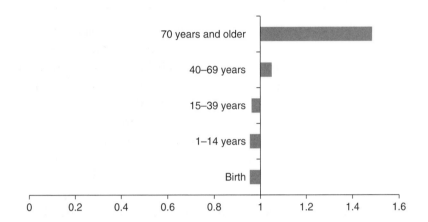

FIGURE 4.7 Female-to-male ratio in the United States, 2007. Deviation bar chart.
Data from: Surveillance, Epidemiology, and End Results (SEER) Program (www.seer.cancer.gov). SEER*Stat Database: Mortality—All COD, Aggregated with State, Total U.S. (1969–2008) <Katrina/Rita Population Adjustment>, National Cancer Institute, DCCPS, Surveillance Research Program, Cancer Statistics Branch, released September 2011. Underlying mortality data provided by NCHS (www.cdc.gov/nchs).

PIE CHART

A pie chart shows components of the whole. The proportional mortality ratio and the death-to-case ratio are statistics that can effectively be presented using pie charts. The *proportional mortality ratio* is the number of deaths from a specific cause in a specific time per 100 deaths from all causes during the same time period. *The death-to-case ratio* is the number of deaths attributed to a particular disease during a specified time period divided by the number of new cases of that disease identified during the same time period.

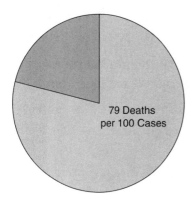

FIGURE 4.8 Death-to-case ratio for pancreatic cancer in Hawaii, 2007.
Data from: Surveillance, Epidemiology, and End Results (SEER) Program (www.seer.cancer.gov). SEER*Stat Database: Mortality—All COD, Aggregated with State, Total U.S. (1969–2008) <Katrina/Rita Population Adjustment>, National Cancer Institute, DCCPS, Surveillance Research Program, Cancer Statistics Branch, released September 2011. Underlying mortality data provided by NCHS (www.cdc.gov/nchs).

Definitions

Outbreak carries the same definition as *epidemic* but is typically used when the event is confined to a more limited geographic area. *Outbreak* is sometimes the preferred word, as it may escape the sensationalism associated with the word *epidemic.*

An **epidemic curve** is a histogram that shows the course of a disease outbreak or epidemic by plotting the number of cases by the date of onset.

EXAMPLE 4.5

The death-to-case ratio for pancreatic cancer in Hawaii during 2007 is shown in **Figure 4.8**.[2] In other words, there were 79 deaths from pancreatic cancer per 100 new diagnosed cases of the disease in 2007.

HISTOGRAM

A histogram is commonly used in epidemiology to reflect the frequency of health-related states or events over time. In epidemiology, a histogram that shows the course of a disease outbreak is called an *epidemic curve.* An epidemic curve can characterize an outbreak by pattern of spread, magnitude, outliers, time trend, and exposure and/or disease incubation period. The overall shape of the epidemic curve can reveal whether the outbreak involves a common source exposure, a point source exposure, or a propagated exposure.

A *common source outbreak* is one in which people are exposed continuously or intermittently to a harmful source. The period of exposure may be brief or long. An intermittent exposure in a common source outbreak often results in an epidemic curve with irregular peaks that reflect the timing and extent of the exposure.

EXAMPLE 4.6

Figure 4.9 shows a common source outbreak with intermittent exposure. The irregular peaks reflect the timing and dose of exposure. A continuous exposure resulting in an outbreak will often cause cases to rise gradually and plateau instead of peak.

EXAMPLE 4.7

Figure 4.10 is an example of a disease outbreak with a continuous exposure. The duration of exposure for this type of outbreak is typically relatively long.

An epidemic curve with a sharp upward slope and a gradual downward slope typically describes a point source

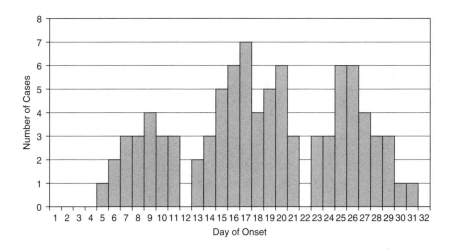

FIGURE 4.9 Common source outbreak of disease with intermittent exposure.

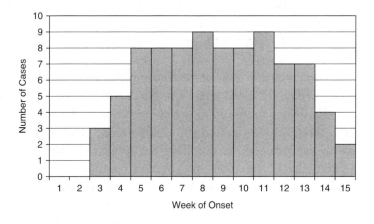

FIGURE 4.10 Common source outbreak of disease with continuous exposure.

outbreak. A *point source outbreak* is a common source outbreak in which the exposure period is relatively brief and all cases occur within one incubation period (e.g., contaminated food at a picnic leading to salmonella poisoning).

EXAMPLE 4.8

Figure 4.11 shows an epidemic curve that is characteristic of a point source epidemic.

A *propagated outbreak* is one that involves a disease that is spread from person to person. Propagated outbreaks typically last longer than common source outbreaks,

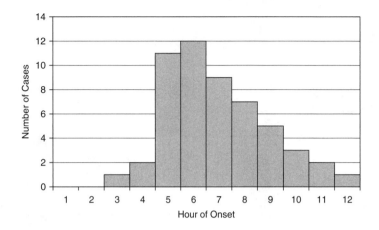

FIGURE 4.11 Point source outbreak of disease.

and they can result in multiple waves of infection if secondary and tertiary cases occur. The classic propagated epidemic curve has a series of progressively taller peaks, each an incubation period apart, but the pattern of the epidemic curve may vary a bit according to the type of illness.

An epidemic curve can also indicate the magnitude of the outbreak. A comparison of the number of cases reported relative to the size of the population from which the cases occurred provides a more meaningful indication of the extent of the public health problem. Additional information about the magnitude of the outbreak within subpopulations can be obtained by stratifying the epidemic curve by characteristics such as gender, age, clinical symptoms, or geographic location.

The epidemic curve allows us to obtain meaningful information about the time trend involved. We are interested in the date of illness onset for the first case, the date when the outbreak peaked, and the date of the illness onset for the last case. Cases at the very beginning or end of the epidemic curve are called outliers. Outlier cases that are not a coding error may indicate baseline levels of illness, outbreak source, a case exposed earlier than the others, an unrelated case, a case exposed later than the others, or a case with a long incubation period.

If the time of the suspected exposure is known, the epidemic curve can be used to estimate the incubation period of the disease. The time from the exposure to the peak of the epidemic curve represents the median incubation period. An understanding of the incubation period helps narrow our search for a cause. Lists of incubation periods for several communicable diseases can be found in the literature.[3] For instance, the incubation period for chickenpox is 2 to 3 weeks. Therefore, if you were diagnosed with chickenpox about 2 weeks after visiting your cousins, you may know the source of the illness.

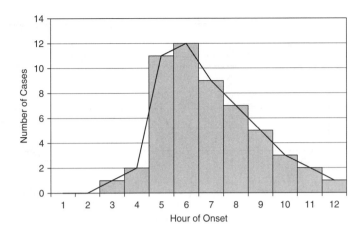

FIGURE 4.12 Frequency polygon.

FREQUENCY POLYGON

A frequency polygon is a graphical display of a frequency table. The polygon outlines the shape of the histogram. A cumulative frequency polygon is a running total of frequencies.

EXAMPLE 4.9

Examples of a frequency polygon, a cumulative frequency polygon, and a cumulative relative frequency polygon are presented in **Figure 4.12**, **Figure 4.13**, and **Figure 4.14**,

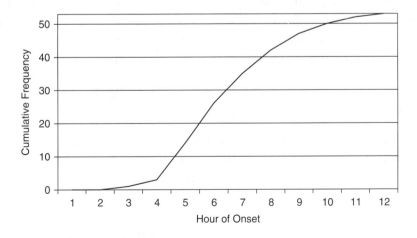

FIGURE 4.13 Cumulative frequency polygon.

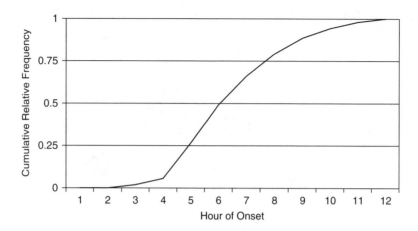

FIGURE 4.14 Cumulative relative frequency polygon.

respectively. Most of the cases occurred around 5–7 hours. Twenty-five percent of the cases (quartile 1) occurred within 5 hours, 50% (quartile 2) within 6 hours, and 75% (quartile 3) between 7 and 8 hours. All the cases were identified within 12 hours.

AREA MAP

An area map is an effective way of presenting the number or rate of a health-related state or event by place. This type of graph uses different colors or shadings to represent the various levels of the health-related state or event. For example, researchers have used area maps to identify disparities in the infant mortality rate,[4] variation in the world birth rate,[5] differences in cancer rates,[6] and for many other uses.

EXAMPLE 4.10

Obesity levels in the United States and elsewhere in the world have been at epidemic levels. Epidemiologic research has shown that obesity increases a person's risk of illness and death due to diabetes, stroke, coronary artery disease, hypertension, high cholesterol, and kidney and gallbladder disorders. Obesity also increases the risk for certain types of cancer and for the development of osteoarthritis and sleep apnea. Hence, monitoring obesity levels is of primary interest. Obesity levels among adults in the United States are shown for three time periods in **Figure 4.15**.[7]

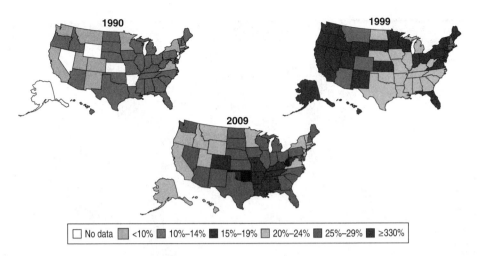

1990

1999

2009

No data   <10%   10%–14%   15%–19%   20%–24%   25%–29%   ≥330%

FIGURE 4.15 Obesity among adults in the United States.
Source: Division of Nutrition, Physical Activity, and Obesity, National Center for Chronic Disease Prevention and Health Promotion. (2010). U.S. Obesity Trends. In Overweight and Obesity. http://www.cdc.gov/obesity/data/trends.html#National. Accessed October 17, 2011.

SPOT MAP

Another type of graph, which gained popularity because of the work of John Snow, is a spot map (see the following History box).

History

John Snow (1813–1858), an English physician, used statistics to help lay the groundwork for descriptive and analytic epidemiologic approaches found useful in epidemiology today. Throughout his medical career, Snow established a link between cholera and water as its vector. Cholera is a disease characterized by watery diarrhea, loss of fluid and electrolytes, dehydration, and collapse. In the later part of his career, Snow conducted two major investigative studies of cholera. The first involved a descriptive epidemiologic investigation of a cholera outbreak in 1848 in the Soho and Golden Square district of London. Within 250 yards of the intersection of Cambridge Street and Broad Street, about 500 fatal attacks of cholera occurred in 10 days. Many more deaths were averted because of the flight of most of the population. Snow was able to identify incubation times, length of time from infection until death, modes of transmission of the disease, and the importance of the flight of the population from the dangerous areas. Snow gathered information about those with cholera in the area, recording their residence and place of work. He then developed a spot map showing the distribution of cholera cases in relation to the water pumps (**Figure 4.16**). He found that nearly all deaths had taken place within a short distance of the Broad Street pump. When he checked with the families of the victims, he confirmed that they had all used the Broad Street pump. Toward the end of the epidemic, as a control measure and a political statement to the community, Snow removed the handle from the Broad Street pump.[8–10]

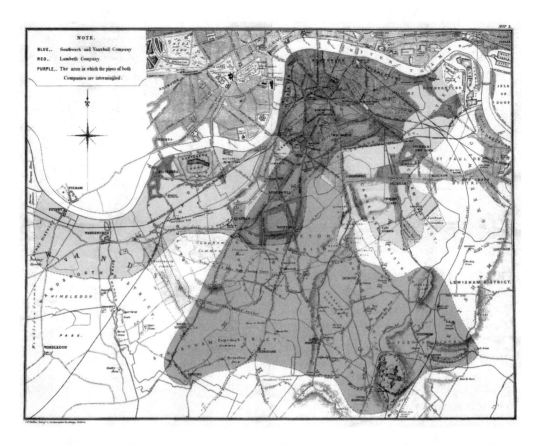

FIGURE 4.16 Original map by Dr. John Snow showing the cluster of cholera cases in the London epidemic of 1848.
Source: John Snow website/UCLA. http://www.ph.ucla.edu/epi/snow.html. Accessed October 24, 2011.

STEM-AND-LEAF PLOT

For numerical data, the stem-and-leaf plot and the box plot provide ways for summarizing the distribution of data. A stem-and-leaf plot resembles a bar chart. The strength of a stem-and-leaf plot is that it retains the actual data.

EXAMPLE 4.11

Consider the data in **Table 4.2**, which presents the percentage of adults with diabetes and who are obese according to state in the United States.[11] Stem-and-leaf plots for diabetes and for obesity are shown in **Figure 4.17**.

TABLE 4.2	Adults in the United States with Diabetes and Who Are Obese by State, 2010	
Geographic Region	**Told by a Doctor You Have Diabetes (%)**	**Obese (%)**
Alabama	13.2	33
Alaska	5.3	25.2
Arizona	11.4	24.7
Arkansas	9.6	30.9
California	8.6	24.7
Colorado	6	21.4
Connecticut	7.3	23
Delaware	8.7	28.7
District of Columbia	10.9	22.7
Florida	10.4	27.2
Georgia	9.7	30.4
Guam	11	27.6
Hawaii	8.3	23.1
Idaho	7.9	26.9
Illinois	8.7	28.7
Indiana	9.8	30.2
Iowa	7.5	29.1
Kansas	8.4	30.1
Kentucky	10	31.8
Louisiana	10.3	31.7
Maine	8.7	27.4
Maryland	9.3	27.9
Massachusetts	7.4	23.6
Michigan	10.1	31.7
Minnesota	6.7	25.4
Mississippi	12.4	34.5
Missouri	9.4	31.4
Montana	7	23.5

(continues)

TABLE 4.2   Adults in the United States with Diabetes and Who Are Obese by State, 2010 (*continued*)

Geographic Region	Told by a Doctor You Have Diabetes (%)	Obese (%)
Nebraska	7.7	27.5
Nevada	8.5	23.1
New Hampshire	7.9	25.5
New Jersey	9.2	24.8
New Mexico	8.5	25.6
New York	8.9	24.5
North Carolina	9.8	28.6
North Dakota	7.4	27.9
Ohio	10.1	29.7
Oklahoma	10.4	31.3
Oregon	7.2	27.6
Pennsylvania	10.3	29.2
Puerto Rico	12.8	27.5
Rhode Island	7.8	26
South Carolina	10.7	32
South Dakota	6.9	27.7
Tennessee	11.3	31.7
Texas	9.7	31.7
Utah	6.5	23
Vermont	6.8	23.9
Virgin Islands	9.1	30
Virginia	8.7	26.4
Washington	7.6	26.2
West Virginia	11.7	32.9
Wisconsin	7.1	26.9
Wyoming	7.2	25.7

Data from: Centers for Disease Control and Prevention. Behavior Risk Factor Surveillance System. Prevalence and Trend Data. http://apps.nccd.cdc.gov/BRFSS/. Accessed July 1, 2011.

Diabetes		Obesity	
Stem	Leaf	Stem	Leaf
13	2	34	5
12	8	33	0
12	4	32	09
11	7	31	3477778
11	034	30	01249
10	79	29	127
10	0113344	28	677
9	67788	27	245566799
9	1234	26	02499
8	55677779	25	24567
8	34	24	5778
7	567899	23	0011569
7	0122344	22	7
6	5789	21	4
6	0		
5			
5	3		

FIGURE 4.17 Stem-and-leaf plots of obesity and diabetes among adults in the United States, 2010.
Data from: Centers for Disease Control and Prevention. Behavior Risk Factor Surveillance System. Prevalence and Trend Data. http://apps.nccd.cdc.gov/BRFSS/. Accessed July 1, 2011.

BOX PLOT

A box plot (also called a box-and-whisker plot) provides a graphical depiction of numerical data through six-number summaries (mean, minimum value, the first quartile, the median, the third quartile, and the maximum value). The box portion of the plot is the middle 50% of the data. The box plot is useful for describing the distribution of the data.

EXAMPLE 4.12

Six summary measures are presented for the diabetes and obesity data presented in **Table 4.3**. A side-by-side box plot depicting these summary measures is shown in **Figure 4.18**. Because the mean and median are very similar, the distributions are fairly normally distributed (symmetric).

TABLE 4.3	Summary Measures for Adults in the United States with Diabetes and Who Are Obese by State, 2010	
	Diabetes	**Obesity**
Mean	9.0	27.7
Minimum	5.3	21.4
Quartile 1	7.5	25.2
Median	8.7	27.6
Quartile 3	10.1	30.2
Maximum	13.2	34.5

Data from: Centers for Disease Control and Prevention. Behavior Risk Factor Surveillance System. Prevalence and Trend Data. http://apps.nccd.cdc.gov/BRFSS/. Accessed July 1, 2011.

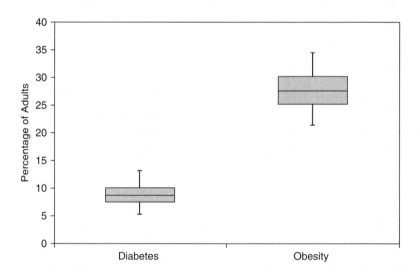

FIGURE 4.18 Side-by-side box plots of the distribution of obesity and diabetes among adults in the United States, 2010.
Data from: Centers for Disease Control and Prevention. Behavior Risk Factor Surveillance System. Prevalence and Trend Data. http://apps.nccd.cdc.gov/BRFSS/. Accessed July 1, 2011.

SCATTER PLOT

To compare two numerical variables graphically, we can use a scatter plot.

EXAMPLE 4.13

A scatter plot showing the association between diabetes and obesity is presented in **Figure 4.19**. For the ecological U.S. state level data depicted in the graph, a positive association is shown between the percentage of adults with diabetes and the percentage of adults who are obese. This visual summary of the association between two numerical variables could be further assessed using statistical measures such as the correlation coefficient or the least-squares regression line.

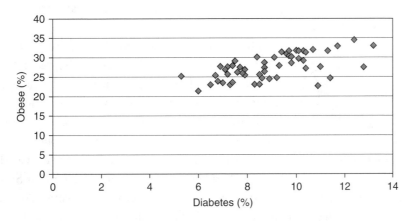

FIGURE 4.19 Scatter plot of the association between obesity and diabetes among adults in the United States, 2010.
Data from: Centers for Disease Control and Prevention. Behavior Risk Factor Surveillance System. Prevalence and Trend Data. http://apps.nccd.cdc.gov/BRFSS/. Accessed July 1, 2011.

POPULATION PYRAMID

A *population pyramid* is a graphical illustration that shows the distribution of age groups for male and female populations (also called an age–sex pyramid). This type of graph is useful for tracking and comparing changes in population age distributions over time. It is effective for depicting the age and sex distribution of a population because

Definition

An **expansive pyramid** is a population pyramid showing a broad base, indicating a high proportion of children, a rapid rate of population growth, and a low proportion of older people.

of the simple, clear way the pyramids are presented. A population pyramid may show that a population is expanding, stationary, or constricting.

The U.S. Census Bureau's interactive site on inter-national demographic data is a nice source for generating population pyramids according to country and calendar year.[12]

EXAMPLE 4.14

Population pyramids showing populations expanding, stationary, and constricting are presented in **Figure 4.20**.

The ability of a population to support itself economically is of concern in public health. The dependency one group has on another can be measured by a dependency ratio. The dependency ratio is calculated by dividing the population aged 0–14 years and 65 and older by the population aged 15–64 years. This ratio is then multiplied by 100.

The dependency ratio represents the number of dependents for every 100 people of working age. For example, in Afghanistan, China, and the United States, the dependency ratio is 84, 36, and 50, respectively. Therefore, for every 100 people of working age, there are 84 dependents in Afghanistan, 36 in China, and 50 in the United States. In the United States, as an increasing percentage of the age distribution is in the older age groups, the dependency ratio is expected to increase. In 2025, for example, 0.196 of the population is expected to be aged 0–14 years and 0.181 of the population is expected to be aged 65 years and older. The dependency ratio is therefore:

$$Dependency\ Ratio = \frac{0.196 + 0.181}{1 - (0.196 + 0.181)} \times 100 = \frac{0.377}{0.623} \times 100 = 61$$

Thus, from 2012 to 2025, the number of dependents for every 100 people of working age is expected to increase from 50 to 61.

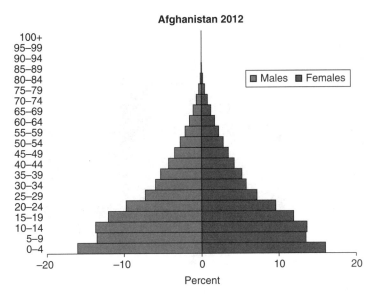

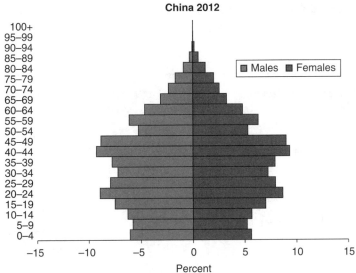

FIGURE 4.20 Population pyramids for Afghanistan, China, and the United States.

Data from: U.S. Census Bureau, Population Division. http://www. census.gov/population/international/data/idb/informationGateway.php. Accessed October 25, 2011.

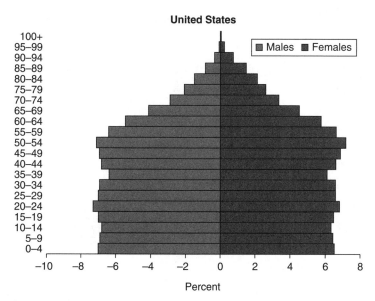

FIGURE 4.20 (*continued*) Population pyramids for Afghanistan, China, and the United States.

EXERCISES

Age-Group Specific Deaths and Populations in Florida and Utah, 2007[2]				
	Florida		**Utah**	
Ages (years)	**All deaths**	**Population**	**All deaths**	**Population**
0–19	3,181	4,466,929	531	912,374
20–39	6,481	4,640,902	892	843,838
40–59	24,039	5,009,290	2,116	583,098
60–79	57,652	3,085,897	4,390	263,995
80+	76,733	996,508	6,213	65,620
Total	168,086	18,199,526	14,142	2,668,925

1. Based on the preceding table, use a graph to compare the age-specific rates between Florida and Utah.

2. Match the types of data in the left column with the types of graph/chart in the right column. (You may use more than one letter for each type of data.)

A. bar chart
___ nominal data
B. histogram
___ ordinal data
C. box plot
___ discrete data
D. stem-and-leaf plot
___ continuous data
E. spot map/area map

3. Construct a stem-and-leaf plot for the data 28.2, 29.1, 26.1, 22, 22.8, 24.5, 26.7, 24.9, 22.3, and 28.7 (presented originally in Chapter 2, Exercise 2.21).

4. Construct a box plot using the same data as in the previous question.

The following table reflects five-year observed survival rates for colon cancer patients in the United States by year of diagnosis.[2]

	White males	White females	Black males	Black females
1973	34.3%	39.8%	41.1%	36.8%
1974	35.8%	39.6%	34.5%	38.9%
1975	37.8%	40.8%	34.9%	36.7%
1976	38.7%	43.3%	35.8%	41.3%
1977	39.0%	42.1%	33.6%	38.6%
1978	39.3%	43.3%	31.8%	40.3%
1979	39.0%	44.4%	40.3%	45.3%
1980	39.9%	42.5%	38.4%	40.6%
1981	43.3%	44.4%	36.7%	44.0%
1982	42.2%	44.2%	32.2%	41.4%
1983	44.1%	43.7%	35.7%	44.6%
1984	42.8%	46.3%	29.2%	39.5%
1985	46.9%	47.0%	44.2%	40.1%
1986	48.2%	47.4%	38.8%	44.4%
1987	47.8%	47.9%	43.8%	41.9%
1988	47.3%	47.9%	38.5%	44.9%

(continues)

	White males	White females	Black males	Black females
1989	47.3%	47.8%	36.1%	47.6%
1990	48.4%	49.4%	43.4%	39.5%
1991	49.8%	49.8%	44.5%	45.9%
1992	49.4%	49.1%	43.5%	43.2%
1993	47.8%	48.5%	39.6%	43.3%
1994	48.1%	47.3%	41.5%	44.3%
1995	47.3%	47.1%	44.0%	43.3%
1996	49.7%	49.0%	44.7%	38.8%
1997	49.8%	47.6%	42.0%	48.1%
1998	49.7%	49.7%	42.4%	42.5%
1999	52.5%	51.0%	44.3%	44.5%
2000	51.6%	50.5%	44.4%	41.6%
2001	52.3%	50.7%	41.7%	44.9%
2002	51.2%	50.5%	47.1%	47.1%
2003	53.0%	51.3%	45.0%	45.7%
2004	51.7%	51.3%	40.9%	44.8%

5. For this data, construct an arithmetic-scale line graph for white and black males and describe the results.

6. For this data, construct an arithmetic-scale line graph for white and black females and describe the results.

The following table reflects five-year observed survival rates for white and black colon cancer patients in the United States diagnosed between 2000 and 2004, according to age at diagnosis.[2]

	Whites observed	Blacks observed
20–24 years	42.2%	44.2%
25–29 years	44.1%	43.7%
30–34 years	42.8%	46.3%
35–39 years	46.9%	47.0%

	Whites observed	Blacks observed
40–44 years	48.2%	47.4%
45–49 years	47.8%	47.9%
50–54 years	47.3%	47.9%
55–59 years	47.3%	47.8%
60–64 years	48.4%	49.4%
65–69 years	49.8%	49.8%
70–74 years	49.4%	49.1%
75–79 years	47.8%	48.5%
80–84 years	48.1%	47.3%
85+ years	47.3%	47.1%

7. Construct an arithmetic-scale line graph for whites and blacks and describe the results.

8. Plot the data on a logarithmic scale and interpret the results.

   The following table reflects estimated incidences of liver cancer in the United States for white and black males and females, between 2006 and 2008, by state of disease at diagnosis.[2]

	White males	White females	Black males	Black females
Local	3,488	1,267	596	209
Regional	2,114	643	383	111
Distant	1,386	450	311	99
Unstaged	1,268	557	179	65

9. Construct a 100% component bar chart using the data.

10. Construct a pie chart for the data 4,755 (local), 2,757 (regional), 1,836 (distant), and 1,825 (unstaged), that reflects all cases of liver cancer diagnosed between 2006 and 2008 for white males and females.[2]

11. Suppose that in a certain small company of 30 employees, the number of days absent from work in a given year because of illness is as follows: 8, 12, 31, 7,

0, 4, 2, 26, 18, 1, 0, 22, 17, 8, 5, 9, 22, 5, 13, 12, 2, 16, 9, 4, 0, 3, 1, 14, 8, 23. Construct a histogram for this data.

12. For the data in the previous question, assume the corresponding body mass index (BMI) scores: 25, 30, 43, 30, 23, 23, 24, 38, 25, 22, 18, 37, 23, 28, 22, 18, 37, 31, 35, 36, 35, 27, 22, 26, 21, 21, 27, 23, 27, 49. Construct a scatter plot for this data.

Midyear Population by Age and Gender for the United Kingdom, 2010[13]			
Age	Both sexes' population	Male population	Female population
Total	62,348,447	30,924,685	31,423,762
0–4	3,793,324	1,943,340	1,849,984
5–9	3,448,501	1,768,998	1,679,503
10–14	3,596,295	1,842,751	1,753,544
15–19	3,989,674	2,039,985	1,949,689
20–24	4,327,763	2,208,825	2,118,938
25–29	4,180,180	2,140,080	2,040,100
30–34	3,830,300	1,965,243	1,865,057
35–39	4,175,625	2,143,012	2,032,613
40–44	4,728,020	2,406,814	2,321,206
45–49	4,708,869	2,344,827	2,364,042
50–54	4,073,241	2,046,493	2,026,748
55–59	3,573,855	1,767,867	1,805,988
60–64	3,765,928	1,842,113	1,923,815
65–69	2,901,739	1,396,827	1,504,912
70–74	2,419,895	1,137,504	1,282,391
75–79	1,943,279	867,725	1,075,554
80–84	1,464,179	596,096	868,083
85–89	924,209	326,743	597,466
90–94	366,515	107,801	258,714
95–99	116,063	27,732	88,331
100+	20,993	3,909	17,084

13. Construct a population pyramid for this data and describe what the shape of the pyramid is telling us about the population distribution.

14. Construct a deviation bar chart to show the ratio of females to males in the United Kingdom in 2010. Use the age groups 0–14, 15–39, 40–69, and 70 years and older.

15. The U.S. National Cancer Institute has an interactive site where you can select certain options and generate your own cancer mortality map. Go to the site http://ratecalc.cancer.gov/ and generate your own area map of cancer mortality.

REFERENCES

1. U.S. Census Bureau. http://www.census.gov. Accessed August 4, 2011.
2. Surveillance, Epidemiology, and End Results (SEER) Program (www.seer.cancer.gov). SEER* Stat Database: Mortality—All COD, Aggregated with State, Total U.S. (1969–2007) <Katrina/Rita Population Adjustment>, National Cancer Institute, DCCPS, Surveillance Research Program, Cancer Statistics Branch. Underlying mortality data provided by NCHS. www.cdc.gov/nchs. Published June 2010. Accessed August 2, 2011.
3. Merrill RM. *Introduction to Epidemiology.* 5th ed. Sudbury, MA: Jones and Bartlett Publishers; 2010.
4. Mathews TJ, MacDorman MS, MacDorman, MF. Division of vital statistics: Infant mortality statistics from the 2007 period linked birth/infant death data set. *National Vital Statistics Report.* 2009;59(6): Figure 2. http://cdc.gov/nchs/data/nvsr/nvsr59/nvsr59_06.pdf. Accessed July 3, 2011.
5. Central Intelligence Agency. The World Factbook. https://www.cia.gov/library/publications /the-world-factbook/fields/2054.html. Accessed August 4, 2011.
6. U.S. National Cancer Institute. Cancer mortality maps. http://ratecalc.cancer.gov/. Accessed July 24, 2011.
7. Centers for Disease Control and Prevention. Overweight and obesity. http://www.cdc.gov /obesity/data/trends.html. Published July 21, 2011. Accessed December 20, 2011.
8. Benenson AS, ed. *Control of Communicable Diseases in Man.* 15th ed. Washington, DC: American Public Health Association; 1990:367–373.
9. Snow J. *On the Mode of Communication of Cholera.* 2nd ed, 1855. Reprinted by Commonwealth Fund, New York, NY; 1936.
10. Snow J. On the mode of communication of cholera. In: Buck C, Llopis A, Najera E, Terris M, eds. *The Challenge of Epidemiology: Issues and Selected Readings.* Washington, DC: World Health Organization; 1988:42–45.
11. Centers for Disease Control and Prevention. Behavior risk factor surveillance system. Prevalence and trend data. http://apps.nccd.cdc.gov/BRFSS/. Published 2011. Accessed July 1, 2011.
12. U.S. Census Bureau, Population Division. International Programs. http://www.census.gov/ipc /www/idb/informationGateway.php. Published June 27, 2011. Accessed July 19, 2011.
13. U.S. Census Bureau, International Programs. http://www.census.gov/population/international /data/idb/country.php. Published June 27, 2011. Accessed August 9, 2011.

CHAPTER 5

Life Tables

Since the days of John Graunt in the 1600s, life tables have been used to summarize the health status of populations. Life tables fall under descriptive epidemiology and identify the death rates experienced by a population for a specified time period. In addition to using life tables to compute life expectancy for a particular population, they may also be used to calculate survival curves for the population.

A life table applies cross-sectional mortality data to a hypothetical cohort of individuals, usually 100,000 or 1,000,000, from birth until the last individual has died. It is useful for describing the mortality experience of the group for a specified time period. The selected cohort size at the beginning of the age span is called the radix. We typically choose a radix of 10 to the nth power because it simplifies the calculations.

In this chapter, we will show the computation of the life table and use the life table to derive years of potential life lost.

History

John Graunt (1620–1674), a British merchant, is considered one of the first experts in epidemiology because of his work involving the "Bills of Mortality," a systematic recording of deaths in London, which began in 1603. In his book entitled *Natural and Political Observations Made upon the Bills of Mortality*, first published in 1662, he presented human statistical and census methods, which provided a framework for modern demography. Graunt used the Bills of Mortality to describe deaths according to age, sex, residence, season, and whether they were related to acute or chronic conditions. He also used the mortality data to develop life tables and to attach probabilities of survival to each age group.[1,2]

About 200 years later, William Farr (1807–1883), a British epidemiologist, was appointed registrar general in England. At the time, the concept of "political arithmetic" was replaced by a new term called *statistics*. Farr was responsible for collecting official medical statistics in England and Wales. He extended the use of statistics for describing births and deaths. He also organized and developed a modern vital statistics system, much of which is still in use today.[3]

CALCULATION OF THE PROBABILITY OF DYING (q_x)

The complete life table is derived from the probability of death (q_x), which is based on the number of deaths (D_x), and the midyear population (P_x) for each year of age (x) experienced during the calendar year of interest. To calculate q_0 we use the birth cohort method with a separation factor (f), which is the proportion of infant deaths in year t among infants born in the previous year ($t - 1$). The value of f is obtained by classifying infant deaths by date of birth. For example, the number of deaths in 2005 involving infants born in 2004 or 2005 was 28,440. Of this number, 3,550 were born in 2004. Hence, $f = 3,550/28,440 = 0.125$.[4]

$$q_0 = \frac{D_0(1-f)}{B^t} + \frac{D_0(f)}{B^{t-1}}$$

where D_0 is the number of infant deaths, B^t is the number of births in year t, and B^{t-1} is the number of births in year $t - 1$.

For ages 1–99, we assume that l_x, which is the number of survivors at exact age x in the life table population, declines linearly between x and $x + 1$. Thus, the deaths between x to $x + 1$ occur on average at age $x + 1/2$. Then, $l_x = L_x + \frac{1}{2}d_x$, where L_x is the average life table population at risk of dying in the age range x to $x + 1$ and d_x is the number of deaths occurring in the age range x to $x + 1$. The value of q_x is then:

$$q_x = \frac{d_x}{L_x + \frac{1}{2}d_x} = \frac{R_x}{1 + \frac{1}{2}R_x}$$

where $R_x = \frac{d_x}{L_x}$.[4] This is a conditional probability of death; that is, it represents the probability of death in a given age interval given survival to that age interval. The *National Vital Statistics Reports* provide probability of dying estimates each year for the United States.[4,5] A list of q_x corresponding to the first 20 single-year age intervals is shown in **Table 5.1**. As we have seen, q_x is calculated slightly differently than the overall death rate for a given age interval. This quantity is also known as the *hazard function*, which is the instantaneous rate of death relative to being alive at age x. We will use the estimates of q_x to calculate the remaining life table.

CALCULATION OF THE REMAINING LIFE TABLE

To calculate the remaining life table, we consider the survival function (l_x), the decrement function (d_x), person-years lived (L_x), person-years lived at and above age x (T_x), and life expectancy at age x (e_x).

TABLE 5.1   Probability of Dying between Ages *x* to *x* + 1 in the United States, 2006

Age	q_x
0–<1	0.006713
1–2	0.000444
2–3	0.000300
3–4	0.000216
4–5	0.000179
5–6	0.000168
6–7	0.000156
7–8	0.000143
8–9	0.000125
9–10	0.000103
10–11	0.000086
11–12	0.000088
12–13	0.000125
13–14	0.000206
14–15	0.000317
15–16	0.000438
16–17	0.000552
17–18	0.000657
18–19	0.000747
19–20	0.000825

Data from: Arias E. United States life tables, 2006. *National Vital Statistics Reports*. 2010;58(21). Hyattsville, MD: National Center for Health Statistics.

Life Table Notation

The number alive at the beginning of x is l_x, which is the life table population at risk for the interval x to $x + 1$. The life table radix, l_0, is set at 100,000. For ages greater than 0, the number of survivors remaining at exact age x is calculated as[6]:

$l_x = l_{x-1}(1 - q_{x-1})$.

$d_x = l_x - l_{x+1} = q_x \times l_x$ is the number of deaths occurring between age x and $x + 1$.[7]

Note that $_\infty d_{100} = {_\infty}l_{100}$ because $_\infty d_{100} = 1$.

$L_x = (l_x - d_x) + \frac{1}{2}d_x$ is the person-years lived. For ages 1 to 99 years, we assume that the survivor function declines linearly between age x and $x + 1$.[8] For $x = 0$, L_0 is calculated using the separation factor f[9]:

$$L_0 = f \times l_0 + (1 - f)l_1$$

$_\infty L_{100}$ is estimated as the sum of the extrapolated L_x values for ages 100 to 130 years.

$T_x = \sum_{x=0}^{\infty} L_x$ is the person-years lived at and above age x.[10]

$e_x = \dfrac{T_x}{l_x}$ is life expectancy at age x.[11]

With the estimates of q_x, we can now apply these formulas to complete the life table (**Table 5.2**). The iterative process through the life table begins with the hypothetical cohort, $l_0 = 100{,}000$. The number of deaths in the first interval is $d_0 = 0.006713 \times 100{,}000 = 671$. The number alive at the beginning of age interval 1 to 2 is $l_1 = 100{,}000 - 671 = 99{,}329$. The number of deaths in this age interval is $d_1 = 0.000444 \times 99{,}329 = 671$. The person-years lived in the first two age intervals is derived as:

$$L_0 = 0.119 \times 100{,}000 + (1 - 0.119)99{,}329 = 99{,}409$$

$$L_1 = (99{,}329 - 44) + \frac{1}{2}44 = 99{,}307$$

We continue sequentially through the life table. The person-years lived at and above age x are then computed. The total number of person-years lived for our cohort of 100,000 aged through the life table is 7,770,850. The total person-years divided by the cohort size gives 77.7 years of life expected, on average.

ABRIDGING THE COMPLETE LIFE TABLE

For the sake of convenience, abridged or collapsed life tables are used most often in practice. Summarizing the life table by using age intervals of typically 5 years, the

	Probability of dying between ages x and x + 1	Number surviving to age x	Number dying between ages x and x + 1	Person-years lived between ages x and x + 1	Total number of person-years lived about age x	Expecta-tion of life at age x
Age	q_x	l_x	d_x	L_x	T_x	e_x
0–<1	0.006713	100,000	671	99,409	7,770,850	77.7
1–2	0.000444	99,329	44	99,307	7,671,441	77.2
2–3	0.000300	99,285	30	99,270	7,572,134	76.3
3–4	0.000216	99,255	21	99,244	7,472,864	75.3
4–5	0.000179	99,233	18	99,225	7,373,620	74.3
5–6	0.000168	99,216	17	99,207	7,274,396	73.3
6–7	0.000156	99,199	15	99,191	7,175,188	72.3
7–8	0.000143	99,184	14	99,177	7,075,997	71.3
8–9	0.000125	99,169	12	99,163	6,976,820	70.4
9–10	0.000103	99,157	10	99,152	6,877,657	69.4
10–11	0.000086	99,147	9	99,143	6,778,505	68.4
11–12	0.000088	99,138	9	99,134	6,679,363	67.4
12–13	0.000125	99,130	12	99,123	6,580,229	66.4
13–14	0.000206	99,117	20	99,107	6,481,105	65.4
14–15	0.000317	99,097	31	99,081	6,381,999	64.4
15–16	0.000438	99,065	43	99,044	6,282,918	63.4
16–17	0.000552	99,022	55	98,995	6,183,874	62.4
17–18	0.000657	98,967	65	98,935	6,084,879	61.5
18–19	0.000747	98,902	74	98,865	5,985,945	60.5
19–20	0.000825	98,828	82	98,788	5,887,079	59.6
...						
98–99	0.282188	3,475	981	2,985	9,009	2.6
99–100	0.303810	2,494	758	2,115	6,024	2.4
100 and over	1.00000	1,737	1,737	3,909	3,909	2.3

TABLE 5.2   Life Table for the Total Population in the United States, 2006

Data from: Arias E. United States life tables, 2006. Hyattsville, MD: National Center for Health Statistics. *National Vital Statistics Reports*, 2010;58(21).

abridged life table saves space and is more easily communicated. To abridge the complete life table, we will change the notation for 3 of the 6 life table functions. The q_x, d_x, and L_x functions describe the age interval x to $x + n$ (n denotes the length of the age interval). The notation for these functions is modified in the abridged life table to $_nq_x$, $_nd_x$, and $_nL_x$. For example, $_5d_{40}$ is the probability of dying in the age range 40 through 44. We do not change the notation for l_x, T_x, and e_x because these functions describe exact age x at the beginning of the age interval.

In the abridged life table (**Table 5.3**), we recalculate $_nq_x$, $_nd_x$, and $_nL_x$ for the age groups 1 through 99. We do this by simply summing the values in Table 5.2 for the number of intervals. Then, T_x, and e_x are computed as before. Note that:

$$_nd_x = l_x - l_{x+n}$$

$$_nq_x = \frac{_nd_x}{l_x}$$

$$_nL_x = T_x - T_{x+n}$$

Note that for the open-ended interval beginning at age 100, $_\infty d_{100} = l_{100}$, $q_{100} = 1$, and $_\infty L_{100} = T_{100}$.

Life expectancy according to age is presented in **Figure 5.1** for white and black males and females in the United States in 2006.[5] At birth, average life expectancy is 75.7 for white males, 80.6 for white females, 69.7 for black males, and 76.5 for black females. For a person surviving to age 25, for example, average years of life remaining are 50.7 for white males, 55.6 for white females, 44.7 for black males, and 51.5 for black females. If a white man married a white woman, both aged 25, on average the woman would be a widow for 4.9 years at the end of her life. If a black man married a black woman, both aged 25, on average the woman would be a widow for 6.8 years at the end of her life.

From 1900 to 1902, life expectancy in the United States was 49.2.[5] In 2011, it was estimated to be 78.4.[12] Improving life expectancy in the United States and elsewhere has been primarily attributed to cultural adaptations.[13,14] Research has indicated that longer life spans are more common in recent human evolution.[14,15] For example, in the early 1600s, life expectancy was about 35 years in England because about two-thirds of children died within the first 3 years of life.[16] In Colonial times in the United States, life expectancy was under 25 years in the Virginia colony,[17] and roughly 40% of children in New England never reached adulthood.[18] Life expectancy increased considerably during the Industrial Revolution.[19] More recent increases in life expectancy have been attributed to advances in public health (e.g., nutrition, housing conditions, sanitation, water supply, antibiotics, and immunization programs).[20]

TABLE 5.3   Abridged Life Table for the Total Population in the United States, 2006

Age	Probability of dying between ages x and x + n	Number surviving to age x	Number dying between ages x and x + n	Person-years lived between ages x and x + n	Total number of person-years lived about age x	Expectation of life at age x
	$_nq_x$	l_x	$_nd_x$	$_nL_x$	T_x	e_x
0–<1	0.00671	100,000	671	99,409	7,769,651	77.7
1–4	0.00114	99,329	113	397,089	7,670,242	77.2
5–9	0.00069	99,216	69	495,906	7,273,153	73.3
10–14	0.00082	99,147	81	495,530	6,777,247	68.4
15–19	0.00321	99,065	318	494,531	6,281,717	63.4
20–24	0.00500	98,747	494	492,501	5,787,186	58.6
25–29	0.00503	98,253	495	490,031	5,294,686	53.9
30–34	0.00558	97,759	546	487,430	4,804,655	49.1
35–39	0.00739	97,213	718	484,270	4,317,225	44.4
40–44	0.01138	96,495	1,098	479,729	3,832,955	39.7
45–49	0.01726	95,397	1,647	472,866	3,353,227	35.2
50–54	0.02558	93,750	2,398	462,754	2,880,361	30.7
55–59	0.03606	91,352	3,295	448,523	2,417,607	26.5
60–64	0.05458	88,057	4,806	428,272	1,969,084	22.4
65–69	0.07917	83,251	6,591	399,781	1,540,811	18.5
70–74	0.12170	76,661	9,330	359,980	1,141,031	14.9
75–79	0.19501	67,331	13,130	303,831	781,051	11.6
80–84	0.30251	54,201	16,396	230,015	477,220	8.8
85–89	0.44721	37,805	16,907	146,757	247,205	6.5
90–94	0.61764	20,898	12,907	72,221	100,448	4.8
95–99	0.78268	7,991	6,254	24,318	28,227	3.5
100 and over	1.00000	1,737	1,737	3,909	3,909	2.3

Data from: Arias E. United States life tables, 2006. Hyattsville, MD: National Center for Health Statistics. 2010. *National Vital Statistics Reports*, 2010;58(21).

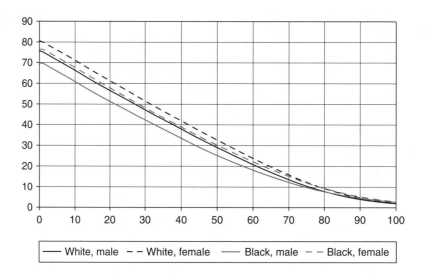

FIGURE 5.1 Age-conditional life expectancy in the United States for white and black males and females, 2006.
Data from: Arias E. United States life tables, 2006. Hyattsville, MD: National Center for Health Statistics. *National Vital Statistics Reports*, 2010;59(21).

Considerable variation in life expectancy throughout the world may be attributed to differences in wealth, public health, nutrition, and medical care. To illustrate, ecological data involving life expectancy and GDP per capita is shown for 219 countries in **Figure 5.2**. A positive relationship between GDP per capita and life expectancy is seen. However, once GDP per capita reaches $20,000 or so, there is not much improvement in life expectancy associated with greater GDP per capita.

MULTIPLE CAUSE LIFE TABLE

A multiple cause life table is used to describe in a single life table the mortality patterns of multiple diseases in the population. This table organizes and displays the age structure of people dying of specific causes. The components of the multiple-cause life table are total deaths, cause-specific deaths, and the midyear population for specific age groups.

Multiple Cause Life Table Notation
D_x = total number of deaths in the age interval x to $x + n$
D_x^i = total number of deaths from the ith cause in the age interval x to $x + n$
P_x = total number of people at risk in the age interval x to $x + n$ at midyear

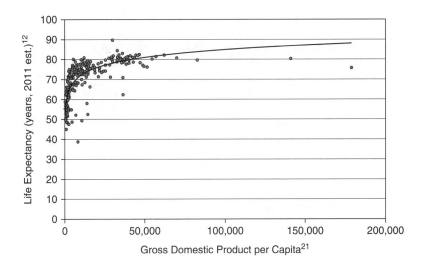

FIGURE 5.2 Life expectancy versus GDP per capita in 2011.
Data from: Central Intelligence Agency. The World Factbook. https://www.cia.
gov/library/publications/the-world-factbook/rankorder/2004rank.html. Accessed
August 3, 2011.

Average age-specific mortality rates for the age interval x to $x + n$ are computed as:

$$R_x = \frac{D_x}{P_x}$$

$$_n q_x = \frac{nR_x}{1 + \frac{1}{2}nR_x}$$

Recall that this is a conditional probability of death in which the probability of death between x to $x + n$ is for those people alive at age x. The length of the interval starting at age x is denoted by n. Note that for the first interval, the separation factor could be used to provide a better estimate of average time lived by those who died, but this has little impact on the final calculation for the entire life span.

To compute cause-specific conditional probabilities of death, we use the formula:

$$q_x^i = \frac{D_x^i}{D_x} q_x$$

Age- and cause-specific deaths for males in Texas during 2007 are shown in **Table 5.4**.[22] Applying these data to the formulas result in the conditional probabilities appearing in **Table 5.5**.

TABLE 5.4   Deaths from Four Causes among Males in Texas, 2007

	P_x	D_x^1	D_x^2	D_x^3	D_x^4
Age	Population	Malignant cancer	Accidents and adverse effects	Suicide and self-inflicted injury	All other
0–<1	206,445	4	51	0	1,346
1–4	806,533	17	127	0	147
5–9	929,284	25	56	0	69
10–14	890,203	22	70	10	71
15–19	897,008	43	377	108	255
20–24	913,310	52	644	190	494
25–29	942,508	62	530	153	522
30–34	862,549	87	430	189	558
35–39	874,370	145	444	167	852
40–44	851,611	284	495	190	1,433
45–49	851,879	661	539	214	2,327
50–54	752,071	1,224	483	177	3,206
55–59	619,431	1,727	398	147	3,750
60–64	474,973	2,130	256	112	4,178
65–69	334,352	2,359	168	69	4,322
70–74	253,950	2,484	220	58	5,243
75–79	194,504	2,689	249	60	6,734
80–84	132,392	2,410	278	39	7,819
85+	102,646	2,136	365	49	11,619

Data from: Surveillance, Epidemiology, and End Results (SEER) Program (www.seer.cancer.gov). SEER*Stat Database: Mortality—All COD, Aggregated with State, Total U.S. (1969–2007) <Katrina/Rita Population Adjustment>, National Cancer Institute, DCCPS, Surveillance Research Program, Cancer Statistics Branch, released June 2010. Underlying mortality data provided by NCHS (www.cdc.gov/nchs).

TABLE 5.5 Conditional Probabilities of Death for Four Causes among Males in Texas, 2007

Age	q_x Total	q_x^1 Malignant cancer	q_x^2 Accidents and adverse effects	q_x^3 Suicide and self-inflicted injury	q_x^4 All other
0–<1	0.00676	0.00002	0.00025	0.00000	0.00650
1–4	0.00144	0.00008	0.00063	0.00000	0.00073
5–9	0.00081	0.00013	0.00030	0.00000	0.00037
10–14	0.00097	0.00012	0.00039	0.00006	0.00040
15–19	0.00436	0.00024	0.00210	0.00060	0.00142
20–24	0.00753	0.00028	0.00351	0.00104	0.00269
25–29	0.00670	0.00033	0.00280	0.00081	0.00276
30–34	0.00730	0.00050	0.00248	0.00109	0.00322
35–39	0.00915	0.00083	0.00253	0.00095	0.00485
40–44	0.01400	0.00166	0.00289	0.00111	0.00835
45–49	0.02172	0.00384	0.00313	0.00124	0.01351
50–54	0.03328	0.00800	0.00316	0.00116	0.02096
55–59	0.04746	0.01361	0.00314	0.00116	0.02955
60–64	0.06789	0.02166	0.00260	0.00114	0.04249
65–69	0.09837	0.03354	0.00239	0.00098	0.06145
70–74	0.14610	0.04533	0.00402	0.00106	0.09569
75–79	0.22236	0.06144	0.00569	0.00137	0.15386
80–84	0.33214	0.07590	0.00876	0.00123	0.24626
85+	1.00000	0.15075	0.02576	0.00346	0.82003

Data from: Surveillance, Epidemiology, and End Results (SEER) Program (www.seer.cancer.gov). SEER*Stat Database: Mortality—All COD, Aggregated with State, Total U.S. (1969–2007) <Katrina/Rita Population Adjustment>, National Cancer Institute, DCCPS, Surveillance Research Program, Cancer Statistics Branch, released June 2010. Underlying mortality data provided by NCHS (www.cdc.gov/nchs).

Parallel to the single-cause life table, an arbitrary number of, say, $l_x = 1,000,000$ people can be distributed according to the conditional probabilities of death; that is, the distribution of life table deaths for a population can be obtained from the pattern of age-specific mortality described by the estimated q^i_x values. The life table deaths are obtained using the formula:

$$d^i_x = l_x q^i_x$$

where l_x is the number of individuals alive at the beginning of age interval x. Thus, we can calculate the data as shown in **Table 5.6**.

The cumulative number of deaths at and above age x is:

$$W^i_x = \sum_{x=0}^{\infty} d^i_x$$

Cumulative numbers of deaths for males in Texas during 2007, according to the selected causes, are shown in **Table 5.7**.

Because 1,000,000 males make up the population at risk, the probability of dying of cancer is 23% ($225,567/1,000,000 \times 100$), of an accident or adverse event is 5% ($48,837/1,000,000 \times 100$), from suicide is 1% ($13,780/1,000,000 \times 100$), and from all other causes is 71% ($711,817/1,000,000 \times 100$). A person's probability of dying from a specific cause changes as he lives to a given age. For example, the probability of dying from cancer after age 70 is 22% ($153,445/713,518 \times 100$).

With the cumulative number of deaths, we have the values needed to estimate the probability of death before age x for each cause:

$$F^i_x = 1 - \frac{W^i_x}{W^i_0}$$

These results are presented in **Table 5.8**. For example, among males in Texas dying of cancer, the probability of dying before age 50 is about 3.4%; among people dying of accidents and adverse events, the probability of dying before age 50 is about 41.8%; and among males in Texas dying of suicide, the probability of dying before age 50 is about 48.4%.

YEARS OF POTENTIAL LIFE LOST

The methodology of life tables can be used to quantify the level of premature death. A frequently used measure of the relative impact of various health-related states or events on the population is years of potential life lost (YPLL). This measure identifies the loss of expected years of life because of premature death in the population. Death due to causes that tend to affect younger people (e.g., homicide) will result in more

TABLE 5.6   Death for Four Causes among Males in Texas, 2007

Age	l_x Total	d_x^1 Malignant cancer	d_x^2 Accidents and adverse effects	d_x^3 Suicide and self-inflicted injury	d_x^4 All other
0–<1	1,000,000	19	246	0	6,498
1–4	993,237	84	625	0	724
5–9	991,804	133	299	0	368
10–14	991,004	122	389	56	395
15–19	990,042	237	2,076	595	1,404
20–24	985,730	280	3,462	1,021	2,656
25–29	978,311	321	2,741	791	2,700
30–34	971,757	488	2,413	1,061	3,132
35–39	964,663	796	2,438	917	4,678
40–44	955,833	1,583	2,758	1,059	7,986
45–49	942,448	3,617	2,949	1,171	12,732
50–54	921,979	7,378	2,911	1,067	19,325
55–59	891,298	12,130	2,795	1,032	26,339
60–64	849,001	18,390	2,210	967	36,073
65–69	791,361	26,544	1,890	776	48,632
70–74	713,518	32,347	2,865	755	68,275
75–79	609,275	37,433	3,466	835	93,744
80–84	473,797	35,962	4,148	582	116,676
85+	316,429	47,702	8,151	1,094	259,481

Data from: Surveillance, Epidemiology, and End Results (SEER) Program (www.seer.cancer.gov). SEER*Stat Database: Mortality—All COD, Aggregated with State, Total U.S. (1969–2007) <Katrina/Rita Population Adjustment>, National Cancer Institute, DCCPS, Surveillance Research Program, Cancer Statistics Branch, released June 2010. Underlying mortality data provided by NCHS (www.cdc.gov/nchs).

TABLE 5.7   Expected Number of Deaths after Age x among Males in Texas, 2007

	W_x^1	W_x^2	W_x^3	W_x^4
Age	Malignant cancer	Accidents and adverse effects	Suicide and self-inflicted injury	All other
0–<1	225,567	48,837	13,780	711,817
1–4	225,547	48,590	13,780	705,319
5–9	225,464	47,965	13,780	704,595
10–14	225,330	47,666	13,780	704,227
15–19	225,208	47,277	13,725	703,832
20–24	224,971	45,201	13,130	702,428
25–29	224,692	41,739	12,108	699,772
30–34	224,371	38,997	11,317	697,072
35–39	223,883	36,584	10,256	693,940
40–44	223,086	34,146	9,339	689,262
45–49	221,504	31,387	8,280	681,276
50–54	217,887	28,438	7,110	668,544
55–59	210,509	25,527	6,043	649,219
60–64	198,379	22,732	5,010	622,880
65–69	179,989	20,521	4,043	586,808
70–74	153,445	18,631	3,267	538,176
75–79	121,098	15,766	2,512	469,900
80–84	83,664	12,300	1,676	376,157
85+	47,702	8,151	1,094	259,481

Data from: Surveillance, Epidemiology, and End Results (SEER) Program (www.seer.cancer.gov). SEER*Stat Database: Mortality–All COD, Aggregated with State, Total U.S. (1969–2007) <Katrina/Rita Population Adjustment>, National Cancer Institute, DCCPS, Surveillance Research Program, Cancer Statistics Branch, released June 2010. Underlying mortality data provided by NCHS (www.cdc.gov/nchs).

	F_x^1	F_x^2	F_x^3	F_x^4
TABLE 5.8	**Cumulative Probabilities of Death for Four Causes among Males in Texas, 2007**			
Age	Malignant cancer	Accidents and adverse effects	Suicide and self-inflicted injury	All other
0–<1	0.00000	0.00000	0.00000	0.00000
1–4	0.00009	0.00504	0.00000	0.00913
5–9	0.00046	0.01784	0.00000	0.01015
10–14	0.00105	0.02396	0.00000	0.01066
15–19	0.00159	0.03193	0.00404	0.01122
20–24	0.00264	0.07444	0.04719	0.01319
25–29	0.00388	0.14534	0.12132	0.01692
30–34	0.00530	0.20147	0.17875	0.02071
35–39	0.00747	0.25089	0.25573	0.02511
40–44	0.01100	0.30081	0.32227	0.03169
45–49	0.01801	0.35729	0.39911	0.04290
50–54	0.03405	0.41768	0.48408	0.06079
55–59	0.06675	0.47730	0.56150	0.08794
60–64	0.12053	0.53454	0.63642	0.12494
65–69	0.20206	0.57980	0.70660	0.17562
70–74	0.31974	0.61851	0.76294	0.24394
75–79	0.46314	0.67717	0.81775	0.33986
80–84	0.62909	0.74815	0.87836	0.47155
85+	0.78852	0.83309	0.92059	0.63547

Data from: Surveillance, Epidemiology, and End Results (SEER) Program (www.seer.cancer.gov). SEER*Stat Database: Mortality–All COD, Aggregated with State, Total U.S. (1969–2007) <Katrina/Rita Population Adjustment>, National Cancer Institute, DCCPS, Surveillance Research Program, Cancer Statistics Branch, released June 2010. Underlying mortality data provided by NCHS (www.cdc.gov/nchs).

years of life lost than deaths that predominately affect older people (e.g., heart disease). The YPLL equation is:

$$YPLL = \sum_{i=1}^{n}(Endpoint - age\ at\ death\ before\ endpoint)$$

The endpoint is generally predetermined at the retirement age of 65 years or the average life expectancy, and n is the number of people in the sample. Using age 65 as the endpoint may represent seeing the data from a strictly economic point of view. However, we may wish to consider social and humane aspects as well. Thus, the average life expectancy rather than the age of retirement may be the more appropriate endpoint.

To illustrate, suppose five workers ($n = 5$) died because of exposure to high levels of radiation. The YPLL for these five workers, given that their ages at death were 20, 25, 30, 35, and 40 years, and based on age 65 as the endpoint, is:

$$YPLL = (65 - 20) + (65 - 25) + (65 - 30) + (65 - 35) + (65 - 40) = 175$$

In other words, the YPLL among these 5 workers due to exposure to high levels of radiation in the workplace is 175 years. The average YPLL is:

$$Average\ YPLL = \frac{1}{n}\sum_{i=1}^{n}(Endpoint - age\ at\ death\ before\ endpoint) = \frac{175}{5} = 35$$

Therefore, the average number of years of premature death among these 5 workers who died is 35 years.

Now refer to the data in **Table 5.9**.[22] In a situation like this where data are grouped into 5-year age categories, YPLL is calculated slightly differently. In particular, we begin by determining the average age of death for each age interval. The equation is as follows:

$$Mid\ Age = \frac{Age\ group's\ youngest\ age + oldest\ age + 1}{2}$$

The 1 is added in the numerator to include people in the last age year for the selected age interval. For example, the mid age in the age group 0 through 4 is:

$$Mid\ Age = \frac{0 + 4 + 1}{2} = 2.5$$

The table also contains the mid age values for age groups up through 64, as well as the average years of life lost up through age 64 for people dying in each age group. Thus, persons who died in the first age group lost, on average, 62.5 years of life.

TABLE 5.9 Deaths from Malignant Cancer in the United States, 2003–2007, by Age and Gender

Age group (years)	Mid age	Years to 65	Males			Females		
			Deaths	Population	YPLL	Deaths	Population	YPLL
0–4	2.5	62.5	1,248	51,808,329	78,000	1,033	49,488,057	64,563
5–9	7.5	57.5	2,426	91,520,322	139,495	1,949	87,431,717	112,068
10–14	12.5	52.5	2,726	103,520,121	143,115	2,235	98,749,126	117,338
15–19	17.5	47.5	3,480	106,987,680	165,300	2,515	101,775,679	119,463
20–24	22.5	42.5	5,035	107,377,885	213,988	3,339	101,617,180	141,908
25–29	27.5	37.5	6,458	104,488,614	242,175	5,054	99,400,573	189,525
30–34	32.5	32.5	8,821	101,345,911	286,683	9,273	98,273,176	301,373
35–59	37.5	27.5	14,677	103,408,313	403,618	19,229	101,938,156	528,798
40–44	42.5	22.5	31,251	109,193,431	703,148	40,752	109,360,546	916,920
45–49	47.5	17.5	68,218	111,512,286	1,193,815	77,481	113,511,130	1,355,918
50–54	52.5	12.5	127,088	104,160,607	1,588,600	123,181	107,704,652	1,539,763
55–59	57.5	7.5	200,284	90,639,986	1,502,130	175,172	95,313,986	1,313,790
60–64	62.5	2.5	270,611	72,985,863	676,528	225,902	78,519,633	564,755
65–69			327,835	55,000,713		266,469	61,469,823	
70–74			382,357	42,887,901		312,774	50,858,188	
75–79			435,127	34,719,609		370,183	45,116,238	
80–84			433,573	26,298,068		395,047	38,750,702	
85+			389,441	18,707,645		426,450	34,714,939	

Data from: Surveillance, Epidemiology, and End Results (SEER) Program (www.seer.cancer.gov). SEER*Stat Database: Mortality—All COD, Aggregated with State, Total U.S. (1969–2007) <Katrina/Rita Population Adjustment>, National Cancer Institute, DCCPS, Surveillance Research Program, Cancer Statistics Branch, released June 2010. Underlying mortality data provided by NCHS (www.cdc.gov/nchs).

Because 1,248 males and 1,033 females died of malignant cancer, the estimated YPLL from 2003 to 2007 in the United States from malignant cancer in the age group 0–4 is:

$$YPLL_{M,0-4} = 62.5 \times 1,248 = 78,000$$

$$YPLL_{F,0-4} = 62.5 \times 1,033 = 64,563$$

This same approach can be taken for each age group through the age group 60–64 in order to obtain the age-group-specific YPLL. The total YPLL for all age groups combined is the sum of the YPLL across the age groups: 7,336,593 for males and 7,266,178 for females.

To make more meaningful comparisons of nominal data among groups, rates may be used instead of raw numbers. Similarly, the YPLL rate is preferred when making comparisons among groups because it takes into account the size of the populations in which the deaths occurred (**Table 5.10**). The age-group-specific

TABLE 5.10	Age-Group-Specific YPLL Rates (per 100,000) for Malignant Cancer in the United States According to Gender, 2003–2007	
Age group (years)	**Males**	**Females**
0–4	151	130
5–9	152	128
10–14	138	119
15–19	155	117
20–24	199	140
25–29	232	191
30–34	283	307
35–59	390	519
40–44	644	838
45–49	1,071	1,195
50–54	1,525	1,430
55–59	1,657	1,378
60–64	927	719
0–64	583	585

Data from: Surveillance, Epidemiology, and End Results (SEER) Program (www.seer.cancer.gov). SEER*Stat Database: Mortality–All COD, Aggregated with State, Total U.S. (1969–2007) <Katrina/Rita Population Adjustment>, National Cancer Institute, DCCPS, Surveillance Research Program, Cancer Statistics Branch, released June 2010. Underlying mortality data provided by NCHS (www.cdc.gov/nchs).

YPLL is greater for females than males in each age category from 30 through 49. This is most likely because of deaths due to female breast cancer. The age-group-specific YPLL is greater for males than females in the age groups beginning with 50, most likely because of deaths from lung and prostate cancer. Although the YPLL is greater for males than females, the YPLL rate is slightly higher for females than males. When computing the total rate, divide the total YPLL through age 64 by the total population through the same age. Do not use the population for the entire age span.

EXERCISES

Age-Group-Specific Probability of Death in the United States, 2007[23]	
	Probability of dying between ages x to $x + n$
Age	$_nq_x$
0–<1	0.006760
1–4	0.001140
5–9	0.000683
10–14	0.000839
15–19	0.003089
20–24	0.004907
25–29	0.004958
30–34	0.005524
35–39	0.007251
40–44	0.011003
45–49	0.016870
50–54	0.025217
55–59	0.035858
60–64	0.052469
65–69	0.077793
70–74	0.119029
75–79	0.191290
80–84	0.297734

(continues)

Age-Group-Specific Probability of Death in the United States, 2007[23] (*continued*)

Age	Probability of dying between ages x to $x + n$ $_nq_x$
85–89	0.441765
90–94	0.612438
95–99	0.778825
100+	1

1. From this data, complete the life table. To simplify your calculations, use a separation factor of 0.5 in each age group.
2. Graph the age-conditional life expectancy data obtained in your life table.

Deaths from Four Causes among Females in Texas, 2007[22]

Age	P_x Population	D_x^1 Malignant cancer	D_x^2 Accidents and adverse effects	D_x^3 Suicide and self-inflicted injury	D_x^4 All other
0–<1	197,736	4	35	0	1,124
1–4	771,419	12	65	0	129
5–9	886,569	21	40	0	54
10–14	850,680	19	41	0	63
15–19	844,815	20	159	26	118
20–24	832,569	40	181	29	153
25–29	876,216	40	165	41	267
30–34	824,416	99	120	41	310
35–39	856,043	211	149	50	498
40–44	839,219	394	212	64	744
45–49	855,627	715	263	71	1,219
50–54	773,939	1,032	223	62	1,736
55–59	655,083	1,422	144	37	2,131
60–64	513,329	1,679	126	33	2,723
65–69	379,124	1,894	102	9	3,239

	P_x	D_x^1	D_x^2	D_x^3	D_x^4
Deaths from Four Causes among Females in Texas, 2007[22] *(continued)*					
Age	Population	Malignant cancer	Accidents and adverse effects	Suicide and self-inflicted injury	All other
70–74	310,299	2,071	112	13	4,424
75–79	263,955	2,318	176	12	6,763
80–84	207,471	2,172	284	4	9,420
85+	214,904	2,350	610	7	23,582

3. Calculate the cause-specific probabilities of death for the three specific causes for females in Texas in 2007.

4. Calculate the distribution of life table deaths for the population with a pattern of age-specific mortality described by the estimated conditional probabilities that you derived in question 3. Use $l_0 = 1,000,000$.

5. From your answer in question 4, calculate the expected number of deaths after age x.

6. From your answer in question 5, calculate the cumulative probabilities of death for the selected causes.

7. Calculate the years of potential life lost (YPLL) for malignant cancer, accidents and adverse effects, and suicide and self-inflicted injury.

8. In which age-group is the YPLL greatest for malignant cancer, accidents and adverse effects, and suicide and self-inflicted injury?

9. Calculate the YPLL rate for malignant cancer, accidents and adverse effects, and suicide and self-inflicted injury.

10. What is the rationale for using age 65 as the endpoint?

REFERENCES

1. Garrison FH. *History of Medicine*. Philadelphia, PA: Saunders; 1926.
2. Rosen G. *A History of Public Health*. New York, NY: MD Publications; 1958.
3. Fox JP, Hall CE, Elveback LR. *Epidemiology: Man and Disease*. New York, NY: Macmillan Company; 1970.
4. Arias E, Rostron BL, Tejada-Vera B. United States life tables, 2005. *National Vital Statistics Reports* 2010;58(10). Hyattsville, MD: National Center for Health Statistics.
5. Arias E. United States life tables, 2006. *National Vital Statistics Reports* 2010;58(10). Hyattsville, MD: National Center for Health Statistics.
6. Ingram DD, Weed JA, Parker JD, Hamilton B, Arias E, Madans JH. U.S. Census 2000 with bridged race categories. National Center for Health Statistics. *Vital Health Stat.* 2003;2(135):1–56.

7. Sirken MG. Comparison of two methods of constructing abridged life tables by reference to a "standard" table. National Center for Health Statistics. *Vital Health Stat.* 1966;2(4):1–13.

8. Arias E, Curtin LR, Wei R, Anderson RN. U.S. decennial life tables for 1999–2001, United States life tables. *National Vital Statistics Reports* 2008;57(1). Hyattsville, MD: National Center for Health Statistics.

9. Heron M, Hoyert DL, Murphy SL, et al. Deaths: final data for 2006. *National Vital Statistics Reports* 2009;57(14). Hyattsville, MD: National Center for Health Statistics.

10. National Center for Health Statistics. U.S. decennial life tables for 1989–91. Vol. 1, no. 3. *Some Trends and Comparisons of United States Life Table Data: 1900–91.* Hyattsville, MD: National Center for Health Statistics; 1999.

11. Kung HC, Hoyert DL, Xu J, Murphy SL. Deaths: final data for 2005. *National Vital Statistics Reports* 2008;56(10). Hyattsville, MD: National Center for Health Statistics.

12. Central Intelligence Agency. The world factbook. https://www.cia.gov/library/publications/the-world-factbook/rankorder/2102rank.html. Published 2011. Accessed August 3, 2011.

13. Jones S, Martin R, Pilbeam D, eds. *The Cambridge Encyclopedia of Human Evolution.* Cambridge UK: Cambridge University Press; 1994:242.

14. Caspari R, Lee S-H. Is human longevity a consequence of cultural change or modern biology? *Am J Phys Anthropol.* 2006;129(4):512–517.

15. Caspari R, Lee S-H. Older age becomes common late in human evolution. Proceedings of the National Academy of Sciences. 2004;101(20):10,895–10,900.

16. Rorabaugh WJ, Critchlow DT, Baker PC. *America's Promise: A Concise History of the United States.* Lanham, MD: Rowman & Littlefield; 2004:47.

17. Stratford Hall. Medicine & health. http://www.stratfordhall.org/learn/teacher/medicine.php. Published 2005. Accessed August 4, 2011.

18. Digital History. Death in early America. http://www.digitalhistory.uh.edu/historyonline/usdeath.cfm. Published 2011. Accessed August 4, 2011.

19. Britannica Academic Edition. Modernization—population change. http://www.britannica.com/EBchecked/topic/387301/modernization/12022/Population-change. Published 2011. Accessed August 4, 2011.

20. Centers for Disease Control and Prevention. Ten great public health achievements—United States, 1900–1999. *MMWR.* 1999;48 (12):241–243. http://cdc.gov/mmwr/preview/mmwrhtml/00056796.htm. Reprinted in: From the Centers for Disease Control and Prevention. Ten great public health achievements—United States, 1900–1999. *JAMA.* 1999;281(16):1481.

21. Central Intelligence Agency. The world factbook. https://www.cia.gov/library/publications/the-world-factbook/rankorder/2004rank.html. Published 2011. Accessed August 3, 2011.

22. Surveillance, Epidemiology, and End Results (SEER) Program (www.seer.cancer.gov). SEER*Stat Database: Mortality—All COD, Aggregated with State, Total U.S. (1969–2007) <Katrina/Rita Population Adjustment>, National Cancer Institute, DCCPS, Surveillance Research Program, Cancer Statistics Branch. Underlying mortality data provided by NCHS. www.cdc.gov/nchs. Released June 2010. Accessed July 10, 2010.

23. Jiaquan X, Kochanek KD, Murphy SL, Tejada-Vera B; Division of Vital Statistics. Deaths: final data for 2007. *National Vital Statistics Reports* 2010;58(19). Hyattsville, MD: National Center for Health Statistics.

CHAPTER 6

Probability

A primary component of the life table is the probability of death within a specific age interval x to $x + n$, conditional on having survived to age x. Probability is the second major topic in the area of biostatistics. Probability provides a basis for evaluating the reliability of the conclusions we reach and the inferences we make when applying statistical techniques to the collection, analysis, and interpretation of quantitative data. In other words, the foundation of statistical inference is probability. In this chapter, we will cover the meaning of probability in terms of random experiments, outcomes, sample space, and events; present formulas for computing probabilities for various types of events; and discuss common methods of sampling.

PROBABILITY CONCEPTS

Most of us are familiar with the word probability. *Probability* is used when discussing the chance or likelihood that a given event will occur. An event is the result of an experiment, an observation, or the description of a particular outcome. For example, an event may be an adverse reaction to a drug, that a man is diagnosed with prostate cancer before he turns 80, that a woman diagnosed with pancreatic cancer will be alive in one year, or that a medical procedure will successfully treat a disease. Events may involve a single outcome or a set of outcomes.

Probability may be subjective or objective. A personal conception of probability is subjective. For example, a doctor may indicate a probability that a patient will respond favorably to treatment, or a public health official may give a probability that an epidemic will be contained within the next week. In contrast, objective

Definitions

Subjective probability is a person's degree of belief in the occurrence of an event based on previous observation and experience.

Objective probability is the likelihood of the outcome of any event based upon repeated random experiments or measurements rather than subjective assessment.

probability is the likelihood or chance of a specific occurrence, based on repeated random experiments or measurements. For example, in a randomized, placebo controlled clinical trial, researchers can indicate a probability of 5-year survival among patients receiving a new drug. Objective probability is considered more accurate than subjective probability.

In the context of objective probability, the term *experiment* is any planned process of data collection. An experiment consists of a number of independent trials under the same conditions, such as treating 10 cancer patients with a new drug and evaluating whether they respond favorably or measuring the amount of dissolved oxygen in a polluted river. Thus, you can see that to qualify as an experiment, the operation need only produce observations or measurements. All possible outcomes from an experiment make up the sample space.

Events are represented by upper case letters such as *A*, *B*, and *C*. Within a sample space, there is usually a smaller set of events. There are three basic operations that can be performed on events: intersection, union, and complement. The intersection of *A* and *B*, for example, is denoted $A \cap B$, and is the event *both A and B*. The union of *A* and *B* is denoted by $A \cup B$ and is the event of *either A or B*. The complement of an event *A* is denoted by $\bar{A}$ and is the event *not A*. Each of these operations is illustrated for two events, *A* and *B*, in **Figure 6.1**.

The probability of an event *A* is the proportion of times it occurs out of a large number of trials repeated under virtually identical conditions. This is called the frequentist definition of probability and will be applied in this text. The probability of a particular event—say, *A*—is written as $P(A)$. If *A* is any event, then:

$$0 \le P(A) \le 1$$

Thus, the probability of an event may be 0, 1, or any value between 0 and 1. In addition, because the sample

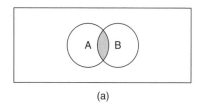

(a)

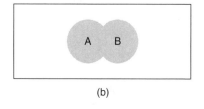

(b)

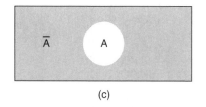

(c)

FIGURE 6.1 Venn diagrams representing the basic operations on events.

space S contains all possible events resulting from the experiment,

$$P(S) = 1$$

EXAMPLE 6.1

For the data appearing in **Table 6.1**,[1] the sample space is the set of all 16 possible outcomes. The probability of being staged with localized disease among the female breast cancer patients is:

$$P(Local) = 0.6187$$

> **Definition**
>
> The **frequentist definition** of probability is that if an experiment is repeated n times under the same conditions, and if the event A occurs m times, then as n grows large, the ratio m/n approaches a fixed limit that is the probability of A. $P(A) = \dfrac{m}{n}$.

Sometimes we want to know the probability that an event will not happen; that is, what is the event opposite to the event of primary interest? This is called a complementary event. The probability of a complementary event is found by calculating one minus the probability of the event.

> **Rule for Complementary Events**
>
> If $\bar{A}$ is the complement of event A, then:
>
> $$P(\bar{A}) = 1 - P(A)$$

TABLE 6.1   Sample Space for Female Breast Cancer in the United States According to Tumor Stage at Diagnosis and Race, 2005–2008

	Probabilities				
Stage	**White**	**Black**	**American Indian or Alaska Native**	**Asian or Pacific Islander**	**Total**
Local	0.4841	0.0623	0.0083	0.0640	0.6187
Regional	0.2238	0.0410	0.0043	0.0299	0.2990
Distant	0.0458	0.0114	0.0010	0.0053	0.0635
Unknown Stage	0.0147	0.0025	0.0002	0.0014	0.0188
Total	0.7684	0.1172	0.0138	0.1006	1

Data from: Surveillance, Epidemiology, and End Results (SEER) Program (www.seer.cancer.gov) SEER*Stat Database.

EXAMPLE 6.2

What is the complement of locally staged female breast cancer, based on the data in Table 6.1?

$$P(\overline{Local}) = 1 - P(Local) = 1 - 0.6187 = 0.3813$$

MUTUALLY EXCLUSIVE EVENTS VERSUS INDEPENDENT EVENTS _____

The outcomes presented in Table 6.1 are mutually exclusive because the occurrence of one outcome precludes the occurrence of the other. There is a link between mutually exclusive events in that they cannot both happen at once. However, there is no link between independent events. For example, exposure status is a mutually exclusive event because a single person cannot be exposed and not exposed. On the other hand, being exposed and developing an illness are not mutually exclusive events because a single person can be both exposed and ill. Now suppose I select a child from a preschool class and evaluate his/her weight status, then return the student to the class, and then select a student again and evaluate his/her weight status. The sample space remains the same for both selections because the first student was returned to the class. If the first student was not returned to the class, and he/she was overweight, then there is one fewer student and one fewer overweight student in the class. Therefore, the probability for the second selection has changed—the sample space is different. Thus, mutually exclusive events are contrasted with nonmutually exclusive events, wherein we determine whether one event excludes the other. Independent events are contrasted with dependent events, wherein we determine whether one event influences the probability of the other.

> **Definition**
>
> Two sets of outcomes are **mutually exclusive** if there is no outcome that belongs to both sets.

Complementary events are mutually exclusive, but mutually exclusive events are not necessarily complementary if three or more events are involved.

CONDITIONAL PROBABILITIES _____

> **Definition**
>
> The **conditional probability** of an event B given another event A, is:
>
> $$P(B|A) = \frac{P(A \text{ and } B)}{P(A)} \text{ where } P(A) > 0$$

In this section, we consider conditional probability. The definition of *conditional probability* allows us to develop a general equation that uses multiplication to compute probabilities for joint events. Using the vertical line | to mean "given," we can express the probability of one event given another as $P(B|A)$.

EXAMPLE 6.3

Among a group of female breast cancer patients, what is the probability of having distant staged disease given the patient's race is black? The sample space is reduced to the black female population, and we solve the problem using the following definition for conditional probabilities:

$$P(Distant\ Stage|Black) = \frac{0.0114}{0.1173} = 0.097$$

Thus, among our group of female breast cancer patients, the probability of having distant staged cancer given their race is black is 0.097 or 9.7%.

RULE FOR MULTIPLYING PROBABILITIES

When two of the three terms in the previous equation are known, we can solve the third. For instance, multiplying both sides of the equation by $P(A)$ gives the following multiplication rule, wherein we may compute the joint probability:

General Rule for Multiplication of Probabilities
$P(A\ and\ B) = P(B|A) \times P(A)$

It also holds that because $P(A\ and\ B) = P(B\ and\ A)$, that $P(A\ and\ B) = P(A|B) \times P(B)$. In Table 6.1, the probabilities in the total column or total row are called marginal probabilities because they appear on the margins of the probability table. The probability of two events $P(A\ and\ B)$ is a joint probability.

INDEPENDENT EVENTS

Now let us think of the situation where the events are independent.

EXAMPLE 6.4

The distribution of blood types is presented according to Rh status in **Table 6.2**.[2] If we let the notation B be the

> **Definition**
>
> A and B are **independent events** if:
>
> $$P(B|A) = P(B)$$
>
> So A gives no information about the probability of B.

TABLE 6.2 Blood Type by Rh Status			
Blood type	**Rh positive**	**Rh negative**	**Total**
O	0.374	0.066	0.44
A	0.357	0.063	0.42
B	0.085	0.015	0.10
AB	0.034	0.006	0.04
Total	0.85	0.15	1

Data from: Blood types in the U.S. http://bloodcenter.stanford.edu/about_blood/blood_types.html.

event that blood type is AB and the notation A the event of Rh status is positive, then the event A and B is 0.034. Because P(A) is 0.85,

$$P(B|A) = \frac{0.034}{0.85} = 0.04$$

In the case where A and B are independent events, conditional and unconditional probabilities are equal; $P(Blood\ Type\ AB) = P(Blood\ type\ AB|Rh\ positive) = 0.04$. That is, Rh status does not influence blood type.

EXAMPLE 6.5

The probability of Rh negative given blood type O is:

$$P(Rh\ negative|Blood\ type\ O) = \frac{0.066}{0.44} = 0.150$$

If the outcome of one event has no influence on the outcome of a second event, the two events are independent. In this case, the product of the marginal probabilities will equal the joint probability.

Rule for Multiplication of Independent Events

If A and B are independent events, then:

$$P(A\ and\ B) = P(A) \times P(B)$$

EXAMPLE 6.6

Blood type and Rh status are independent events because the product of each combination of marginal probabilities equals the corresponding joint probability; for example,

$$P(Blood\ Type\ AB\ and\ Rh\ positive) = P(Blood\ Type\ AB) \times P(Rh\ positive)$$

$$= 0.85 \times 0.04 = 0.034$$

In contrast, for the data in Table 6.1 where cancer stage is not independent of race, the product of any combination of marginal probabilities does not equal the corresponding joint probability. In other words, the distribution of stage differs according to racial group, and, thus, we are interested in the conditional probabilities.

Recall that the probability of two mutually exclusive events occurring is the probability that one or the other event occurs. To find this probability, we apply the addition rule for probabilities.

> **Rule for Addition of Probabilities of Mutually Exclusive Events**
>
> If events *A* and *B* are mutually exclusive, then,
>
> $$P(A\ or\ B) = P(A) + P(B)$$

EXAMPLE 6.7

Among female breast cancer patients, the probability of having local or regional staged disease (see Table 6.1) is:

$$P(Local\ or\ Regional) = P(Local) + P(Regional) = 0.6187 + 0.2990 = 0.9177$$

The addition rule also applies for more than two mutually exclusive events.

EXAMPLE 6.8

The probability of blood type A, B, or AB (see Table 6.2) is:

$$P(A\ or\ B\ or\ AB) = P(A) + P(B) + P(AB) = 0.42 + 0.10 + 0.04 = 0.56$$

If two events are not mutually exclusive, we use a modified addition rule.

Rule for Probabilities That Are Not Mutually Exclusive Events

If events A and B are not mutually exclusive, then,

$$P(A \text{ or } B) = P(A) + P(B) - P(A \text{ and } B)$$

EXAMPLE 6.9

Blood type and Rh factor are not mutually exclusive events because the occurrence of one does not preclude the occurrence of the other. The probability of having blood type O is 0.44 and the probability of being Rh positive is 0.85. However, the probability of having blood type O or of being Rh positive is not $0.44 + 0.85$, because in this sum, those with blood type O who are Rh positive have been counted twice. Hence, the joint probability of having blood type O and being Rh positive, 0.374, must be subtracted. So:

$$P(Type\ O\ or\ Rh\ Positive) = P(Type\ O) + P(Rh\ Positive) - P(Type\ O\ and\ Rh\ positive)$$

$$= 0.44 + 0.85 - 0.374 = 0.916$$

If we did not known that $P(Type\ O\ and\ Rh\ positive) = 0.374$, we could determine this probability using the multiplication rule (for independent events).

BAYES' THEOREM

Thomas Bayes (1702–1761), an English theologian and mathematician, researched probability and statistical inference and developed the law of inverse probability known as Bayes' Theorem. Bayes' Theorem relates the probability of the occurrence of an event to the presence or nonpresence of an associated event; that is, it shows that if we know the conditional probability of B given A, we can identify the conditional probability of A given B. In Bayes' Theorem, $P(A|B)$ is the conditional probability of A given B; $P(B)$ is the prior probability (or marginal probability) of B. It is "prior" in that it does not take into account any information about A. $P(B|A)$ is the conditional probability of B given A. It is also called the posterior probability because it is derived from or depends upon the specific value of A.

Bayes' Theorem

$$P(B|A) = \frac{P(A|B) \times P(B)}{P(A|B) \times P(B) + P(A|\bar{B}) \times P(\bar{B})}$$

where $P(B) > 0$.

TABLE 6.3	Test Results and True Disease Status	
	True disease status	
Test result	**Present**	**Not present**
Positive	TP	FP
Negative	FN	TN
	TP + FN	FP + TN

TP = true positive; FP = false positive; FN = false negative; TN = true negative

Bayes' Theorem may be used to evaluate the validity of a screening test. The validity of a test is shown by how well the test actually measures what it is supposed to measure. Validity is determined by the sensitivity and specificity of the test. In **Table 6.3**, the top represents the true disease status, whether the disease is present or not. The left side represents our test results. If a person has the disease and tests positive, he/she is classified as a true positive (*TP*); if a person does not have the disease and tests negative, he/she is classified as a true negative (*TN*); if a person has the disease and tests negative, he/she is classified as a false negative (*FN*); and if a person does not have a disease and tests positive, he/she is classified as a false positive (*FP*). Sensitivity is the proportion of people with the disease who have a positive test. Specificity is the proportion of people without the disease who have a negative test.

Definitions

$$Sensitivity = \frac{TP}{TP + FN}$$

$$Specificity = \frac{TN}{FP + TN}$$

Now suppose we are interested in knowing the probability that an individual with a positive test (T^+) actually has the disease (D). The equation for the predictive value of a positive test, based on Bayes' Theorem, is:

$$P(D|T^+) = \frac{P(T^+|D) \times P(D)}{P(T^+|D) \times P(D) + P(T^+|\bar{D}) \times P(\bar{D})}$$

We may also be interested in knowing the probability that an individual with a negative test (T^-) does not have the disease (D). The equation for the predictive value of a negative test is:

$$P(\bar{D}|T^-) = \frac{P(T^-|\bar{D}) \times P(\bar{D})}{P(T^-|\bar{D}) \times P(\bar{D}) + P(T^-|D) \times P(D)}$$

Note:

$P(T^+|D) = \text{Sensitivity}$

$P(T^-|\bar{D}) = \text{Specificity}$

$P(T^-|D) = 1 - \text{Sensitivity}$

$P(T^+|\bar{D}) = 1 - \text{Specificity}$

$P(D) = \text{Prior (or marginal)probability}$

$P(\bar{D}) = 1 - \text{Prior probability}$

EXAMPLE 6.10

Consider the prostate specific antigen (PSA) screening test for prostate cancer (**Table 6.4**). Assume that a PSA score of at least 4 is a positive test. Suppose the prior probability (or prevalence) of prostate cancer is 0.15.

$$Sensitivity = \frac{110}{131} = 0.84$$

$$Specificity = \frac{524}{1,310} = 0.40$$

$$P(D|T^+) = \frac{0.84 \times 0.15}{0.84 \times 0.15 + (1 - 0.40) \times (1 - 0.15)} = 0.20$$

$$P(\bar{D}|T^-) = \frac{0.40 \times (1 - .15)}{0.40 \times (1 - .15) + (1 - 0.84) \times 0.15} = 0.93$$

TABLE 6.4   Prostate Specific Antigen Screening for Prostate Cancer

Test Result	True prostate cancer status	
	Present	Not present
PSA ≥ 4	110	786
PSA < 4	21	524
Total	131	1,310

Thus, using the PSA cutoff of 4 produced a sensitivity value of 84% (i.e., 84% of participants with prostate cancer were correctly classified as having the disease), a specificity of 40% (i.e., 40% of participants without prostate cancer were correctly classified as not having the disease), a predictive value positive of 20% (i.e., of those with a positive test, 20% had prostate cancer), and a predictive value negative of 93% (i.e., of those with a negative test, 93% did not have prostate cancer).

If the prior probability is not known, the following simplified equations may be used:

$$P(D|T^+) = \frac{TP}{(TP + FP)}$$

$$P(\bar{D}|T^-) = \frac{TN}{(FN + TN)}$$

which yields 0.12 and 0.96, respectively.

In a general sense, a valid screening test minimizes the threat of a false positive test, which may cause unnecessary stress, anxiety, and treatment. It also minimizes the threat of a false negative, which may cause an individual to not receive needed treatment. Screening is intended to improve the prognosis of a diagnosed case. It is particularly important for chronic disease, in which there is often a high prevalence of individuals in the presymptomatic phase of the disease.

> **Definition**
>
> A **prognosis** is a prediction of the likely course and outcome of a disease. It is generally based on selected prognostic indicators (signs, symptoms, and circumstances). Clinical exams and laboratory findings provide prognostic information.

CLINICAL EPIDEMIOLOGY

Clinical epidemiology involves the application of epidemiologic methods in a clinical setting. It specifically involves the application of epidemiology for evaluating patient screening and diagnosis, treatment, and prognosis. The concepts and methods already presented in this chapter provide the tools for evaluating the accuracy of screening and diagnostic tests; identifying the level of risk associated with screening, diagnostic testing, and treatment; and identifying the lethality and survival probability of the illness.

As discussed, measures of validity include sensitivity, specificity, and overall accuracy. Predictive value positive and predictive value negative, which are derived using Bayes' Theorem, are also commonly used measures of screening and diagnostic accuracy. Accurate screening and diagnostic testing are important for ensuring that a patient is properly treated.

A simple measure of prognosis is the *case-fatality rate*, which is the proportion of all people with a disease who die from that condition. When the course of an illness is long, prognosis is often measured using the survival rate, which is the proportion of patients surviving regardless of the cause of death. The efficacy of treatment options may be evaluated by comparing the case fatality rate or the survival rate among treatment options.

METHODS OF SAMPLING

Often the number of people who meet the criteria for selection into a study is too large, making it necessary to select a sample for study from the population. Keep in mind the word *inference* means "to infer or generalize from a sample to a larger population." This subset of the population may be a convenience sample or a probability sample.

In clinical research, a convenience sample is made up of people who meet the selection criteria and are easily accessible. This type of sampling is often less logistically difficult and less expensive. A convenience sample is a good choice for answering many research questions. It is valid if the sample sufficiently represents the target population, which requires a subjective judgment. Selection bias should always be considered as a possible threat in convenience samples.

There is often a need to generalize the results from the study sample to the population. Ensuring that the sample represents the population can be accomplished using statistical methods based on probability. The best way to obtain a sample wherein the results produce valid inferences is to use probability samples. Four commonly used probability sampling methods that use the random process will be presented in this section: simple random sampling, systematic sampling, stratified random sampling, and cluster sampling.

> **Definition**
>
> A **simple random sample** is a sample that is selected from a finite population in such a way that all samples of the same size have the same probability of being chosen.

A simple random sample is obtained by assigning a number to each unit of the population and selecting a subset such that each has an equal chance of being selected. This process may be thought of as a random experiment. We recommend selecting a simple random sample from a computer-generated list of random numbers.

EXAMPLE 6.11

To take a random sample of all liver cancer patients recorded by the Iowa cancer registry during 2004–2008, a list of all patients identified for the study period were obtained.

During this time, there were 700 patients. To take a random sample of 100 of these patients, assign each individual a number and then obtain a computer-generated list of 100 patients.

Computing Random Numbers in Excel

Once the spreadsheet is open, put the curser in any given cell. Then type "=RANDBETWEEN ([Bottom number], [Top number])" (inserting the lowest and highest numbers from the data) and press the Enter key. This will give a random number, somewhere from the bottom to the top number specified. Then, copy this formula and paste it down the column for the number of cells for which you are interested in obtaining random numbers.

A systematic sample is one where every kth item is selected. To determine k, we divide the number of items in the sampling frame by the desired sample size.

EXAMPLE 6.12

Continuing with the previous example, $700/100 = 7$, so every 7th patient is sampled using a systematic sampling approach. However, we must first select a number randomly between 1 and 7, and then select every 7th patient. Using Excel, suppose we get a random number of 3. Then, the systematic sample consists of patients with assigned numbers 10, 17, 24, 31, and so on. Systematic sampling should only be used when a cyclic repetition is not inherent in the sampling frame. Had our patients been numbered according to the time they were diagnosed, this approach may not be appropriate. However, if they were numbered according to their last name, then we would not be concerned that time of diagnosis is influencing the sample.

A stratified random sample is used when we want to highlight a specific subgroup within the population because it ensures the presence of the particular subgroup within the sample. It is also useful if we want to observe existing relationships between two or more

Definitions

A **systematic sample** involves selecting elements from an ordered sampling frame. It resembles the simple random sample in that there is a random starting point, but every kth member is selected thereafter from the total population.

A **sampling frame** is the actual set of units from which a sample will be drawn. It is a list that contains every member of the population from which a sample with be selected.

Definition

A **stratified random sample** (also sometimes called *proportional* or *quota* random sampling) involves dividing the population into homogeneous subgroups and then taking a simple random sample in each subgroup (e.g., age, gender, socioeconomic status, religion, nationality, and educational attainment).

subgroups. Even small and less accessible subgroups of the population can be representatively sampled. This sampling technique yields a higher statistical precision compared to simple random sampling because the variability within the subgroups is lower. In addition, a smaller sample size is required. In studying the incidence of hypertension in pregnancy, for example, we could stratify the population according to race and age groups and then sample equal numbers from each stratum.

Cluster sampling occurs when a population is divided into groups (clusters) and a subset of groups is selected. Clusters of populations may include blocks, neighborhoods, villages, or other easily definable areas. Each cluster must be mutually exclusive, and together the clusters must include the entire population. Once the groups are chosen, all or a sample of individuals in each group (e.g., households, hospitals, doctors) are selected for inclusion in the study. This sampling approach is more common in epidemiology than clinical studies because clusters are commonly based on geographic areas. For example, a sample for a hospital survey taken in a state may be selected by using census tracts as clusters; a sample is then taken of hospitals in each census tract. To ensure that subgroups are fully represented in each area, cluster sampling may be combined with other forms of sampling (e.g., random sampling). In multicenter trials, the institutions selected to participate in the study constitute the clusters. Then, patients from each institution can be selected using another method of probability sampling.

The primary reason for using cluster sampling is that it is usually less expensive and more convenient to sample the population in clusters than to do so randomly. It is a less expensive approach when the population units cover a wide area. For example,

Definition

A **cluster sample** involves a form of probability sample where respondents are drawn from a random sample of mutually exclusive groups (clusters) within a total population.

suppose you want to survey homeless women who are of reproductive age in a specific region. If you conducted a simple random sample of all these women, you might have to visit all homeless shelters in the region to interview the sample. With cluster sampling, we could first select the homeless shelters to be included in the sample, and then select homeless women within each of the chosen homeless shelters. That would probably reduce the number of homeless shelters we would need to visit and, consequently, reduce the cost of data collection. In addition, a smaller number of areas required to visit could also improve the quality of data collection (e.g., it could make more efficient supervision possible).[3] In this example, the homeless shelters are what are sometimes referred to as *natural clusters*.

In cluster sampling, we refer to the clusters as the primary sampling units, and the units within the clusters as the secondary sampling units. Making this distinction is important when calculating standard errors from cluster samples. If we treated the cluster sample as though it were a simple random sample, the estimated standard errors would be biased downward, giving a misleading picture of precision. The reason for this is that units in a cluster are generally more similar than units selected at random from the whole population. For cluster sampling to provide the same precision as simple random sampling, it is usually necessary to increase the sample size.[3]

EXERCISES

1. What is the frequentist definition of probability?
2. What are the three basic operations that can be performed on events?
3. Describe the difference between mutually exclusive and independent events.
4. When does the additive rule of probability apply?
5. If two events are not mutually exclusive, how would you express $P(A \cup B)$?
6. Suppose that the probability of hypertension if you are obese is 0.15 and the probability of hypertension if you are overweight is 0.10. What is the probability that either of these events will occur?
7. When does the multiplication rule of probability apply?
8. If two events are not independent, how would you express $P(A \cap B)$?
9. Among seniors competing at the World Senior Games, 461 completed a survey investigating the relationship between selected quality of life indicators and a history of voice disorders. Individuals were asked whether they had ever had a voice problem in which their voice did not work, perform, or sound as they felt it normally should, such that it interfered with their communication. Apply probability and then comment on the dependence or independence of the event being a man and not having a previous voice disorder for these data.

History of Voice Disorders in a Group of Elderly Adults[4]			
	Previous voice disorder		
Classification	**Yes**	**No**	**Total**
Man	30	189	219
Women	47	195	242
Total	77	384	461

10. What is the probability that both babies in a set of fraternal twins will be girls? Refer to the data in the following table to answer questions 11–17.

Birth Statistics for the U.S. Population, 2009[5]						
	Married		Unmarried		Total	
Age	Frequency	Relative frequency	Frequency	Relative frequency	Frequency	Relative frequency
<15	5,030	0.001	4,980	0.003	10,010	0.002
15–19	409,840	0.099	357,510	0.211	767,350	0.132
20–24	1,006,055	0.244	624,354	0.369	1,630,409	0.280
25–29	1,166,904	0.282	394,616	0.233	1,561,520	0.268
30–34	955,300	0.231	198,183	0.117	1,153,483	0.198
35–39	474,143	0.115	89,873	0.053	564,016	0.097
40–54	113,747	0.028	24,332	0.014	138,079	0.023
Total	4,131,019	1	1,693,848	1	5,824,867	1

11. What is the probability that a woman who gave birth in 2009 is unmarried?
12. If a woman who gave birth is < 15 years of age, what is the probability that she is unmarried?
13. Is marital status independent of age?
14. What is the probability that a woman giving birth is less than 30 years of age?
15. Given that the mother of a particular child was under 30 years of age, what is the probability that she was less than 20 years of age?
16. What is the joint probability of being married and age 20–29?
17. From your answer in question 10, what is the marginal probability of being married?

Test Result	Abused	Not Abused	Total
Positive	285	970	1,255
Negative	15	8,730	8,745
Total	300	9,700	10,000

18. Describe Bayes' theorem.
    Consider the following data that reflects physical abuse from parents and a physical exam conducted under the direction of school officials.
19. Calculate the sensitivity and specificity of the physical exam to detect abuse and interpret your results.
20. Assuming the prior probability of abuse is 3%, what is the predictive value positive and negative for these data? Interpret your results.
21. Which sampling method involves drawing respondents from a random sample of mutually exclusive groups?
22. Which sampling method is useful if you want to ensure the presence of a particular subgroup within the sample?
23. Can you think of a situation in which a systematic sample would be inappropriate?
24. When would a convenience sample be as good as a random sample?
25. Suppose you have a sampling frame of 500 from which you want to select a random sample of 100. Use Excel to obtain your 100 random numbers.

REFERENCES

1. Surveillance, Epidemiology, and End Results (SEER) Program (www.seer.cancer.gov) SEER*Stat Database: Mortality—All COD, Aggregated with State, Total U.S. (1969–2007) <Katrina/Rita Population Adjustment>, National Cancer Institute, DCCPS, Surveillance Research Program, Cancer Statistics Branch, released June 2010. Underlying mortality data provided by NCHS (www.cdc.gov/nchs).
2. Blood types in the U.S. http://bloodcenter.stanford.edu/about_blood/blood_types.html.
3. Sarndal CE, Swenson B, Wreman JH. Model assisted survey sampling, Springer-Verlag, New York, 1992.
4. Merrill RM, Anderson AE, Sloan A. Quality of life indicators according to voice disorders and voice-related conditions. *Laryngoscope.* 2011;121:2,004–2,011.
5. Hamilton BE, Martin JA, Ventura SJ. Births: preliminary data for 2009. *National Vital Statistics Reports.* 2010;59(3). Hyattsville, MD: National Center for Health Statistics.

CHAPTER 7

Random Variables and Probability Distributions

Parameters represent characteristics from a population and are typically not known. Statistics represent characteristics from a sample. To obtain a representative sample, such that measures characterizing the sample data may be generalized to the total population, we use probability sampling. However, even if the sample is based on random selection, for example, the sample size must be sufficiently large. It is possible that a finding based on a sample may not be representative of the overall population but is unique to the specific sample taken; that is, due to the luck of the draw. For this reason, when we use sample statistics to estimate parameters, we attach a level of confidence to the statistic. The purpose of this chapter is to introduce and discuss random variables, selected probability distributions, the concept of sampling distributions, confidence intervals, and the central limit theorem.

RANDOM VARIABLES

Most random variables of interest arise from random sampling. Examples include the number of people exposed to a chemical in a sample; the number of people who became ill among a sample of exposed workers; or the sex, age, race, marital status, and income in a sample of cancer patients. Random variables are classified according to the set of values that the variable can take.

A discrete random variable is a whole number. It usually has a definite distance from any possible value of the random variable to the next possible value. For example, the number of children in a sample of women is discrete. Other examples of discrete random variables include the number of patients reacting negatively to a

> **Definition**
>
> A **random variable** is a variable whose numerical value is determined by a chance mechanism. We denote random variables by X, Y, and so on.

> **Definition**
>
> A **discrete random variable** has a numerical scale and can take on a countable number of values in an interval; it is a number without a fraction.

drug during the course of a study period or the number of individuals visiting the emergency room during a given hour.

> **Definition**
>
> A **continuous random variable** has a numerical scale and can take on any value in an interval.

Continuous random variables are numbers that involve a fraction. With complete accuracy, they can take on any positive value, such as height, weight, temperature, pressure, and time. In practice, however, we are limited to the level of precision of the measure. For example, a person's height is rounded to the nearest inch, weight is rounded to the nearest pound.

PROBABILITY DISTRIBUTIONS FOR DISCRETE RANDOM VARIABLES

> **Definition**
>
> A **probability distribution for a discrete random variable** is a collection of probabilities along with the associated values that the distribution can take.

A discrete random variable can be described as the probability associated with each of its distinct, discrete values when an experiment is conducted. A probability distribution for a discrete random variable is often presented as a table, graph, or formula.

In equations for computing discrete random variables, the expected value of a discrete random variable X is denoted by $E(X)$. This is the weighted mean of the possible values of X, where the weights are the probabilities of these values:

$$E(X) = \mu = \sum_{i=1}^{n} f_i X_i / n$$

The word *expected* means "on average." The expected value of X is also called the mean of X or μ (Greek mu).

The variance of a discrete random variable is:

$$Variance(X) = E(X - \mu)^2 = \sigma^2 = \frac{1}{\left(\sum_{i=1}^{n} f_i - 1\right)} \sum_{i=1}^{n} f_i \left(X - \bar{X}\right)^2$$

Notice that the formula $(X - \mu)^2$ is always positive. The expected value of $(X - \mu)^2$ is a measure of the amount the distribution is spread around the mean μ.

The variance is typically denoted by σ^2 (Greek sigma, squared), and the standard deviation by σ.

Two discrete probability distributions that will now be presented are the binomial distribution and the Poisson distribution.

THE BINOMIAL PROBABILITY DISTRIBUTION _____

The conditions that must be met for us to use the binomial probability formula are called Bernoulli trials, named after the mathematician Jakob Bernoulli (1654–1705). There are three conditions:

1. A fixed number of trials n of an experiment occur with only two possible mutually exclusive outcomes for each trial ("success" or "failure").
2. The probability of a success on any given trial, designated as π, remains constant from trial to trial. Therefore, the probability of failure is $1 - \pi$.
3. The trials are independent of one another in that the probabilities associated with the outcomes in one trial are not influenced by the outcomes in another trial.

Note that the fraction of successes observed in a sample is denoted by f. Of interest is the probability of r success given a fixed number of trials n.

EXAMPLE 7.1

Five full-term pregnancies can be considered as a series of trials with only two possible outcomes for each trial with respect to the child's sex. In this example, we will first call a female a "success" and a male a "failure." (Note that the terms *success* and *failure* have no moral connotations, but merely denote the two possible outcomes.) Second, the chance of success remains constant from pregnancy to pregnancy. Let's say the chance of a female is 0.5. Third, each of the pregnancies is independent of one another.

The general principle is that we repeat an experiment with an event we call success. Let

π = probability of a success for a single trial
$1 - \pi$ = probability of a failure for a single trial
n = number of trials
X = number of success

We are interested in finding the probability that a random variable for a number of successes, X, takes on a value r; that is, the probability that a success occurs exactly r times in n trials at chance π.

Equation for Binomial Probability

$$P(X = r \mid n, \pi) = \binom{n}{r} \pi^r (1 - \pi)^{n-r} \quad r = 0, 1, 2, \ldots, n$$

For our pregnancy example, we calculate this probability using the equation for binomial probability.

$$P(X = 0|5,\ 0.5) = \binom{5}{0} 0.5^0 (1 - 0.5)^{5-0} = 0.031$$

We read $P(X = r|n,\pi)$ as the binomial probability of r success given n trials, where the chance of success in each trial is 0.5. The number of different sequences that contain r success and $n - r$ failures (i.e., combinations of n things taken r at a time) is denoted by:

$$\binom{n}{r} = \frac{n!}{r!(n-r)!}$$

The symbol $n!$ is read "n factorial" and is the product of n down to 1. In our example,

$$\binom{5}{0} = \frac{5!}{0!(5-0)!} = \frac{5 \times 4 \times 3 \times 2 \times 1}{1 \times 5 \times 4 \times 3 \times 2 \times 1} = \frac{120}{120} = 1$$

Thus, the probability of 0 females out of 5 pregnancies, assuming the probability of having a female is 0.5, is 0.031 or 3.1%. The probability of 1 female is 0.156, of 2 females is 0.312, of 3 females is 0.312, of 4 females is 0.156, and of 5 females is 0.031. The probability of having 0 or 1 females is $0.031 + 0.156 = 0.187$. The probability of at least 2 females is $1 - 0.187 = 0.813$.

We can use equations to find the mean, variance, and standard deviation of a binomial-distributed random variable, using the equations that follow.

Equation for the Mean of the Binomial-Distributed Random Variable

$$E(X) = n\pi$$

Equation for the Variance of the Binomial-Distributed Random Variable

$$Variance(X) = n\pi(1 - \pi)$$

Equation for the Standard Deviation of the Binomial-Distributed Random Variable

$$Standard\ Deviation(X) = \sqrt{n\pi(1 - \pi)}$$

The expected number, variance, and standard deviation of females for 5 pregnancies is 2.5, 1.25, and 1.12, respectively.

A binomial probability distribution can have many shapes, depending on the values of n and f. The distribution is skewed right when π is less than 0.5, skewed left when π is greater than 0.5, and more symmetric when π gets close to 0.5. In addition, as n increases, the mean increases and the variance increases.

THE POISSON PROBABILITY DISTRIBUTION

The Poisson probability distribution is named after the French mathematician Simeon Poisson (1781–1840), who developed it. Characteristics of the Poisson probability distribution are:

1. Sampling is conducted over an interval on some continuous medium, such as area, distance, or time.
2. Events occur independently from one interval of the medium to another.
3. The probability of the occurrence of an event increases if the interval increases.
4. The probability of more than one event occurring in a very small interval is negligible.

The Poisson probability distribution is particularly useful in epidemiology in determining the probability of rare events, such as the occurrence of selected exposures or diseases. It can be used to model things such as the emission of radioactive particles from a specified source, the number of arrivals at an emergency room during a specific period, the number of cells in a given volume of fluid, or the number of bacterial colonies growing in a certain amount of medium. The mean and variance of the Poisson probability distribution both equal λ (the lowercase Greek letter lambda). Thus, only one piece of information, λ, is needed to characterize any Poisson distribution.

Equation for Poisson Probability

$$P(X = r|\lambda) = \frac{e^{-\lambda}\lambda^r}{r!} \quad r = 0,1,2,\ldots$$

where λ is the mean number of Poisson-distributed events over the sampling medium that is being examined. λ is also the variance. The number e is a mathematical constant equal to 2.71828.

EXAMPLE 7.2

The rate of acute lymphocytic leukemia in the United States for a given year is 1.7 per 100,000. A given city has approximately 500,000 people. Let us find the probability that the city will have no cases of acute lymphocytic leukemia in the current year. The sampling medium is 500,000 person-years. Thus, the expected number of cases in this city is $\lambda = 1.7 \times 5 = 8.5$. Then,

$$P(X = 0|8.5) = \frac{e^{-8.5}8.5^0}{0!} = 0.0002$$

The probability of 1, 2, 3, 4, or 5 cases is 0.0017, 0.0074, 0.0208, 0.0443, and 0.0752, respectively. The probability of up to 5 cases is 0.1496. The probability of 6 or more cases is 0.8504.

Poisson distributions are skewed to the right. When the number of trials n is large and the chance of success f for each trial is small, then the binomial probability is approximately equal to the Poisson probability. Then $\lambda = nf$, the mean for the binomial distribution.

PROBABILITY DISTRIBUTIONS FOR CONTINUOUS RANDOM VARIABLES

Unlike the discrete random variable, where probabilities are available for its various possible values, there are infinitely many possible values for a continuous variable. Because we cannot list all those values in a table, as we have for probability distributions for discrete random variables, the distribution for a continuous random variable X must be given by a continuous curve. The curve is referred to as a *frequency curve* or a *probability density curve*. The area under the curve between two values on the horizontal scale is the probability of the random variable between those two limits. The relative probability (i.e., the relevant area under the curve) is determined by integral calculus. These calculations are beyond the scope of this text.

> **Definition**
>
> A **probability distribution for a continuous random variable** is specified by a probability density curve (also called a frequency curve). Areas under the probability density curve are probabilities.

NORMAL PROBABILITY DISTRIBUTION

The probability that a measurement on a continuous scale, such as height, weight, or time, lies within a particular range of values can be determined using the normal distribution. The normal distribution is a symmetric bell-shaped curve, with 50%

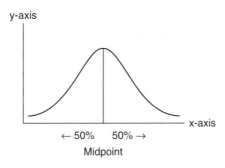

FIGURE 7.1 The normal distribution.

of the scores above and 50% below the midpoint of the distribution. The curve is asymptotic to the x-axis, and the mean, median, and mode are located at the midpoint of the x-axis (**Figure 7.1**).

The equation for the normal distribution is shown in the following box. In the equation, π is the mathematical constant 3.14159, which you will note is different than the definition of π used in the section on the Binomial Probability Distribution. The values of μ and σ are parameters.

Equation for the Normal Distribution

$$\frac{1}{\sqrt{2\pi\sigma^2}} exp\left[-\frac{1}{2}\left(\frac{X-\mu}{\sigma}\right)^2\right]$$

There is a normal distribution for each pair of μ and σ^2, where μ is the mean and σ^2 is the variance of the distribution, respectively. There are many continuous random variables in epidemiology and clinical medicine with distributions wherein the normal distribution is a good approximation. For example, body mass index tends to be normally distributed. Rather than applying integral calculus to answer questions about probabilities for each specific variable, we will find probabilities for normally distributed variables by converting to the standard normal distribution. Although constructing a table for each possible pair of μ and σ^2 is impossible, we can use the standard normal table to estimate probabilities by transforming any normally distributed variable.

Definition

The **standard normal distribution** is the normal distribution with a mean of 0 and a variance of 1.

Definition

If X is a random variable with a mean of μ and a variance of σ^2, then the **standard normal variable**

$$Z = \frac{X - \mu}{\sigma}$$

has a mean of 0 and a variance of 1. If X is normally distributed, then Z is a standard normal variable.

The standard normal distribution is symmetric, has a single peak, has a mean of 0 and a variance of 1, and ranges from $-\infty$ to $+\infty$.

The z transformation allows us to use the standard normal table (see Appendix B, Table 3).

To illustrate, let us assume that the systolic blood pressure in a healthy population is normally distributed with $\mu = 120$ and $\sigma^2 = 100$ mm Hg.

What area under the curve is above 120?

$$P(X > 120) = P\left(Z > \frac{120 - 120}{10}\right) = P(Z > 0) = 0.5$$

What area under the curve is above 130?

$$P(X > 130) = P\left(Z > \frac{130 - 120}{10}\right) = P(Z > 1) = 0.159$$

What area under the curve is less than 140?

$$P(X < 140) = P\left(Z > \frac{140 - 120}{10}\right) = P(Z < 2) = 0.5 + 0.477 = 0.977$$

What area under the curve is between 110 and 130?

$$P(110 < X < 130) = P\left(\frac{110 - 120}{10} < Z < \frac{140 - 120}{10}\right) = P(-1 < Z < 2)$$

$$= 0.341 + 0.4772 = 0.818$$

NORMAL APPROXIMATION TO THE BINOMIAL

The equation for the binomial probability distribution was presented earlier in this chapter as a way to compute the binomial probability of X successes in n trials, with π representing the probability of a success for each trial. However, this equation is cumbersome to compute when n is large. In this case, the normal distribution can be used to find approximate binomial probabilities. In this section, we will discuss the normal approximation of the binomial.

When the number of trials n is large and π is close to 0.5, the binomial distribution is "approximately equal to" (represented by the symbol $\approx$) a normal distribution. Even when the probability of success is not very close to 0 or 1 but if n is large, the binomial distribution still becomes close to a normal distribution.

Equation for Standardized Binomial Variable

$$Z = \frac{X - n\pi}{\sqrt{n\pi(1-\pi)}}$$

How large does n need to be and how far can p depart from 0.5 before the normal distribution fails to approximate binomial probabilities? A conservative rule of thumb is that the variance of the binomial distribution must be at least 5. Specifically,

$n\pi(1-\pi) \geq 5$.

EXAMPLE 7.3

Of the 2,086 cases seen by a medical examiner during a year-long study period in Utah, 420 involved unintentional drug overdose as the cause of death.[1] Among the drug-related deaths, 273 (65%) consisted of nonillicit drugs only. Researchers took a random sample of 100 of these cases and interviewed family members to investigate the background of the cases. Let's label a drug-related death that only involved nonillicit drugs as a "success." The mean, variance, and standard deviation are:

$\mu = n\pi = 100 \times 0.65 = 65$

$\sigma^2 = n\pi(1-\pi) = 100 \times 0.65 \times 0.35 = 22.75$

$\sigma = \sqrt{n\pi(1-\pi)} = \sqrt{22.75} = 4.77$

The standardized formula is:

$Z = \dfrac{X - 65}{4.77}$

The letter Z represents a random variable with a standard normal distribution. Now suppose we wanted to know the probability that the number of X successes is between 60 and 70, inclusive. Then,

$$P(60 \le X \le 70) = P\left(\frac{60-65}{4.77} \le \frac{X-65}{4.77} \le \frac{70-65}{4.77}\right)$$

$$\approx P\left(\frac{60-65}{4.77} \le Z \le \frac{70-65}{4.77}\right)$$

$$= P(-1.05 \le Z \le 1.05)$$

From the table for normal probabilities in Appendix B (Table 3) we get

$$P(-1.05 \le Z \le 1.05) = 0.3531 + 0.3531 = 0.7062$$

In some situations, rather than working with the number X of successes in n trials, we are dealing with the fraction of success, $f = \dfrac{X}{n}$. The standardized binomial fraction of success is:

Equation for Standardized Binomial Variable

$$Z = \frac{f - \pi}{\sqrt{\pi(1-\pi)/n}}$$

The standardized binomial fraction of success approximates the standard normal when n is large. This is because f has a mean, variance, and standard deviation as follows:

Equation for the Mean of the Binomial Fraction of Success

$$E(f) = \pi$$

Equations for the Variance and the Standard Deviation of the Binomial Fraction of Success

$$Variance(f) = \frac{\pi(1-\pi)}{n}$$

$$Standard\ Deviation(f) = \sqrt{\frac{\pi(1-\pi)}{n}}$$

EXAMPLE 7.4

Now suppose that n is 100 and π is 0.65. Let us compute the probability that the fraction f of successes will lie between 0.60 and 0.70, inclusive. First, the mean, variance, and standard deviation of f are:

$$E(f) = \pi = 0.65$$

$$Variance(f) = \frac{\pi(1-\pi)}{n} = \frac{0.65 \times 0.35}{100} = 0.002275$$

$$Standard\ deviation(f) = \sqrt{\frac{\pi(1-\pi)}{n}} = 0.048$$

The standardized formula is:

$$Z = \frac{X - 0.65}{0.048}$$

Then,

$$P(0.60 \leq X \leq 0.70) = P\left(\frac{0.60 - 0.65}{0.048} \leq \frac{X - 0.65}{0.048} \leq \frac{0.70 - 0.65}{0.048}\right)$$

$$\approx P\left(\frac{0.60 - 0.65}{0.048} \leq Z \leq \frac{0.70 - 0.65}{0.048}\right)$$

$$= P(-1.05 \leq Z \leq 1.05) = 0.3531 + 0.3531 = 0.7062$$

Further accuracy is possible by applying a continuity correction, which is an adjustment that we make by adding or subtracting ½ to a discrete value when we use a continuous distribution to approximate a discrete distribution.

Rule for Applying the Continuity Correction
Subtract ½ from the lower value of the number of successes, add ½ to the upper value, and then proceed as previously shown.

$$P(59.5 \leq X \leq 70.5) = P\left(\frac{59.5 - 65}{4.77} \leq \frac{X - 65}{4.77} \leq \frac{70.5 - 65}{4.77}\right)$$

$$\approx P\left(\frac{59.5 - 65}{4.77} \leq Z \leq \frac{70.5 - 65}{4.77}\right)$$

$$= P(-1.15 \leq Z \leq 1.15) = 0.3749 + 0.3749 = 0.7498$$

In this chapter, we complete our discussion of probability by presenting an important concept in statistics called sampling distributions. Probability distributions for sample statistics are called sampling distributions. Our focus will be on sampling distributions for the sample mean ($\bar{X}$). An important theorem in statistics called the central limit theorem will also be presented.

SAMPLING DISTRIBUTION

Now that we have learned how the binomial, Poisson, and normal distribution can be used to determine the likelihood that a specific measurement is in the population, we will consider another distribution involving sample statistics called a sampling distribution. A sampling distribution is a theoretical distribution of all possible values of a given statistic taken from all possible samples of a given size obtained from a population. This distribution is distinct from the distribution of individual observations.

> **Definition**
>
> A **sampling distribution** is the probability distribution of a given statistic based on a random sample of size *n*; it is the distribution of the statistic for all possible samples of a given size.

Features of the sampling distribution are: (1) the statistic of interest (e.g., mean, standard deviation, or proportion), (2) the random selection of the sample, (3) the size of the random sample, and (4) the specification of the population being sampled. The sampling distribution of the mean plays a very important role in statistics and will be used as the statistic of interest in our discussion.

SAMPLING DISTRIBUTION OF THE MEAN

Let $\bar{X}$ be the sample mean for an independent sample of size *n*. As previously seen, the population mean and variance are μ and σ^2. In addition,

$$E(\bar{X}) = \mu$$
$$Variance(\bar{X}) = \frac{\sigma^2}{n}$$

The sampling distribution of the sample mean is normally distributed if the population distribution is normal. If the parent population is normal, then $\bar{X}$ is normally distributed with mean μ and variance $\frac{\sigma^2}{n}$. The variance of a sampling distribution is smaller than the variance of the population distribution, and decreases as the sample size increases.

Sample Means from Normal Populations
If the population for X is normally distributed with mean μ and variance σ^2, the sample mean $\bar{X}$ is normally distributed with mean μ and variance $\dfrac{\sigma^2}{n}$.

The following equation is used to standardize a sample mean $\bar{X}$ for a sampling distribution.

Equation for the Standardized Sample Mean
Because $\bar{X}$ has a mean of μ and a standard error of $\dfrac{\sigma}{\sqrt{n}}$, the standardized sample mean is:

$$Z = \frac{\bar{X} - \mu}{\sigma/\sqrt{n}}$$

The mean of the standardized sample is 0 and the variance is 1. If the population is normal, then Z is a standard normal variable. In this case, we may use the standard normal distribution table to calculate probabilities for the sample mean.

It is important to note that it would be very tedious to take many samples in order to estimate the variability of the mean. In reality, we only take one sample. Therefore, among the several desirable characteristics of the sampling distribution, it allows us to answer questions about the mean based on only one sample.

EXAMPLE 7.5

In the United States in 2010, the percentage of adults who were obese in each of the 50 states and 4 territories was normally distributed around a mean of $\mu = 27.7$. The standard deviation around the mean was $\sigma = 3.2$.[2] We took a random sample of $n = 10$ and obtained $\bar{X}$ for the sample of 28.1. Now let's calculate the probability of getting a sample mean this high or higher if the true mean is $\mu = 27.7$.

$$P\left(\bar{X} \geq 28.1\right) = P\left(Z \geq \frac{28.1 - 27.7}{3.2/\sqrt{10}}\right) = P(Z \geq 0.40)$$

In Table 3 in Appendix B, this value is $0.5000 - 0.1554 = 0.3446$.

THE CENTRAL LIMIT THEOREM

The central limit theorem involves the approximate normality of means of random samples. A mathematical proof of the central limit theorem will not be given in this text, but some empirical arguments will be presented to show that the theory is valid.

For a population with a mean of μ and a standard deviation of σ, the sampling distribution of the mean with repeated random samples of size n has the following properties:

1. The mean of the sampling distribution of $\bar{X}$ equals the mean of the population μ from which the sample is taken.
2. The standard deviation in the sampling distribution of $\bar{X}$ equals the standard deviation of the sampled population divided by the square root of the sample size, $\dfrac{\sigma}{\sqrt{n}}$, which is called the standard error of the mean.
3. If the distribution in the population is normal, then the sampling distribution of the mean is also normal. However, regardless of the shape of the original population distribution, if the sample size is sufficiently large, the sampling distribution of the mean is approximately normally distributed.

Central Limit Theorem

If n is large, then

$$Z = \frac{\bar{X} - \mu}{\sigma/\sqrt{n}}$$

has approximately a standard normal distribution; that is, $\bar{X}$ has approximately a normal distribution with a mean of μ and a variance of $\dfrac{\sigma^2}{n}$.

A sample of 30 is sufficiently large so that regardless of the original population distribution, the sampling distribution of the means will be normally distributed. However, a sample size this large is not necessary if the original population distribution is normally distributed or close to it.

To summarize, whatever the parent population may be, the standardized variable has a mean of 0 and a standard deviation of 1. In addition, if the parent population is normal, then the variable in the previous equation has exactly a standard normal distribution. A remarkable fact is that even if the parent population is not normally distributed, the standardized mean is approximately normal if n is sufficiently large. Thus, the central limit theorem indicates that we can use normal theory for inferences about the population mean, regardless of the form of the parent population, if the sample size is large enough. A sample size of 30 or more is sufficiently large in all cases, but we may use a sample size smaller than 30, depending on how close the parent population is to being normal.

Another important consequence of the central limit theorem is the empirical rule, which is a statistical rule stating that for any normal distribution, 68% of the data lie

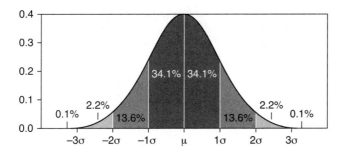

FIGURE 7.2 Empirical rule for normally distributed data.

within ± 1 standard deviation of the mean, 95% of the data lie within ± 2 standard deviations of the mean, and 99.7% of the data lie within ± 3 standard deviations of the mean (**Figure 7.2**). For smaller sample sizes in which the data are not normally distributed, Chebyshev's inequality can be used to summarize the distribution of data. Chebyshev's inequality says that for any number k that is greater than or equal to 1, at least one $[1 - (1/k)^2]$ of the measurements in the data set lie within k standard deviations of the mean.[3] If k is 2, for example, then $[1 - (1/2)^2] = 0.75$, meaning that 75% of the values lie within two standard deviations of the mean (i.e., $\bar{X} \pm 2s$ includes at least 75% of the observations). If k is 3, then $[1 - (1/3)^2] = 0.889$, meaning that 88.9% of the values lie within three standard deviations of the mean (i.e., $\bar{X} \pm 3s$ includes at least 88.9% of the observations).

EXERCISES

1. What is a random variable?
2. How is a probability distribution related to a random variable?
3. How does a parameter compare with a statistic?
4. What are three properties of the binomial probability distribution?
5. What are four characteristics of the Poisson probability distribution?
6. Under which two conditions will the binomial probability be approximately equal to the Poisson probability?
7. Describe the properties of the normal distribution.
8. What is the practical value of the standard normal distribution?

In one study, cancer-related claims were presented according to type of service rendered. Let X be a discrete random variable that represents the number of three specific combinations of services. The probability distribution for X appears as follows.[4]

Cancer-Related Claims According to Type of Service Rendered				
Non–Skin Cancer–Related Claims*				
Physician services	Nonphysician professional health services	Hospital services	Number	P(X = x)
Yes	Yes	Yes	698	0.310
Yes	Yes	No	151	0.067
Yes	No	Yes	788	0.349
Yes	No	No	526	0.233
No	Yes	Yes	10	0.004
No	Yes	No	13	0.006
No	No	Yes	69	0.031
No	No	No	0	0.000

Data source: DMBA enrollees during 1998–2006, aged 15–64.
*First ICD-9-CM cancer code assigned 140–208, excluding 172.0–173.9 (skin cancer).

9. Construct a graph of the probability distribution given the cancer claim data.
10. What is the probability that a cancer patient receives all three types of services?
11. What is the probability that the cancer patient received both physician and hospital services only?
12. What is the probability of receiving nonphysician professional health services?
13. In the United States in 2010, the prevalence of asthma in adults was 8.8%; the prevalence of adults who were limited in any activities because of physical, mental, or emotional problems was 20.6%; and the prevalence of adults who did not have any kind of health care coverage was 15%.[5] If you selected repeated samples of size 10 from the U.S. population, what would the mean number of individuals per sample be of asthma, disability, and no health care coverage?
14. Referring to question 13, what are the standard deviations that correspond to these expected values?
15. Referring to question 13, what is the probability of finding exactly two people who have asthma? What is the probability of finding two people who are disabled? What is the probability of finding two people who do not have health care coverage?

16. Referring to question 13, what is the probability of finding more than two people with no health care coverage?

17. In 2008, the rate of prostate cancer among white men in Salt Lake county, Utah, ages 70–79, was 967.4 per 100,000.[6] In a sample of 100 men in this age range, what is the expected number of cases?

18. Referring to question 17, what is the probability that no one in this sample will have prostate cancer?

19. Referring to question 17, what is the probability that exactly one person will have prostate cancer?

20. Referring to question 17, what is the probability that two or more men will have prostate cancer?

21. Define the empirical rule and state when it may be used.

22. When would you use Chebyshev's inequality to summarize a distribution of values?

23. What are the properties of the central limit theorem?

24. Let X be a random variable that represents the Beck Depression Inventory score. For a population of people aged 24–81 years, the mean Beck Depression Inventory score is approximately normally distributed with a mean of 4.35 and a standard deviation of 4.64.[7] What change in the curve results when this is transformed to the standard normal curve?

25. Referring to question 24, what is the area of the population curve above 13.63? Below −0.29?

26. Referring to question 24, what is the area of the population curve between −0.29 and 8.99?

27. Referring to question 24, what value in the population corresponds with $Z = -0.5$?

28. In 2010, within a sample of 1,000 individuals aged 65 years and older in the United States, 67.4% had a flu shot within the past year.[5] We may consider the selection of a person having had a flu shot within the past year as a "success." Find the probability that the number of X successes will lie above 70%.

29. Referring to question 28, what would your result have been had you used the continuity correction?

30. Referring to question 24, find the probability that in a sample of $n = 75$, the mean Beck Depression Inventory score will be less than 4.

31. The number of people that an emergency room doctor sees on his shift each week averages 35. The number of people the doctor sees varies from week to

week, with a standard deviation of 12. What is the probability that during a sample of $n = 30$ shifts, the mean number of people the doctor sees will be at least 30?

32. The distribution of parity for women in a breast cancer study found that the mean number of children was 3.2 and the median number of children was 3. Most of the women had 2 children. The standard deviation for this data was 1.9.[8] Summarize this skewed distribution using Chebyshev's inequality.

REFERENCES

1. Merrill RM, Johnson E, Sloan A, Lanier WA. Characterizing decedents involving unintentional nonillicit and illicit drugs. (Submitted).

2. Centers for Disease Control and Prevention. Behavioral risk factor surveillance system. Prevalence and trends data, 2010. http://apps.nccd.cdc.gov/brfss/list.asp?cat=OB&yr=2010&qkey=4409&state=US. Published 2011. Accessed July 4, 2011.

3. Papoulis A. *Probability, Random Variables, and Stochastic Processes.* 2nd ed. New York, NY: McGraw-Hill; 1984:149–151.

4. Merrill RM, Baker RK, Lyon JL, Gren LH. Healthcare claims for identifying the level of diagnostic investigation and treatment of cancer. *Med Sci Monit.* 2009;15(5):PH25–31.

5. Centers for Disease Control and Prevention. Prevalence and trend data. Nationwide (States, DC, and Territories). Current asthma prevalence, 2010. http://apps.nccd.cdc.gov/brfss/display.asp?cat=AS&yr=2010&qkey=4416&state=US. Published 2011. Accessed August 10, 2011.

6. Surveillance, Epidemiology, and End Results (SEER) Program (www.seer.cancer.gov). SEER*Stat Database: Mortality—All COD, Aggregated with State, Total U.S. (1969–2007) <Katrina/Rita Population Adjustment>, National Cancer Institute, DCCPS, Surveillance Research Program, Cancer Statistics Branch. Underlying mortality data provided by NCHS. www.cdc.gov/nchs. Published June 2010. Accessed August 5, 2011.

7. Merrill RM, Aldana SG, Greenlaw RL, Diehl HA. The coronary health improvement project's impact on lowering eating, sleep, stress, and depressive disorders. *Am J Health Educ.* 2008;39(6):337–344.

8. Daniels M, Merrill RM, Lyon JL, Stanford JB, White GL. Associations between breast cancer risk factors and religious practices in Utah. *Prev Med.* 2004;38:28–38.

CHAPTER 8

Estimation and Hypothesis Testing

We often use data from samples or experiments to estimate the values of unknown parameters or for tests of hypotheses concerning these values. The process of drawing conclusions from sample data about characteristics of a population is called statistical inference. Inferential statistics is the third of four general areas of biostatistics, as presented in the outset of this text. In this chapter, we cover several aspects of statistical inference, including estimators and hypothesis testing.

ESTIMATORS

In the context of sampling from a population, the aim is to construct a sample quantity that will estimate the unknown parameter. We call this sample quantity an *estimator*. The actual numerical value obtained for an estimator is called an *estimate*, or *point estimate*. An estimator is a statistic that is a measure from a sample. For instance, the sample mean $\bar{X}$ is an estimator of the population mean μ and the sample variance s^2 is an estimator of the population variance σ^2. Both $\bar{X}$ and s^2 are also unbiased estimators, since it can be shown that their expected values equal the corresponding population parameters.

Definitions

An **estimator** is a random variable or a sample statistic that is used to estimate an unknown population parameter.

A **confidence interval** is an interval, bounded on the left by L and on the right by R, that is used to estimate an unknown population parameter.

L and R are referred to as **confidence limits.** Reliability of the estimate may be evaluated objectively by the use of a confidence statement.

CONFIDENCE INTERVALS FOR NORMAL MEANS AND KNOWN VARIANCE

Instead of presenting a point estimate, we may want to identify a measure that indicates the likelihood of the value. We can associate a probability with interval estimates. Confidence intervals define an upper limit and a lower limit with an associated probability. The ends of the confidence interval are called the *confidence limits*. An interval estimate is called a *confidence interval*.

Definition

The $100(1 - \alpha)\%$ **confidence interval for the population mean μ when the population is normally distributed and the variance σ^2 is known** is the interval bounded by the confidence limits

$$L = \bar{X} - Z_{\alpha/2}\frac{\sigma}{\sqrt{n}}$$

and

$$R = \bar{X} + Z_{\alpha/2}\frac{\sigma}{\sqrt{n}}$$

The value of Z is obtained from Table 3 in Appendix B.

Confidence intervals can be calculated for any population parameter, such as the mean, rate, odds ratio, or risk ratio. Confidence intervals for many of these measures will be presented throughout this text. For now, we will present the confidence interval for the population mean μ when the population variance is known.

The value $1 - \alpha$ is called the *confidence coefficient*, and $100(1 - \alpha)\%$ is referred to as the *confidence level*. If the level of significance $\alpha = 0.05$, then the confidence level is $100(1 - 0.05)\% = 95\%$.

EXAMPLE 8.1

Suppose 10 patients were given a drug to improve their sleep. We know from experience that the increase in sleep (minutes) is normally distributed with some mean and a population variance of 1.7. For the 10 patients, mean improvement in sleep was 65 minutes. The 95% confidence interval for the mean is:

$$L = 65 - 1.96\frac{1.7}{\sqrt{10}} = 63.9 \; and \; R = 65 + 1.96\frac{1.7}{\sqrt{10}} = 66.1$$

Thus we can feel 95% confident that the population mean improvement in sleep lies between 63.9 and 66.1 minutes.

The reason why we are 95% confident is because if we were to take 100 different samples from the sample population and calculate the confidence limits for each sample, we would expect that 95 out of these 100 intervals would contain the true value of μ. We would also expect 5 of the 100 intervals would not contain the true value of μ. Because we only have one confidence interval based on a single sample, we do not know whether the interval is one of the 95 or of the 5. It is in this sense that we are 95% confident.

t DISTRIBUTION

Recall that the sampling distribution of the mean assumes that the value of the population standard deviation σ is known. In reality, we rarely know this value, but must estimate it by the sample standard deviation *s*. When *s* is used, the sampling distribution of the mean instead follows a *t* distribution.

Equation for the *t* Statistic

$$t = \frac{\bar{X} - \mu}{s/\sqrt{n}}$$

The *t* distribution is a theoretical probability distribution that is symmetric, bell-shaped, and has mean 0. It is similar to the standard normal curve, only there is more area in the tails and it is not as high in the middle. The primary difference between the *t* and the *z* is that the *t* distribution is more variable because *s* will vary more from sample to sample for small samples, but *s* remains constant for large samples. The variability in the sampling distribution of *t* depends on the sample size *n*. A convenient way of expressing this dependence is to say that the *t* statistic has *n* − 1 degrees of freedom (number of independent pieces of data being used to make a calculation). The smaller the number of degrees of freedom associated with the *t* statistic, the more variable its sampling distribution will be.

To assure the validity of a small sample test of a hypothesis about the population mean μ, or to calculate a confidence interval for μ, two conditions should be met. First, a random sample must be taken from the population. Second, the population should be approximately normally distributed. However, it has been shown that the *t* distribution is somewhat insensitive to moderate departures from normality. For small sample sizes and large deviations from normality, a nonparametric statistic is preferred.

CONFIDENCE INTERVALS FOR NORMAL MEANS AND UNKNOWN VARIANCE

To calculate a confidence interval when the population standard deviation σ is unknown, we simply replace σ by its estimator *s* in the equations for constructing confidence intervals.

Small-Sample Confidence Interval for μ

The 100(1 − α)% confidence interval for the population mean μ when the population is approximately normally distributed and the variance σ² is not known is the interval bounded by the confidence limits

$$L = \bar{X} - t_{\alpha/2, n-1} \frac{s}{\sqrt{n}} \text{ and } R = \bar{X} + t_{\alpha/2, n-1} \frac{s}{\sqrt{n}}$$

The value of *t* is obtained from Table 4 in Appendix B, using *n* − 1 degrees of freedom.

EXAMPLE 8.2

In a sample of 10 U.S. states and territories, the mean percentage of obese adults was 28.1. The sample standard deviation was 3.5. Assuming we do not know the population standard deviation, we could use the sample standard deviation to calculate a 95% confidence interval, as follows:

$$L = 28.1 - 2.262\frac{3.5}{\sqrt{10}} = 25.6 \text{ and } R = 28.1 + 2.262\frac{3.5}{\sqrt{10}} = 30.6$$

Thus we can feel 95% confident that the population mean obesity level in the United States lies between 25.6 and 30.6.

CONFIDENCE INTERVALS FOR THE BINOMIAL WITH LARGE SAMPLE SIZES

The fraction of success is $f = \dfrac{X}{n}$, and the expected value of f is π, $E(f) = \pi$. The normal approximation to the binomial provides a method of finding approximate confidence limits for large sample sizes.

Confidence Interval for π

The $100(1 - \alpha)\%$ confidence interval for the population mean μ when the population is approximately normally distributed and the variance σ^2 is not known is the interval bounded by the confidence limits

$$L = f - Z_{\alpha/2}\sqrt{\frac{f(1-f)}{n}} \text{ and } R = f + Z_{\alpha/2}\sqrt{\frac{f(1-f)}{n}}$$

EXAMPLE 8.3

In a study where the cause of death was an unintentional drug overdose, a sample of 100 decedents identified 65 that involved nonillicit drugs only. The 95% confidence interval is:

$$L = 0.65 - 1.96\sqrt{\frac{0.65(1-0.65)}{100}} = 0.56 \text{ and } R = 0.65 + 1.96\sqrt{\frac{0.65(1-0.65)}{100}} = 0.74$$

Thus we can feel 95% confident that the population proportion of unintentional drug overdose deaths involving nonillicit, prescribed drugs only lies between 0.56 and 0.74.

HYPOTHESIS TESTING

Like the confidence interval, a hypothesis test is a means to generalize the population, based on sample information. A hypothesis test makes an assumption about the population. Then, probability is used to estimate the likelihood that the results obtained from the sample meet the assumption about the population. As was the case with confidence intervals, sample data from the population are involved.

Hypotheses are expressed in terms of population parameters, such as $\mu \geq 27$ (a population mean is at least 27) or $\pi \neq 0.7$ (a population proportion does not equal 0.7). A test of hypothesis is a statistical procedure used to make a decision about the value of a population parameter. Hypotheses may apply to a single variable or involve relationships between or among variables.

Hypotheses are shown to be consistent or inconsistent with the facts. If established information or facts are lacking to substantiate a research hypothesis, then more information should be gathered, or we fail to reject the null hypothesis. The null hypothesis usually states what is currently believed or expected, or what has been claimed or has been expected in the past. We assume the null hypothesis is correct unless sufficient evidence can show otherwise. The alternative hypothesis (or research hypothesis) is what the investigator wants to show. Formulation of the hypotheses depends on the research question. The statistical methods for evaluating the hypotheses also depend on the research question.

> **Definitions**
>
> A **hypothesis** is a conjecture about the nature of a population.
>
> The **null hypothesis**, denoted by H_o, specifies the value of a population parameter. We want to show that the null hypothesis is incorrect. The null hypothesis is what is currently believed; it is the status quo.
>
> The **alternative hypothesis**, denoted by H_a, gives an opposing conjecture to that of the null hypothesis. We want to support this hypothesis as being true.
>
> A **test statistic** is a quantity calculated from the sample that is used when making a decision about the hypothesis of interest.

We can summarize the steps taken in hypothesis testing as follows.

1. Formulate the null hypothesis in statistical terms.
2. Formulate the alternative (or research) hypothesis in statistical terms.
3. Select the level of significance α for the statistical test and the sample size. The level of significance is generally 0.05, but if a more conservative test is desired, 0.01 can be used. In exploratory studies, the level of significance may be 0.1 or higher.
4. Select the appropriate test statistics and identify the degrees of freedom and the critical value for rejecting the null hypothesis.

Definitions

A **rejection region** specifies the values of the test statistic wherein the null hypothesis is rejected in favor of the alternative hypothesis.

The **P value of the test involving the mean** is the probability of obtaining a mean as extreme, or more extreme, than the observed sample mean, given that the null hypothesis (i.e., $H_0 : \mu = \mu_0$) is true.

The **P value of an effect** equals the probability that an effect as large, or larger, than that observed in a particular study could have occurred by chance alone, given that the null hypothesis is true (i.e., $H_0 : No\ relationship$).

$\alpha = P(type\ I\ error)$

$= P(reject\ H_0 | H_0\ is\ true)$

$\beta = P(type\ II\ error)$

$= P(accept\ H_0 | H_0\ is\ false)$

5. Collect the data and calculate the test statistic.
6. Reject or fail to reject the null hypothesis.

Before providing specific examples, a few related concepts will be discussed.

THE *P* VALUE

When samples are involved, characteristics of the subjects may vary from sample to sample. As a result, a statistical result may be explained by chance (i.e., the "luck of the draw"). Sample size is directly related to chance. As the sample size increases, the probability that the result is due to chance decreases. The *P* value is a probability that ranges from 0 to 1 and provides a means of evaluating the role of chance. For example, a *P* value of 0.02 means there is a 0.02 probability that the result occurred by chance. When statistical tests are used to draw conclusions about a population, a corresponding *P* value is obtained.

TYPE I AND TYPE II ERRORS

There are different consequences that result from possible decisions. These are summarized in **Table 8.1**. The true state of the population is reflected in the headings of the table, and the decisions made by the investigator are reflected by the rows of the table. For example, if H_0 is true and we fail to reject H_0, then we have made a correct decision. If H_a is true and we reject H_0 and accept H_a, then we have also made a correct decision. However, in hypothesis testing, there is always the concern that we either reject H_0 when it is true (type I error) or we fail to reject H_0 when it is false (type II error).

There is always the possibility of making a type I error or a type II error when using a sample to make inferences. Hence, let us consider the probability of making these errors. The probability of a type I error is denoted by the Greek letter alpha: α. The probability of a type II error is denoted by the Greek letter beta: β.

TABLE 8.1 Possible Decisions and Consequences for a Test of Hypothesis

Possible decisions	True state of the population	
	H_0 is true	H_a is true
Reject H_0 (accept H_a)	Type I error	Correct decision
Fail to reject H_0	Correct decision	Type II error

Although we would prefer α and β to be near 0, this is often not possible. Because the investigator is interested in accepting H_a (rejecting H_0), we are more interested in α having a small probability. By convention, the investigator typically chooses α to equal 0.05. However, if the investigator wishes to lower the chance of a type 1 error, α may be set at a smaller value such as 0.01. In exploratory research, α is typically set at 0.1 or higher. It is important to note that the investigator is free to choose how rare an observation must be in order to reject H_0.

To reject a null hypothesis, we can compare the calculated value of a test statistic with a critical value, based on our chosen α, as done in the previous example. However, we could also compare our P value, which corresponds directly to the calculated test statistic, to our chosen α.

Criteria for Rejecting or Not Rejecting a Null Hypothesis Based on the P Value

If P value $< \alpha$, then reject H_0

If P value $\geq \alpha$, then do not reject H_0

The investigator also chooses the value of β. If β is set at 0.20, then the investigator is willing to accept a 20% chance of incorrectly accepting H_0. Another probability measure that is related to β, the quantity $(1 - \beta)$, is called *power*. Power can also be thought of as the chance that a given study will detect a deviation from the null hypothesis when one really exists. As power increases, the probability of committing a type II error decreases.

> **Definition**
> **Power** is the probability that a statistical test will reject the null hypothesis when H_0 is false.

RESEARCH QUESTION ABOUT THE MEAN IN ONE GROUP

Assumptions: Normal population with the variance σ^2 unknown.

Formulation of hypotheses: Three forms of a null hypothesis for a specified value of the mean μ_0:

$H_0: \mu \geq \mu_0$ $H_a: \mu < \mu_0$

$H_0: \mu \leq \mu_0$ $H_a: \mu > \mu_0$

$H_0: \mu = \mu_0$ $H_a: \mu \neq \mu_0$

Test statistic: t

EXAMPLE 8.4

Suppose that it is commonly believed that the mean percentage of the United States adult population that is obese is 25. On the other hand, based on a recent descriptive study, we believe that the mean percentage of obese adults in this country is greater than 25. Assuming a normal distribution of mean percent scores for each state in the country, let us take a random sample of 10 states and territories. Applying the steps of hypothesis testing gives the following:

1. $H_0: \mu \leq 25\%$
2. $H_a: \mu > 25\%$
3. $\alpha = 0.05, n = 10$
4. t statistic and $(10 - 1) = 9$ degrees of freedom
5. From our sample, suppose $\bar{X} = 28.1\%$ and $s = 3.5$, then:

$$t = \frac{28.1 - 25}{3.5/\sqrt{10}} = 2.8$$

6. On the basis of the alternative hypothesis, we see that the rejection region is in the upper tail of the t distribution. Referring to Table 4 in Appendix B, the critical value is 2.26. So the rejection region is in the area under the tail of the t distribution from 2.26 and above. Because the calculated value is in the rejection region, we reject H_0 and accept that the percentage of adults in the United States who are obese is significantly greater than 25%. (Note that the P value that corresponds to 2.8 and 9 degrees of freedom is between 0.025 and 0.01. Because the P value is smaller than our chosen α of 0.05, we reject the null hypothesis and accept the alternative.)

In some situations, we are interested in means when the same group is measured twice. In this situation, we use a paired design because before-and-after measurements are taken. We use the paired t test to evaluate whether significant change occurs.

Assumptions: The difference score is normally distributed with the variances σ^2 unknown.

Formulation of hypotheses: The statistical hypothesis for a paired design typically involves the Greek letter delta δ with potential forms of the hypotheses as:

$H_0: \delta \geq 0$ *versus* $H_a: \delta < 0$

$H_0: \delta \leq 0$ *versus* $H_a: \delta > 0$

$H_0: \delta = 0$ *versus* $H_a: \delta \neq 0$

Test statistic: The t statistic can be used, with the modification as follows:

$$t = \frac{\bar{d} - 0}{s_d / \sqrt{n}}$$

where sd $s_d = \sqrt{\dfrac{\Sigma(d - \bar{d})^2}{n-1}}$. There are $n - 1$ degrees of freedom, and the denominator is the standard error of the mean differences.

The confidence interval is obtained as described in the following box.

Confidence Interval for the Mean Difference in Paired Design

The $100(1 - \alpha)\%$ confidence interval for the population mean difference in paired design δ when the mean difference in the population is approximately normally distributed and the variance s_d^2 is not known is the interval bounded by the confidence limits:

$$L = \bar{d} - t_{\alpha/2, n-1} \frac{s_d}{\sqrt{n}} \text{ and } R = \bar{d} + t_{\alpha/2, n-1} \frac{s_d}{\sqrt{n}}$$

The value of t is obtained from Table 4 in Appendix B, using $n - 1$ degrees of freedom.

EXAMPLE 8.5

In a study evaluating the efficacy of a coronary heart disease prevention program at improving selected health indicators, researchers wanted to identify whether a decrease in these health indicators occurred from baseline to 6 weeks after beginning the intervention.[1] One of these health indicators was body mass index (BMI). Applying the steps of hypothesis testing gives the following:

1. $H_0: \delta \geq 0$
2. $H_a: \delta < 0$

3. $\alpha = 0.05$, $n = 165$
4. t statistic and $(165 - 1) = 164$ degrees of freedom
5. From our sample, $\bar{d} = -1.23$ and $s = 0.73$, then:

$$t = \frac{-1.23 - 0}{0.73/\sqrt{165}} = -21.6$$

6. On the basis of the alternative hypothesis, we see that the rejection region is in the lower tail of the t distribution. Referring to Table 4 in Appendix B, the critical value is -1.645. Because the calculated value is in the rejection region, we reject H_0 and accept that a significant decrease in BMI occurred over the study period. Note that the P value corresponding to -21.6 is < 0.0001.

The 95% confidence interval is:

$$L = -1.23 - 1.96 \frac{0.73}{\sqrt{165}} = -1.34 \ and \ R = -1.23 + 1.96 \frac{0.73}{\sqrt{165}} = -1.12$$

Because both the lower and upper limits of the interval are both less than 0, this also tells us that at the 0.05 level, the difference score is significantly less than 0. In general, any time the P value is less than 0.05, the 95% confidence interval will also indicate statistical significance.

When the paired difference is not normally distributed, we can use a nonparametric procedure called the *Wilcoxon signed rank test*. There is no disadvantage to using the Wilcoxon signed rank test in terms of power, even if the difference is normally distributed. Prior to statistical software and computers, this test required considerable computational effort. However, nonparametric tests can now be easily derived with the computer.

In the study referred to in the previous example,[1] mean change in calories consumed in a given day from baseline to 6 weeks for those participating in a health education and nutrition intervention was -428. The median was -340. Because the mean is more sensitive to outliers than the median, the large difference between the mean and median indicates deviation from normality. The results of the Wilcoxon signed rank test, computed in SAS using PROC UNIVARIATE, are presented, along with results for the t statistic and another nonparametric test called the sign test, in **Table 8.2**. All three test statistics indicate statistical significance, given that the P values are all much lower than 0.05.

RESEARCH QUESTION ABOUT A PROPORTION IN ONE GROUP _____

Assumptions: When n is large, assume an approximate Z distribution, based on the central limit theorem.

TABLE 8.2   Test Statistics Produced from an SAS Procedure (Partial Output)

	Tests for location: Mu0=0			
Test	**Statistic**		**P value**	
Student's t	t	−6.59	$Pr > |t|$	< 0.0001
Sign	M	−36	$Pr \geq |M|$	< 0.0001
Signed rank	S	−3763	$Pr \geq |S|$	< 0.0001

Formulation of hypotheses: Three forms of a null hypothesis for a specified value of the proportion of success in the population π has a specified value π_0:

$H_0: \pi \geq \pi_0 \; H_a: \pi < \pi_0$

$H_0: \pi \leq \pi_0 \; H_a: \pi > \pi_0$

$H_0: \pi = \pi_0 \; H_a: \pi \neq \pi_0$

Test statistic: $Z = \dfrac{X - n\pi_0}{\sqrt{n\pi_0(1-\pi_0)}} = \dfrac{f - \pi_0}{\sqrt{\pi_0(1-\pi_0)/n}}$, where f is X/n, the fraction of successes in the sample.

EXAMPLE 8.6

A researcher is trying to recruit participants for a clinical trial and offers participation incentives of $25 cash or a gift certificate of equal value to a local restaurant. She wants to know whether there is any difference in the incentives chosen. After 100 people entered the study, 30 chose the gift certificate and 70 chose the cash. Applying the steps of hypothesis testing gives the following:

1. $H_0: \pi = 0.5$
2. $H_a: \pi \neq 0.5$
3. $\alpha = 0.05, n = 100$
4. Z statistic
5. $Z = \dfrac{f - \pi_0}{\sqrt{\dfrac{\pi_0(1-\pi_0)}{n}}} = \dfrac{0.3 - 0.5}{\sqrt{\dfrac{0.5(1-0.5)}{100}}} = -4$
6. This falls well into the lower tail of the rejection region, so we reject the null hypothesis and conclude that the gift certificate incentive is not as effective as the cash. The chance of error in this conclusion is 5% or less.

Investigators may want to evaluate change in proportions when the same group is measured twice. In studies involving a binary (two-level) variable, it may be of interest whether change occurs with the passage of time. In many situations, a proportion is compared before and after an intervention. The appropriate measure of evaluation in this situation is the McNemar test.

Assumptions: Has some characteristic of interest, measured as a binary scale with r "successes," changed over time?

Formulation of hypotheses:

$$H_0 : \pi_B \geq \pi_A \ versus \ H_a : \pi_B < \pi_A$$

$$H_0 : \pi_B \leq \pi_A \ versus \ H_a : \pi_B > \pi_A$$

$$H_0 : \pi_B = \pi_A \ versus \ H_a : \pi_B \neq \pi_A$$

Test statistic:

$$\text{McNemar} = \frac{(|b - c|)^2}{b + c}$$

EXAMPLE 8.7

A study was conducted to assess the effectiveness of the Berkshire Health System Cardiovascular Health Risk Reduction Program.[2] A group of 385 employees who completed an initial and follow-up personal health risk assessment were included in the study. One-on-one nurse coaching occurred, with referrals and recommendations based on screening results. A specific question assessed in the study was whether the proportion feeling depressed or hopeless at least some days in the prior 2 weeks at least some days was lower after a year of program participation. This question was assessed separately for employees aged 18–49 and those 50 and older. Applying the steps of hypothesis testing gives the following:

1. $H_0 : \pi_B \leq \pi_A$
2. $H_a : \pi_B > \pi_A$
3. $\alpha = 0.05$, $n = 385$
4. McNemar test, degrees of freedom $= (r - 1)(c - 1) = (2 - 1)(2 - 1) = 1$
5. Feelings of depression or hopelessness for at least some days in the past 2 weeks (yes versus no):

Ages 18–49	Screening 2		Total
Screening 1	Yes	No	
Yes	$a = 159$	$b = 18$	177
No	$c = 38$	$d = 26$	64
Total	197	44	241

Ages 50–72	Screening 2		Total
Screening 1	Yes	No	
Yes	$a = 104$	$b = 14$	118
No	$c = 11$	$d = 15$	26
Total	115	29	144

$$\text{McNemar}\left(\text{Aged 18–49}\right) = \frac{\left(|18 - 38|\right)^2}{18 + 38} = 7.14$$

$$\text{McNemar}\left(\text{Aged 50–72}\right) = \frac{\left(|14 - 11|\right)^2}{14 + 11} = 0.36$$

6. To obtain the rejection region for the McNemar test, refer to Table 5 in Appendix B, which gives a critical value of 3.84. For those aged 18–49, because 7.14 is greater than the critical value of 3.84, we reject the null hypothesis and conclude that there was a significant decrease in feelings of depression or hopelessness. There is not a significant decrease in feelings of depression or hopelessness for those aged 50–72.

A statistic that is commonly used to measure the level of agreement between two observers on a binary variable is Cohen's kappa (k).[3]

Equation for Kappa

$$k = \frac{Observed\ agreement - Expected\ agreement}{1 - Expected\ agreement}$$

Kappa ranges from −1 (perfect disagreement) to 1 (perfect agreement). When k is zero, agreement is what might be expected by chance. If k is 1, there is perfect agreement between the raters. Expected agreement in each cell is the proportion in that cell's row multiplied by the proportion in that cell's column.

Assumptions: Measuring the agreement between two raters who each classify N items into C mutually exclusive categories.

The following guidelines have been suggested for interpreting k in terms of agreement[4]:

0.93–1.00	Excellent agreement
0.81–0.92	Very good agreement
0.61–0.80	Good agreement
0.41–0.60	Fair agreement
0.21–0.40	Slight agreement
0.01–0.20	Poor agreement
0.00	No agreement

Appropriate test statistic: Cohen's kappa

EXAMPLE 8.8

Suppose two voice specialists assessed 50 selected voice patients for a disorder called spasmodic dysphonia (SD).

Observed Counts

	Specialist 2		
Specialist 1	**Yes**	**No**	**Total**
Yes	13	2	15
No	8	27	35
Total	21	29	50

Specialist 1 indicates that 15 patients, or 30%, have SD, and specialist 2 finds that 21 patients, or 42%, have SD. On the basis of the multiplication rule, the specialists would agree by chance that 30% × 42% = 12.6% of the patients have SD. Further, by chance alone, the specialists would agree that 70% × 58% = 40.6% do not have SD. Thus, the two specialists would agree by chance on 12.6% + 40.6% = 53.2%. In actuality, the specialists agreed on (13 + 27)/50, or 80% of the 50 patients, such that the level of agreement beyond chance is 0.80 − 0.532 = 0.268, which is the numerator of k. Kappa in this situation is therefore:

$$k = \frac{0.80 - 0.532}{1 - 0.532} = \frac{0.268}{0.468} = 0.57$$

Hence, there is fair agreement between the two specialists in diagnosing SD among voice patients.

RESEARCH QUESTION ABOUT MEANS IN TWO SEPARATE GROUPS ————

Assumptions:

1. Assume the samples are independent random samples, such that knowing the values of the observations in one group does not tell us anything about the observations in the other group.
2. Assume the populations are both normally distributed—this is less a concern when the sample size is at least 30, according to the central limit theorem. For smaller sample sizes where the two separate groups are not normally distributed, a nonparametric procedure called the *Wilcoxon rank sum test* is preferred.
3. Assume that the population variances (or equivalently, the standard deviations) for both groups are equal. This assumption follows from the assumption that both populations have equal means, as stated in the null hypothesis (as follows). Further, if the sample sizes are equal between the two groups, the *t* test is robust to deviation in the variances.

Pooled Standard Deviation

$$s_p = \sqrt{\frac{(n_1 - 1)s_1^2 + (n_2 - 1)s_2^2}{n_1 + n_2 - 2}}$$

From the pooled standard deviation, we can obtain the standard error of the difference, as follows:

Standard Error of the Difference

$$SE_{(\bar{x}_1 - \bar{x}_2)} = s_P \sqrt{\frac{1}{n_1} + \frac{1}{n_2}}$$

The standard error of the difference is used in the denominator of the t statistic when evaluating the difference between means from two independent groups.

A common statistical test for the equality of two variances is the F test. To calculate the F test, the larger variance is divided by the smaller variance, and the resulting ratio is compared with the critical value from the F distribution (see Table 6 in Appendix B). Equal variances will result in a ratio of 1. If the ratio is significantly greater than 1, we conclude that the variances are not equal. If the variances are not equal, then the pooled standard error will be underestimated. In this case, the test statistic is:

$$t_v = \frac{(\bar{X}_1 - \bar{X}_2) - 0}{\sqrt{\left(\frac{s_1^2}{n_1} + \frac{s_2^2}{n_2}\right)}}$$

The next step is to calculate the approximate degrees of freedom as:

$$v = \frac{\left[\left(\frac{s_1^2}{n_1}\right) + \left(\frac{s_2^2}{n_2}\right)\right]^2}{\left[\left(\frac{s_1^2}{n_1}\right)^2 \Big/ (n_1 - 1) + \left(\frac{s_2^2}{n_2}\right)^2 \Big/ (n_2 - 1)\right]}$$

Definition

The **F distribution** is an asymmetric probability distribution that ranges from 0 to infinity. It has two degrees of freedom, v_1 for the numerator, v_2 for the denominator. For each combination of these degrees of freedom, there is a different F distribution. The distribution has the greatest spread when the degrees of freedom are small.

If v involves a decimal place, round down to the nearest integer value. Then, the t distribution with v degrees of freedom is identical to the standard normal distribution, and we can use Table 4 in Appendix B. Note that SAS computes the t test for both the pooled and nonpooled approaches, and consultation of the F test for equality of variances will direct you as to which t statistic should be considered.

Hypotheses of Equality of Variances and the Rejection Region for Two-Sided Test

$$H_0 : \sigma_1^2 = \sigma_2^2 \quad H_a : \sigma_1^2 \neq \sigma_2^2$$

If $F > F_{\alpha/2, v_1, v_2}$, then reject H_0, where $F = \dfrac{s_1^2}{s_2^2}$ and the degrees of freedom are $v_1 = n_1 - 1$ and $v_2 = n_2 - 1$.

The largest sample variance is always placed in the numerator of the ratio.

Formulation of Hypotheses:

$H_0: \mu_1 \geq \mu_2 \ H_a: \mu_1 < \mu_2$

$H_0: \mu_1 \leq \mu_2 \ H_a: \mu_1 > \mu_2$

$H_0: \mu_1 = \mu_2 \ H_a: \mu_1 \neq \mu_2$

Test statistic: $t_{n_1+n_2-2} = \dfrac{(\bar{X}_1 - \bar{X}_2) - 0}{s_p\sqrt{\left(\dfrac{1}{n_1} + \dfrac{1}{n_2}\right)}}$

EXAMPLE 8.9

In many clinical studies involving random assignment of participants to an intervention or control group, we are interested in evaluating how well the randomization worked. An effective randomization of participants should produce groups that look similar in terms of demographics and health. In the Coronary Health Improvement Project (CHIP), there were 337 volunteers aged 43 to 81.[5] In this example, we will apply the steps of hypothesis testing to evaluate whether mean age significantly differs between participants in the intervention (I) and control (C) groups.

1. $H_0: \mu_I = \mu_c$
2. $H_a: \mu_I \neq \mu_c$
3. $\alpha = 0.05, n = 337$
4. t statistic, with $(n_1 + n_2 - 2) = 335$ degrees of freedom
5. From our sample:

$n_I = 167, \bar{X}_I = 50.39,$ and $s_I^2 = 10.97$

$n_C = 170, \bar{X}_C = 50.83,$ and $s_C^2 = 11.13$

$t_{n_1+n_2-2} = \dfrac{(50.39 - 50.83)}{11.05\sqrt{\left(\dfrac{1}{167} + \dfrac{1}{170}\right)}} = -0.37$

6. On the basis of the alternative hypothesis, we see that the rejection region is in the lower and upper tails of the t distribution. Referring to Table 4 in Appendix B, the critical values are −1.96 and 1.96. Because −0.37 is not in the rejection region, we fail to reject the null hypothesis of mean ages equal between the intervention and control groups.

> **Definition**
>
> The **100(1 − α)% confidence interval for the difference between two means** is known by the interval bounded by the confidence limits
>
> $L = (\bar{X}_1 - \bar{X}_2) - t_{\alpha/2, \, n_1+n_2-2} SE_{(\bar{X}_1-\bar{X}_2)}$
>
> *and*
>
> $R = (\bar{X}_1 - \bar{X}_2) + t_{\alpha/2, \, n_1+n_2-2} SE_{(\bar{X}_1-\bar{X}_2)}$
>
> The value of t is obtained from Table 4 in Appendix B, using $n_1 + n_2 - 2$ degrees of freedom.

RESEARCH QUESTION ABOUT PROPORTIONS IN TWO INDEPENDENT GROUPS

If we have two binomial populations, we are often interested in testing the hypothesis that the proportions in both groups are equal. For the first sample, the proportion of "success" is $f_1 = X_1/n_1$. For the second sample, the proportion of "success" is $f_2 = X_2/n_2$. The fraction of success for the pooled samples is:

$$f_{pooled} = \frac{X_1 + X_2}{n_1 + n_2}$$

The estimate of the standard error under the assumption that the proportions are the same is:

$$SE_{f_1-f_2} = \sqrt{\frac{f_1(1-f_1)}{n_1} + \frac{f_2(1-f_2)}{n_2}}.$$

If $\pi_1 = \pi_2$, then the variance can be reduced to:

$$SE_{f_1-f_2} = \sqrt{f_{pooled}(1-f_{pooled})\left[\frac{1}{n_1} + \frac{1}{n_2}\right]}.$$

Assumption: Under the null hypothesis, the quantity,

$$Z = \frac{f_1 - f_2}{\sqrt{f_{pooled}(1-f_{pooled})\left[\frac{1}{n_1} + \frac{1}{n_2}\right]}},$$

which has an approximately standard normal distribution if n_1 and n_2 are large.

There are three possible forms of hypotheses:

$H_0 : \pi_1 \geq \pi_2 \ H_a : \pi_1 < \pi_2$

$H_0 : \pi_1 \leq \pi_2 \ H_a : \pi_1 > \pi_2$

$H_0 : \pi_1 = \pi_2 \ H_a : \pi_1 \neq \pi_2$

EXAMPLE 8.10

We saw in the previous example that mean age was similar between those randomly assigned to the intervention (I) and control (C) groups. We may also ask whether the distribution of males ("successes" in this example) to females was similar in both groups. Applying the steps of hypothesis testing gives:

1. $H_0: \pi_I = \pi_C$
2. $H_a: \pi_I \neq \pi_C$
3. $\alpha = 0.05$, $n = 337$
4. Z statistic
5. From our sample:

$$n_I = 167, \, f_I = 0.2695$$
$$n_C = 170, \, f_C = 0.2882$$

$$f_{pooled} = \frac{45 + 49}{167 + 170} = 0.2789$$

$$Z = \frac{0.2695 - 0.2882}{\sqrt{0.2789(1 - 0.2789)\left[\dfrac{1}{167} + \dfrac{1}{170}\right]}} = -0.3827$$

6. Referring to Table 3 in Appendix B, the critical values are -1.96 and 1.96. Because -0.38 is not in the rejection region, we fail to reject the null hypothesis of equal proportions of males to females between intervention and control groups.

Confidence Interval for $\pi_1 - \pi_2$

The $100(1 - \alpha)\%$ confidence interval for the population difference in proportions from two distinct groups is the interval bounded by the confidence limits:

$$L = (f_1 - f_2) - Z_{\alpha/2}\sqrt{f_{pooled}(1 - f_{pooled})\left[\frac{1}{n_1} + \frac{1}{n_2}\right]}$$

$$R = (f_1 - f_2) + Z_{\alpha/2}\sqrt{f_{pooled}(1 - f_{pooled})\left[\frac{1}{n_1} + \frac{1}{n_2}\right]}$$

$$L = (0.2695 - 0.2882) - 1.96\sqrt{0.2789(1 - 0.2789)\left[\frac{1}{167} + \frac{1}{170}\right]} = -0.2003$$

$$R = (0.2695 - 0.2882) + 1.96\sqrt{0.2789(1 - 0.2789)\left[\frac{1}{167} + \frac{1}{170}\right]} = 0.1627$$

Because the 95% confidence interval $(-0.20, 0.16)$ overlaps 0, this also tells us that there is no significant difference in the proportion of males to females between the intervention and control groups.

EVALUATING DIFFERENCES USING ERROR BAR GRAPHS _____

With sample data, an error bar graph shows the mean values of a variable for different groups of individuals. Error bars are connected to the estimated means to show how accurate the measurements are. If the error bars around the mean values are 95% confidence intervals, then three general outcomes may occur (see **Figure 8.1**). In the left panel of the chart, the two graphs do not overlap, so we conclude that the means of the two groups are significantly different. In the middle panel of the chart, the mean value for one group is contained within the error bars of the second graph. Here we can conclude that the means are not significantly different. In the right panel of the chart, the error bars overlap between the two graphs, but not enough to contain either of the means, so we do not know if the means are significantly different. In this latter situation, we need to conduct a statistical test to determine whether the means between the groups are significantly different.

EXAMPLE 8.11

A recent study provided a comprehensive review of the prevalence of selected hepatitis B virus seromarkers in order to identify variability in seroprevalence across the 14 World Health Organization (WHO) subregions and among special groups and populations.[6] The analyses involved 568 papers and 736 population studies. The complete data set includes 21,838,249 individuals and covered the 14 WHO subregions. **Figure 8.2** shows hepatitis B surface antigen (HBsAg) seroprevalence in the general population for selected studies. Mean HBsAg seroprevalence in the first two Nigerian studies is not significantly different, but both studies have significantly greater mean HBsAg seroprevalence than in the third Nigerian study shown in the graph. Mean HBsAg seroprevalence

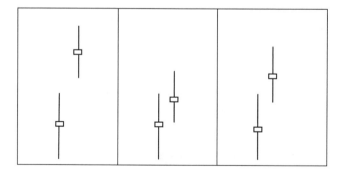

FIGURE 8.1 Visual assessment of differences between two independent groups using 95% confidence intervals.

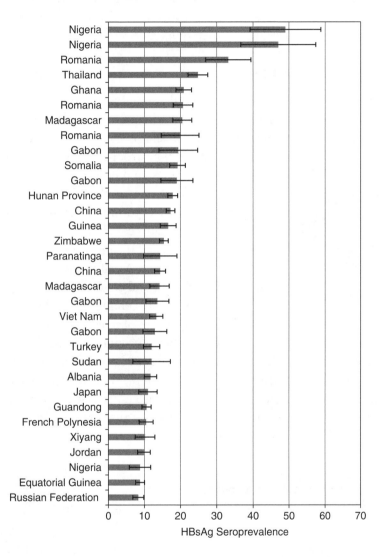

FIGURE 8.2 HBsAg seroprevalence in the general population for several studies.

Data from: Merrill, RM, Hunter, BD. Seroprevalence of markers for Hepatitis B viral infection. *Int J Infect Dis* 2011;15(2):378–121.

is significantly greater in the first Romanian study compared with the two other studies shown in the graph. It is not clear, given the overlapping confidence intervals, whether HBsAg seroprevalence in the two studies involving Gabon are significantly different. Further statistical testing is required to determine this.

CHI-SQUARE DISTRIBUTION

The chi-square test for independence can also be used to compare frequencies or proportions between two groups. The calculations for this test are relatively easy to apply to data in contingency tables. In epidemiology and medicine, many sets of countable data can be grouped according to two or more criteria of groupings, and evaluated to see whether they are independent of one another. If we are interested in comparing whether exposure to a substance is related to disease, exposure status could be represented by the rows in a two-way table, and the disease status could be represented by the columns. A cell of the table represents the intersection of a row and column.

Definition

A **contingency table** is a table showing the distribution of one variable in rows and another in columns, used to study the association between the two categorical variables.

A general two-way contingency table with r rows and c columns has (rows [r] − 1)(columns [c] − 1) degrees of freedom. The χ^2 distribution is used to assess counts in contingency tables. This is a continuous distribution ordinarily derived as the sampling distribution of a sum of squares of independent standard normal variables. It is a (right) skewed distribution such that only nonnegative values of the variable are possible. It depends on a single parameter: the degrees of freedom. As the degrees of freedom increase without limit, the χ^2 distribution goes from being highly skewed to approaching a normal distribution.

Equation for the Chi-Square for a Contingency Table

$$\chi^2 = \sum_{i,j} \frac{(O_{ij} - E_{ij})^2}{E_{ij}}$$

where

O_{ij} = number observed to belong to the ith row and jth column.

E_{ij} = number expected to belong to the ith row and jth column, derived by multiplying the total observed in the ith row by the total observed in the jth column and dividing by the overall sample size.

There are $(r-1)(c-1)$ degrees of freedom.

TABLE 8.3   Low Birth Weight and Residence during Pregnancy

Residence during pregnancy	Low birth weight	Normal weight	Total
Near high-hazard dump site	181	4,268	4,449
Near low-hazard dump site	126	4,236	4,362
Total	307	8,504	8,811

Data from: Gilbreath S, Kass PH. Adverse birth outcomes associated with open dump sites in Alaska Native villages. *Am J Epidemiol.* 2006;164:518–528.

EXAMPLE 8.12

Suppose the rate of low birth weight was greater than expected in a region. Researchers asked whether living near a high-hazard dump site compared with a low-hazard dump site increased the risk of having a low birth weight child. A contingency table representing data from a study investigating this appears in **Table 8.3**.[7]

Applying the steps to hypothesis testing gives the following:

1. H_0: Hazardous dump site residence status is independent of low birth weight status
2. H_a: Hazardous dump site residence status is *not* independent of low birth weight status
3. $\alpha = 0.05$, $n = 8{,}811$
4. χ^2 with $(2 - 1)(2 - 1) = 1$ degree of freedom
5. For the data in Table 8.3, the χ^2 equals:

$$\chi^2 = \frac{(181 - 155)^2}{155} + \frac{(126 - 152)^2}{152} + \frac{(4{,}268 - 4{,}294)^2}{4{,}294} + \frac{(4{,}236 - 4{,}210)^2}{4{,}210} = 9.12$$

Referring to Table 5 in Appendix B, the critical value is 3.84.

6. Because the calculated value lies in the rejection region, we reject the null hypothesis and accept that there is a significant association between living near a hazardous dump site during pregnancy and having a child of low birth weight.

The *P* value that is associated with 9.12 is 0.0025 (provided by SAS). The *P* value is obtain from the chi-square (χ^2) table by going to the first line, which corresponds with 1 degree of freedom, and moving over to 9.12. Then going up to the top of the table, we see that $0.01 > P$ value > 0.001. Since the *P* value is less than 0.05, we reject the null hypothesis.

The chi-square procedure, like the test for evaluating differences in proportions based on the *Z* approximation, is an approximation method. The chi-square test should only be used for evaluating differences in proportions if the expected frequency in any given cell is greater than 5. A less conservative approach sometimes adopted is that if any expected frequency is less than 2 or if more than 20% of the expected frequencies are less than 5, then the chi-square test should not be used. Alternatively, the Fisher's exact test is more appropriate when the sample size is small. Because the computations for this test are complex, it is not presented here. However, SAS and other statistical software packages perform the Fisher's exact test for 2×2 tables, along with the chi-square test.

RESEARCH QUESTION ABOUT MEANS IN THREE OR MORE GROUPS

To test the equality of several means, we can use a procedure called analysis of variance (ANOVA). Similar to the t test, ANOVA is a parametric procedure that has some important assumptions involving independence, normality, and equality of variance. When the sample size is large, the normality assumption is less important than the other assumptions.

Assumptions in ANOVA

- All the samples were randomly selected and are *independent* of one another.
- The populations from which the samples were drawn are *normally distributed*.
- All the populations have the *same variance*.

To conduct an analysis of variance and test the null hypothesis that three or more means are equal, we take independent samples from each of the populations of interest and obtain certain measures that allow us to compute sums of squared deviations. Specifically, suppose we have one factor with j groups. Let

X_{ij} be the *ith* observation in the *jth* group.

$\bar{X}_j$ be the mean of all observations in the *jth* group.

$\bar{\bar{X}}$ be the grand mean of the observations.

Then, the total sum of squares, $SS_T = \Sigma\left(X_{ij} - \bar{\bar{X}}\right)^2$, equals the error sum of squares, $SS_W = \Sigma\left(X_{ij} - \bar{X}_j\right)^2$, plus the sum of squares among groups, $SS_A = \Sigma\left(X_j - \bar{\bar{X}}\right)^2$. In the following formulas, we see that the sums of squares are divided by the degrees of freedom to obtain the mean squares. The degrees of freedom among groups (A) are $j - 1$, and the degrees of freedom within groups (W) are $N - j$. The total degrees of freedom are $N - 1$.

Computational Formulas

$$SS_T = \sum \left(X_{ij} - \bar{\bar{X}} \right)^2 = \sum X_{ij}^2 - \frac{\left(\sum X_{ij} \right)^2}{N}$$

$$SS_A = \sum \left(\bar{X}_j - \bar{\bar{X}} \right)^2 = \sum n_j \bar{X}_j^2 - \frac{\left(\sum X_{ij} \right)^2}{N}$$

$$SS_W = SS_T - SS_A$$

$$MS_A = \frac{SS_A}{j-1}$$

$$MS_W = \frac{SS_W}{N-j}$$

The final step in ANOVA is to obtain the F ratio of MS_A divided by MS_W:

Hypotheses on Equality of Several Population Means and Rejection Region for ANOVA

$$H_0 : \mu_1 = \mu_2 = \cdots = \mu_k$$

H_a : *One or more of the population means is not equal to the others*

If $F > F_{\alpha, v_1, v_{12}}$, then reject H_0, where $F = \dfrac{MS_A}{MS_W}$ and the degrees of freedom are $v_1 = j - 1$ and $v_2 = N - j$.

EXAMPLE 8.13

In a study involving quality-of-life indicators according to voice disorders and voice-related conditions, researchers evaluated the association between a history of voice disorders and voice-related conditions and the Short Form-36 8-scale measures of functional health and well-being as well as psychometrically based physical and mental health summary measures in a senior population.[8] The social functioning measure of health (with the score ranging from 0 to 100, with a higher score reflecting better social functioning) is related to whether the participant in the study indicated he/she had to repeat himself/herself to be understood:

1. never
2. rarely

3. occasionally
4. often

We are interested in whether the mean social functioning score differs among the four groups. Applying the steps of hypothesis testing results in the following:

1. $H_0: \mu_1 = \mu_2 = \mu_3 = \mu_4$
2. $H_a:$ Otherwise
3. $\alpha = 0.05$, $n_1 = 131$, $n_2 = 171$, $n_3 = 84$, $n_4 = 21$.
4. F, $v_1 = j - 1 = 4 - 1 = 3$, $v_2 = N - j = 407 - 4 = 403$.
5.

$$SS_T = \sum\left(X_{ij} - \bar{\bar{X}}\right)^2 = \sum X_{ij}^2 - \frac{\left(\sum X_{ij}\right)^2}{N} = 121265.36$$

$$SS_A = \sum\left(\bar{X}_j - \bar{\bar{X}}\right)^2 = \sum n_j \bar{X}_j^2 - \frac{\left(\sum X_{ij}\right)^2}{N} = 8076.22$$

$$SS_W = SS_T - SS_A = 113189.1$$

$$MS_A = \frac{SS_A}{j-1} = \frac{8076.22}{3} = 2692.07$$

$$MS_W = \frac{113189.1}{403} = 289.87$$

$$F = \frac{MS_A}{MS_W} = \frac{2692.07}{280.87} = 9.58$$

6. Referring to Table 6 in Appendix B, the critical value is 2.60. Hence, we reject the null hypothesis and conclude otherwise.

When the F test is significant, we can say that the population means are not all equal, but we cannot conclude more than that. We do not know whether all the means are different from one another or only some of them are different. If we reject the null hypothesis, we then need to do further testing to find out where the differences lie. We could perform the following number of two-sample t-tests:

$$\binom{k}{2} = \frac{k!}{2!(k-2)!}$$

However, performing multiple tests increases the probability of making a type I error. This problem may be avoided by reducing the individual α levels so that the overall level of significance is kept at a predetermined level. In order for the overall probability of making a type I error to be 0.05, for example, we should use the following adjust-ment to our α level if we had planned on making k comparisons prior to data collection:

$$\alpha^* = \frac{0.05}{\binom{k}{2}}$$

This modification is referred to as the Bonferroni correction. For example, if we have three groups, our modified α is:

$$\alpha^* = \frac{0.05}{\binom{3}{2}} = \frac{0.05}{3} = 0.0167$$

Several procedures are available for making post hoc comparisons after the null hypothesis is rejected in ANOVA. Statistical software readily computes these differ-ent procedures. Although we will not cover these in this text, they include Tukey's HSD procedure, Scheffe's procedure, the Student-Newman-Keuls (SNK) procedure, and the Dunnett's procedure. **Table 8.4** is a partial output for the ANOVA, from SAS, where we requested the SNK procedure. Means with the same letter associated with them are not significantly different. In this example, the group "often" has sig-nificantly lower mean than do the other three groups.

Finally, the previous example is a one-way ANOVA model because there was one independent variable. Two-way ANOVA is similar, except that two factors (or two independent variables) are assessed. Suppose we were interested in whether mean social functioning differed according to having a history of a voice disorder (yes versus no) and sex. In this two-way ANOVA, we can ask whether differences exist in social func-tioning between those with and those without a history of voice disorders, whether a

TABLE 8.4   Student-Newman-Keuls Test for Post Hoc Comparisons of Means

SNK Grouping	Mean	N	Variable Level
Means with the same letter are not significantly different.			
A	93.225	131	never
A	88.690	84	occasionally
A	88.231	171	rarely
B	72.619	21	often

difference exists in social functioning between males and females, and whether difference exists because of the combination of factors. In this latter case, we say an interaction effect (or in epidemiology, we would say effect modification) exists between the two factors.

EXERCISES

1. What is the difference between point and interval estimation?
2. Describe the interpretation for a 95% confidence interval for a population mean μ.
3. Which factors influence the length of a confidence interval for the mean μ?
4. How is the t distribution similar to the standard normal distribution?
5. What is a hypothesis?
6. What is a statistical hypothesis test?
7. What is the function of a P value?
8. What relationship does the P value have with the sample size?
9. What role does hypothesis testing have in characterizing whether a study is descriptive or analytic?
10. Define power and relate it to the probability of committing a type II error.
11. Suppose that the current belief is that the mean percentage of the U.S. adult population who visited the dentist in the past year is about 65%. On the other hand, from your experience and observation, you believe this percentage is higher. Assume that based on a random sample of 200 adults in your community, you find $\overline{X} = 69.7\%$ and $s = 32.5\%$. Assuming a normal distribution of mean percent scores, apply the steps to hypothesis testing.
12. Referring to question 11, calculate and interpret the 95% confidence interval for these data.
13. In a study evaluating whether a 6-week coronary heart disease prevention program can lower depression and stress, 348 individuals ages 24 to 81 were sampled.[9] Mean change in the Beck Depression Inventory from baseline to follow-up was −1.53, with a standard deviation of 3.38. Apply the steps of hypothesis testing to these data.
14. Referring to question 13, calculate and interpret the 95% confidence interval for the mean change score in the Beck Depression Inventory.
15. You would like to test the hypothesis that a significant decrease in depression occurred because of an intervention. A random sample of 10 of the 248 Beck Depression Inventory change scores produced −8, −2, −1, 1, −5, 0, −5, 0, −3, and 0. Use an appropriate test to evaluate whether a significant change in scores occurred for these data.

16. It is assumed that the proportion of women in the United States ages 40 years and older that received a mammogram within the past 2 years is 0.80. You believe the actual proportion is less than this. Taking a sample of 50, you get a proportion of 0.75. Apply the steps of hypothesis testing to these data.

17. You believe that a significant change in depression will result from your intervention. Suppose you collect the following data from 348 individuals.[9] Apply the steps of hypothesis testing to this data.

| Baseline | Six weeks | | Total |
	Yes	No	
Yes	34	33	67
No	9	272	281
Total	43	305	348

18. Suppose two students independently assesses whether several peer-reviewed articles in a given medical journal obtain a high-quality rating in terms of study design and the application of appropriate statistical methods. You are interested in the level of agreement in ratings between these two students. Evaluate this data for agreement.

Observed Counts			
Student 1	Student 2		Total
	High quality	Not high quality	
High quality	22	3	25
Not high quality	8	27	35
Total	30	30	60

19. Referring to question 13, the change score reported there represented both intervention and control participants. We really want to know whether a decrease in depression occurred among those in the intervention group compared with those in the control group. We believe that the decrease we observed earlier will only exist among the people in the intervention group. We found the following in the intervention group: $n = 174, \overline{X} = -2.62, s = 3.61$; and for the control group: $n = 174, \overline{X} = -0.44, s = 2.73$. Test the hypothesis of equality of variance.

20. Continuing with the previous question, apply the steps of hypothesis testing with the null hypothesis that there is no difference in means.

21. Calculate a 95% confidence interval for the difference in means.

22. For the data introduced in question 13, we found that at baseline there was no difference in the level of restless sleep patterns between intervention and control group participants. However, we believe the intervention lowered the level of restless sleep. To test this hypothesis we identify 18.39% of those in the intervention group and 30.46% of those in the control group at 6 weeks who complained about restless sleep problems. Apply the steps of hypothesis testing using the Z test.

23. Continuing with the previous problem, calculate the 95% confidence interval for the difference in proportions.

24. Referring to question 22, we were able to use the Z to evaluate this problem because the sample sizes in the intervention and control groups were large. We could have also used the chi-square test because no expected frequency was less than 5. Apply the steps of hypothesis, only this time, use the chi-square test.

| | Restless sleep at 6 weeks | | |
	Yes	No	Total
Intervention	32	53	85
Control	142	121	263
Total	174	174	348

25. For the same data, at baseline we wanted to test whether there was a significant difference in the mean Beck Depression Inventory by weight category. We classified weight as normal, overweight, or obese according to body mass index. What are your null and research hypotheses?

26. Sample size for normal weight is 67, for overweight is 101, and obese is 180. What are the degrees of freedom for the F test?

27. $SS_A = 366.895$; $SS_T = 7469.526$. What is the F Value?

28. What is the critical value for the F test, and what is your conclusion?

29. If you found that the model was significant and you were interested in where the means differed, what approach would you take to discover this?

30. What type of ANOVA was just performed, one-way or two-way? Explain.

REFERENCES

1. Merrill RM, Aldana SG. Improving overall health status through the CHIP intervention. *Am J Health Behav.* 2009;33(2):135–146.
2. Merrill RM, Aldana SG, Ellrodt G, Orsi R, Grelle-Laramee J. Efficacy of the Berkshire Health System Cardiovascular Health Risk Reduction Program. *J Occup Environ Med.* 2009;51(9): 1024–1031.
3. Cohen J. A coefficient of agreement for nominal scales. *Educ Psychol Meas.* 1960;20(1):37–46.
4. Byrt T. How good is that agreement? *Epidemiology.* 1996;7:561.
5. Aldana SG, Greenlaw RL, Diehl HA, et al. Effects of an intensive diet and physical activity modification program on the health risks of adults. *J Am Diet Assoc.* 2005;105(3):371–381.
6. Merrill RM, Hunter BD. Seroprevalence of markers for hepatitis B viral infection. *Int J Infect Dis.* 2011;15(2):378–421.
7. Gilbreath S, Kass PH. Adverse birth outcomes associated with open dump sites in Alaska native villages. *Am J Epidemiol.* 2006;164:518–528.
8. Merrill RM, Anderson AE, Sloan A. Quality of life indicators according to voice disorders and voice-related conditions. *Laryngoscope.* 2011;121:2004–2011.
9. Merrill RM, Aldana SG, Greenlaw RL, Diehl HA. The coronary health improvement project's impact on lowering eating, sleep, stress, and depressive disorders. *Am J Health Educ.* 2008; 39(6):337–344.

CHAPTER 9

Sample Size

An appropriate sample size is critical to the success of any research study. There are several cookbook formulas for calculating sample size in analytic studies. Sample size can also be calculated for descriptive studies. The purpose of this chapter is to present sample size estimates for analytic studies and descriptive studies, and to cover some special issues related to sample size.

SAMPLE SIZE TECHNIQUES FOR ANALYTIC STUDIES

The appropriate formulas depend on the type of data involved. Despite there being several variations in the recipe for estimating sample size, there are certain steps in common:

1. State the null hypothesis.
2. State the alternative hypothesis (one- or two-sided).
3. Identify the anticipated difference or effect size of the exposure (or intervention).
4. Identify the anticipated variability (if necessary).
5. Select the level of significance (α) and one minus the desired power (β).
6. Use the appropriate formula to estimate the sample size.

By selecting the level of significance α for the null hypothesis and β for the alternative hypothesis, we can determine the sample size. Let z_α be the two-tailed value of z related to α, and z_β be the lower one-tailed value of z related to β. Generally $\alpha = 0.05$ and $\beta = 0.20$. The lower one-sided value for β is used because power equals $1 - \beta$ or greater. The two critical ratios are:

$$z_\alpha = \frac{\overline{X} - \mu_0}{\sigma/\sqrt{n}}$$

$$z_\beta = \frac{\overline{X} - \mu_1}{\sigma/\sqrt{n}}$$

Set the two expressions for $\overline{X}$ equal to each other.

$$z_\alpha \sigma / \sqrt{n} + \mu_0 = \overline{X}$$

$$z_\beta \sigma / \sqrt{n} + \mu_1 = \overline{X}$$

$$z_\alpha \sigma / \sqrt{n} + \mu_0 = z_\beta \sigma / \sqrt{n} + \mu_1$$

Solving the sample size n gives the equation that follows:

Equation for Estimating the Sample Size for One Mean

$$n = \left[\frac{(z_\alpha - z_\beta)\sigma}{\mu_1 - \mu_0} \right]^2$$

The values of z_α and z_β depend on the choice of alpha and beta and whether a one- or two-sided hypothesis is being evaluated.

---

z_α = **the standard normal deviate for α**
z_α = 2.576 if α = 0.005, alternative hypothesis, one-sided
z_α = 2.576 if α = 0.01, alternative hypothesis, two-sided
z_α = 1.96 if α = 0.05, alternative hypothesis, two-sided
z_α = 1.645 if α = 0.1, alternative hypothesis, two-sided
z_α = 1.645 if α = 0.05, alternative hypothesis, one-sided
z_α = **the standard normal deviate for β**
z_β = −0.84 if β = 0.20
z_β = −1.282 if β = 0.10

EXAMPLE 9.1

A study evaluated whether selected health indicators, including body mass index (BMI), could be significantly decreased over the course of a 6 week intervention.[1] Suppose that at the beginning of the study, the investigators wanted to know whether mean BMI differed from 30 by 1 or more. Applying the steps of sample size calculation gives:

1. $H_0: \mu = 30$
2. $H_a: \mu \neq 30$
3. 1 or more
4. Assumed to be 5
5. $\alpha = 0.05$, $\beta = 0.20$
6. $n = \left[\dfrac{(1.96 - [-0.84])5}{31 - 30} \right]^2 = 196$

Thus, to conclude that mean BMI of ≤ 29 or ≥ 31 is a significant departure from the assumed BMI of 30 (with standard deviation of 5), investigators need a sample of 176.

In the case of a proportion, using the same logic as with the sample size for the mean, the two critical ratios for z_α and z_β are:

$$z_\alpha = \frac{f - \pi_0}{\sqrt{\pi_0(1 - \pi_0)/n}}$$

$$z_\beta = \frac{f - \pi_1}{\sqrt{\pi_1(1 - \pi_1)/n}}$$

Set the two expressions for f equal to each other.

$$z_\alpha\sqrt{\pi_0(1 - \pi_0)/n} + \pi_0 = f$$

$$z_\beta\sqrt{\pi_1(1 - \pi_1)/n} + \pi_1 = f$$

$$z_\alpha\sqrt{\pi_0(1 - \pi_0)/n} + \pi_0 = z_\beta\sqrt{\pi_1(1 - \pi_1)/n} + \pi_1$$

Solving the sample size n gives the equation that follows:

Equation for Estimating the Sample Size for One Proportion

$$n = \left[\frac{z_\alpha\sqrt{\pi_0(1 - \pi_0)} - z_\beta\sqrt{\pi_1(1 - \pi_1)}}{\pi_1 - \pi_0}\right]^2$$

EXAMPLE 9.2

A study was conducted to evaluate quality-of-life indicators according to voice disorders and voice-related conditions in a group of older adults.[2] Researchers carrying out this study believed a history of voice disorders for this population was at least 25%. Previously it had been assumed to be about 20%. Applying the steps of sample size calculation gives:

1. $H_0: \pi \leq 0.20$
2. $H_a: \pi > 0.20$
3. Assumed truth is 0.25
4. The proportion itself determines the estimated standard deviation: $\pi(1 - \pi)$

5. $\alpha = 0.05, \beta = 0.20$

6. $n = \left[\dfrac{1.645\sqrt{0.20(1-0.20)} - (-0.84)\sqrt{0.25(1-0.25)}}{0.25 - 0.2} \right]^2 = 417.6$

Rounding up gives a required sample size of 418.

Now suppose we are interested in estimating the approximate sample size for a study comparing the means in two groups of people. If $\mu_1 - \mu_2$ is the magnitude of the difference to be detected between the two groups, σ is the standard error for each group, z_α is the two-tailed value of z related to α, and z_β is the lower one-tailed value of z related to β, then the sample size needed in each group is as described in the following box.

Equation for Estimating the Sample Size for Two Means
Let q_1 = proportion of subjects in group 1; q_2 = proportion of subjects in group 2; and s is the standard deviation.

$$n = \frac{\left[(1/q_1 + 1/q_2)s^2(z_\alpha - z_\beta) \right]^2}{(\mu_1 - \mu_0)^2}$$

EXAMPLE 9.3

Two medications are being evaluated to determine their effects on the time it takes patients experiencing depression to complete a task. Assume that this time is normally distributed, with a standard deviation of 10 seconds for each treatment. In a randomized trial to compare treatments A and B, how many patients are needed to determine if one treatment is better than the other by an average of 10 seconds? Applying the steps of sample size calculation gives:

1. $H_0: \mu_1 = \mu_2$
2. $H_a: \mu_1 \neq \mu_2$
3. Difference in means is 10
4. We assume the standard deviations in the two populations are equal to 10
5. $\alpha = 0.05, \beta = 0.10$

6. $n = \dfrac{\left[(1/0.5 + 1/0.5)10^2(1.96 - [-1.282]) \right]^2}{10^2} = 42.04$

Thus the required sample size is 22 per group.

There are also times when we are interested in estimating the approximate sample size for a study comparing the proportions in two groups of people. The formula for n is described in the following box.

Equation for Estimating the Sample Size for Two Proportions

Let q_1 = proportion of subjects in group 1; q_2 = proportion of subjects in group 2; π_1 = proportion of subjects expected to have the outcome in one group; π_2 = in the other group; and $\pi = q_1\pi_1 + q_2\pi_2$

$$n = \frac{\left[z_\alpha \sqrt{\pi(1-\pi)(1/q_1 + 1/q_2)} - z_\beta\sqrt{\pi_1(1-\pi_1)(1/q_1) + \pi_2(1-\pi_2)(1/q_2)}\right]^2}{(\pi_1 - \pi_2)^2}$$

EXAMPLE 9.4

Suppose you are interested in the response rates (in percentages) for two regimens. A power of 80%, a two-sided test, and a level of significance of 0.05 are desired. How many patients are needed to detect a difference between true response rates of 40% and 50%?

Applying the steps of sample size calculation gives:

1. $H_0: \pi_1 = \pi_2$
2. $H_a: \pi_1 \neq \pi_2$
3. Difference from 40% to 50%
4. The null hypothesis assumes the proportion are equal and the proportion itself determines the estimated standard deviation: $\pi(1-\pi)$
5. $\alpha = 0.05, \beta = 0.20$
6. $n = \dfrac{\left[\begin{array}{c}1.96\sqrt{0.45(1-0.45)(1/0.5 + 1/0.5)} \\ -[-0.84]\sqrt{0.5(1-0.5)(1/0.5) + 0.4(1-0.4)(1/0.5)}\end{array}\right]^2}{(0.5-0.4)^2} = 387$

Thus the required sample size is 386 per group.

Some other sample size issues in analytic studies include loss to follow-up, fixed sample size, and ways to minimize sample size and maximize power.

LOSS TO FOLLOW-UP

Participants enrolled in a study who are not available for outcome assessment (e.g., dropouts) are not included in the sample size. When it is anticipated that some of the participants in a cohort or experimental study will be lost to follow-up, the sample size should be increased accordingly.

> **Sample Size Adjustment Factor for Loss to Follow-up**
>
> $$\frac{1}{1-X}$$
>
> where X is the expected proportion to be lost to follow-up.

EXAMPLE 9.5

If 15% of participants are expected to be lost to follow-up, then the sample size should be increased by a multiple of

$$\frac{1}{1-0.15} = 1.18$$

For instance, if the required sample size is 100, 118 participants should be sampled.

FIXED SAMPLE SIZE

If the sample size is fixed before you begin your study, the investigator can take the fixed sample size and estimate the effect size that can be detected at a given power. A power of 80% or greater is typically required to detect a reasonable effect size. The formula to obtain the effect size for a given sample size, standard deviation, and specified z_α is the two-tailed z value related to the null hypothesis, and z_β is the lower one-tailed z value related to the alternative hypothesis.

$$n = 4\left[\frac{(z_\alpha - z_\beta)\sigma}{\mu_1 - \mu_2}\right]^2$$

Solving for $\mu_1 - \mu_2$ gives the following equation for the effect size when the sample size is fixed:

> **Equation for Estimating the Effect Size for Fixed Sample Size**
>
> $$\mu_1 - \mu_2 = \frac{2(z_\alpha - z_\beta)\sigma}{\sqrt{n}}$$

EXAMPLE 9.6

An investigator finds that there are 128 patients available with a coronary event who are willing to participate in a study of whether a 6-week dietary program affects recovery according to selected biometric measures, as compared with a control group of people who continue with their normal diet. If the standard deviation of the change in systolic blood pressure is expected to be 10 points in both the intervention and control groups, what size difference will the investigator be able to detect between the two groups, at α (two-sided) = 0.05 and β = 0.20?

$$\mu_1 - \mu_2 = \frac{2(1.96 - [-0.84])10}{\sqrt{128}} = 4.95$$

Thus, the investigator who has 64 patients per group will be able to detect a difference of about 5 points between the two groups.

WAYS TO MINIMIZE SAMPLE SIZE AND MAXIMIZE POWER

There are various strategies to take if the estimated sample size is greater than the number of participants who are available. These strategies include checking your calculations for mistakes, reviewing the ingredients to the sample size calculation for unreasonably small effect size or too large of standard deviation, determining whether α and/or β could be increased without harm, and deciding whether a one-sided alternative hypothesis is acceptable.[3] In addition, a continuous variable, if available, compared with a nominal variable allows for smaller sample size. Paired data in a cohort or experimental study involving a continuous variable as opposed to nonpaired data often allows a smaller sample size. When the outcome variable is dichotomous, choosing a variable that occurs more frequently, up to a frequency of 0.5, increases power. In a case-control study, multiple controls may be used per case.[3] In a case-control study, a useful formula for determining the sample size of dichotomous risk factors and outcomes using c controls per case is described in the following box.

Equation for Estimating c Controls per Case with Fixed n

$$n' = \frac{c+1}{2c} \times n \quad \text{or} \quad c = \frac{n}{(2n' - n)}$$

EXAMPLE 9.7

An investigator is studying whether exposure to a pesticide called Atrazine is a risk factor for prostate cancer. The original sample size calculation indicated that 27 cases would be required, with one control per case. However, suppose that Atrazine is a chemical used by farmers in a given area and that only 18 farmers in the area have prostate cancer. We can approach this problem using trial and error, such that $c = 1$, 2, 3 gives the following:

$$n' = \frac{1+1}{2 \times 1} \times 27 = 27$$

$$n' = \frac{2+1}{2 \times 2} \times 27 = 20.25 \text{ or } 21$$

$$n' = \frac{3+1}{2 \times 3} \times 27 = 18$$

Wherein, 3 controls per case are sufficient. Alternatively, we can directly identify the number of controls per case as

$$c = \frac{27}{(2 \times 18 - 27)} = 3.$$

SAMPLE SIZE TECHNIQUES FOR DESCRIPTIVE STUDIES

When sample size is estimated for descriptive studies, we take a different approach compared with that presented thus far in this chapter for analytic studies. In descriptive studies, recall that there are not exposure and outcome variables, nor is there a control group for comparison. Hence, the concepts of null and alternative hypotheses and power are not relevant. Instead, the investigator calculates descriptive statistics.

A descriptive statistic is often associated with confidence intervals (i.e., measures of precision of a sample estimate). In this section, three formulas will be presented for determining the sample size needed to obtain confidence levels for the population mean μ and the population proportion of success π.

To determine the sample size needed to obtain a confidence interval prior to taking the sample, three pieces of information are required:

1. The confidence level (such as 90, 95, or 99%)
2. The maximum width of the confidence interval (width = $R - L$)
3. The standard deviation associated with the population from which we are about to sample

Recall that the confidence interval to estimate the population mean μ is:

$$L = \overline{X} - Z_{\infty/2} \frac{\sigma}{\sqrt{n}} \text{ and } R = \overline{X} + Z_{\infty/2} \frac{\sigma}{\sqrt{n}}$$

The width of the confidence interval is thus:

$$width = 2 \times Z_{\infty/2} \frac{\sigma}{\sqrt{n}}$$

If we know items 1–3 above, we can use this equation to solve for n.

Sample Size Equation for Estimating the Mean, σ Known

$$n = \frac{4 \times Z^2_{\infty/2} \sigma^2}{width^2}$$

EXAMPLE 9.8

The standard deviation of IQ among a group of college freshmen is 16 points. We want to estimate the mean IQ to within ± 4 points, at 95% confidence. The three pieces of information for obtaining the sample size are:

1. A confidence level of 95%, $Z_{0.05/2} = 1.96$
2. Width of the confidence interval of 8 (since ± 4 implies a total width of 2×4)
3. The standard deviation equal to 16

$$n = \frac{4 \times 1.96^2 \times 16^2}{8^2} = 61.5$$

The sample size of $n = 62$ will give us an interval that allows us to estimate the population mean IQ to within 4 points at 95% confidence.

If we do not know the population mean μ, it is unlikely we will know the population standard deviation σ. In this situation, we are often required to replace the population variance in the preceding formula with its estimate s^2, obtained from a previous sample of the population or a related sample. We learned earlier that the confidence interval that involves the sample standard deviation requires that we use $t_{\alpha/2,n-1}$ in place of $Z_{\alpha/2}$.

Sample Size Equation for Estimating the Mean, σ Not Known

$$n = \frac{4 \times \left(t_{\alpha/2,n-1}\right)^2 s^2}{width^2}$$

EXAMPLE 9.9

A hospital administrator wants to know the mean length of time (μ) it takes emergency room patients to see a physician during the evening shift. She wishes to estimate μ to within ± 5 minutes with 90% confidence. She does not know the value of σ, the population standard deviation, so she takes a preliminary sample of $n = 10$ emergency room patients and finds the standard deviation of $s = 20$ minutes. How large does the sample size need to be in order to obtain the desired confidence interval?

From the statement of the problem, we know the following:

1. A confidence level of 90%, $t_{0.05,9} = 1.833$
2. Width of the confidence interval of 10
3. The standard deviation equal to 20

$$n = \frac{4 \times (1.833)^2 \, 20^2}{10^2} = 53.8$$

Rounding up a sample size of $n = 54$ will give us an interval that allows us to estimate the population mean time of seeing a physician while attending the emergency room to within 5 points with 90% confidence. If we include the original 10 patients, then $54 - 10 = 44$ additional patients are needed to complete the sample. This process is known as *two-stage sampling*.

In this problem, we used the $t_{0.05,9}$. However, if we had based the t value on the total number of patients needed for this study, then there are $n - 1 = 53$ degrees of freedom. Since $t_{0.05,53} = 1.677 < t_{0.05,9} = 1.833$, the actual confidence interval obtained will be narrower than the ± 5 specified in the problem. Hence, the sample size is conservatively large.

A similar method can be used to estimate the proportion of successes in a binomial population π. The following formula can be used to find the sample size necessary to obtain a confidence interval as long as we are able to specify the desired level of confidence, the width of the interval, and an estimate of the proportion of successes.

Sample Size Equation for Estimating a Proportion

$$n = \frac{4 \times Z_{\alpha/2}^2 f(1-f)}{width^2}$$

The value f can be obtained by (1) using a preliminary sample in a two-stage sampling approach, as described in the previous example, (2) a good estimate of f based on previous experience, or (3) simply using $f = 0.5$ if (1) and (2) are not feasible. Since $f(1 - f) = 0.5(1 - 0.5)$ has a higher value than obtained for any other value of f, this is the most conservative choice, yielding the largest possible value of n.

EXAMPLE 9.10

An investigator wants to determine the sensitivity of a new diagnostic test for liver cancer. Based on a preliminary study involving 25 patients, she finds that 21 (or 84%) test positive. How many patients are needed to estimate a 95% confidence interval for the test's sensitivity of ± 0.05?

From the statement of the problem, we know the following:

1. A confidence level of 95%, $Z_{0.05/2} = 1.96$
2. Width of the confidence interval of 0.1
3. The standard deviation equal to $(0.84)(1 - 0.84) = 0.1344$

$$n = \frac{4 \times 1.96^2 \times 0.1344}{(0.1)^2} = 206.5$$

So the researcher needs to test $207 - 25 = 182$ more patients. If a preliminary study had not been taken, and the value for f was not known, then using the conservative approach where $f = 0.5$ gives:

$$n = \frac{4 \times 1.96^2 \times 0.5(0.5)}{(0.1)^2} = 384.2$$

So the sample size based on the preliminary sample results required $385 - 207 = 178$ fewer patients. Hence, the value of taking a preliminary study when determining sample size is illustrated.

In general, conditions that require larger sample size include: (1) when more confidence is desired, (2) when there is more variation in the population, and (3) when the confidence interval width is smaller.

Finally, in many sampling situations in epidemiology and clinical medicine, the population from which the sample is taken is finite. The term $\sqrt{\frac{(N - n)}{(N - 1)}}$ is called the finite population correction factor, and it is useful whenever the sample represents 10% or more of the total population. Otherwise, it should be omitted. Including the finite population correction factor in the previous equation results in the following equation:

$$n = \frac{4 \times Z_{\alpha/2}^2 f(1 - f)N}{(N - 1)width^2 + 4 \times Z_{\alpha/2}^2 f(1 - f)}$$

Because there are few situations in which the sample size turns out to be more than 10% of the population, we will generally stick with the simpler equations presented earlier.

EXERCISES

1. Suppose that prior to collecting data among adults in a community intervention study, the investigators wanted to assess whether mean Beck Depression Inventory among participants was different than 4 by either plus or minus 1. From a prior study, the standard deviation was 4.6. What is the required sample size?

2. In a study investigating dietary behaviors, researchers wanted to investigate the level of not eating breakfast. Historically, it has been believed that approximately 20% of adults do not eat breakfast. From your own research, you believe the true percentage is at least 30%. Estimate the required sample size with α (one-sided) = 0.05 and power = 0.80.

3. The research question is whether there is a difference in the efficacy of a new drug for treating asthma. The investigator plans a randomized trial to assess the effect of this intervention after 6 weeks. The effect of the new drug compared with a currently used drug is measured using forced expiratory volume in 1 second. The currently used drug has a forced expiratory volume of 1.5 liters with a standard deviation of 1.0 liters. How many participants are required in each group at α (two-sided) = 0.05 and power = 0.80 to detect a difference of 20%?

4. The research question is whether married people have a lower level of depression than nonmarried people. A review of the literature shows that about 15% of adults who are married experience depression. At α (two-sided) = 0.05 and power = 0.90, how many married and nonmarried individuals are needed to determine whether the prevalence of depression is at least 25% in nonmarried?

5. Referring to question 4, what should the sample size be to account for a 10% loss to follow-up?

6. There are 100 cancer patients available who are willing to participate in a study of whether a counseling program can lower depression levels. If the standard deviation is expected to be 4 points on the Beck Depression Inventory, what size difference will the investigator be able to detect between the two groups, at α (two-sided) = 0.05 and β = 0.20?

7. Suppose that a study assessing a new drug requires a sample size of 30 cases. However, the number of cases available is only 20. If multiple controls per case are available, how many controls per case should be collected?

8. Does using paired data (e.g., a baseline and follow-up measure on the same group of subjects) require a larger, smaller, or the same sample size as when independent groups are used in the study? Explain.

9. Suppose you are interested in measuring the mean cholesterol among a group of obese men with a 95% confidence interval of ± 5. The standard deviation is 20. Use the appropriate formula and derive the required sample size.

10. Explain the meaning of two-stage sampling in the context of sample size calculations for descriptive studies.

11. A preliminary study of 10 patients found that 80% had a positive test. How many patients are needed to estimate a 99% confidence interval for the test's sensitivity of ± 0.05?

12. Consider again question 11 but assume a preliminary study had not been conducted, and the value for f was not known. Then, what would the estimated sample size be, taking the conservative approach?

REFERENCES

1. Merrill RM, Aldana SG. Improving overall health status through the CHIP intervention. *Am J Health Behav*. 2009;33(2):135–146.

2. Merrill RM, Anderson AE, Sloan A. Quality of life indicators according to voice disorders and voice-related conditions. *Laryngoscope*. 2011;121:2004–2011.

3. Browner, WS, Newman TB, Hulley SB. *Estimating sample size and power: Applications and examples*. In: Hulley SB, Cummings SR, eds. *Designing Clinical Research*. 3rd ed. Philadelphia, PA: Lippincott Williams & Wilkins; 2007:65–93.

CHAPTER 10

Study Designs

Quantitative data are observations or measurements that are numerical (e.g., data measured on a discrete or continuous scale), and qualitative data are observations that can only be classified into one of a group of nonnumerical categories (e.g., data measured on a nominal or ordinal scale). Other than case studies, there are several statistical measures that are useful for answering questions about relationships in epidemiologic study designs involving quantitative and qualitative data. The purpose of this chapter is to present selected observational epidemiologic study designs that involve data where measures of association can be obtained.

STUDY DESIGN

The *study design* is a plan for data collection, analysis, and interpretation. It is a formal approach to scientific or scholarly investigation. The study design can be simple or complex. There are three general classifications of study designs: observational, experimental, and meta-analyses. In observational studies, researchers observe and describe cases or relationships among variables. In experimental studies, some or all of the study participants are assigned an intervention. A meta-analysis combines the results of several studies that address a set of related research hypotheses.

Observational studies can be descriptive or analytic. Descriptive studies are exploratory, addressing "who," "where," "when," and "what" questions and evaluating relationships among variables. Although descriptive study designs often generate hypotheses, there is no formal hypothesis being tested. On the other hand, the analytic study design is appropriate for testing a research hypothesis that follows from a research question. Analytic study designs are used to address "how" and "why" questions.

Epidemiology frequently involves evaluating research questions and related hypotheses about associations between exposure and health outcome variables. In clinical medicine, we are often interested in evaluating the efficacy of medical interventions. A description of selected observational study designs and their strengths and weaknesses are presented in **Table 10.1**. Although these study designs may sometimes

TABLE 10.1   Observational Epidemiologic Study Designs

	Description	Strengths	Weaknesses
Cross-sectional	Variables measured at a point in time. No distinction between potential risk factors and outcomes.	• Control over study population • Control over measurements • Several associations between variables can be studied at same time • Short time period required • Complete data collection • Exposure and injury/disease data collected from same individuals • Produces prevalence	• No data on the time relationship between exposure and injury/disease development • Potential bias from low response rate • Potential measurement bias • Higher proportion of long-term survivors • Not feasible with rare exposures or outcomes • Does not yield incidence or relative risk
Ecologic	Aggregate data involved (i.e., no information is available for specific individuals). Prevalence of a potential risk factor compared with the rate of an outcome condition.	• Takes advantage of preexisting data • Relatively quick and inexpensive • Can be used to evaluate programs, policies, or regulations implemented at the ecologic level • Allows estimation of effects not easily measurable for individuals	• Susceptible to confounding • Exposures and disease or injury outcomes not measured on the same individuals • Ecologic fallacy (i.e., an error that occurs if one mistakenly assumes that because the majority of a group has a characteristic, the characteristic is associated with those experiencing the outcome)

Case-control	Presence of risk factor(s) for people with a condition is compared with that for people without a condition.	• Effective for rare outcomes • Compared with the cohort study, it requires less time and money • Yields the odds ratio (when the outcome condition is rare, it is a good estimate of the relative risk)	• Limited to one outcome condition • Does not provide incidence, relative risk, or natural history • Less effective than a cohort study at establishing time sequence of events • Potential recall and interviewer bias • Potential survival bias • Does not yield incidence or prevalence
Cohort	People are followed over time to describe the incidence or the natural history of a condition. Assessment can also be made of risk factors for various conditions.	• Establishes time sequence of events • Avoids bias in measuring exposure from knowing the outcome • Avoid Berkson's bias and prevalence-incidence bias • Several outcomes can be assessed • Number of outcomes grows over time • Allows assessment of incidence and the natural history of disease • Yield incidence, relative risk, attributable risk	• Large samples often required • May not be feasible in terms of time and money • Not feasible with rare outcomes • Potential bias caused by loss to follow-up
Nested case-control study	A case-control study conducted within a cohort study. To carry out a nested case-control study, samples or records of interest must be available from before the outcome condition occurred.	• Has the scientific benefits of a cohort design • Less expensive to conduct than cohort studies • Smaller sample size required than a cohort study • Less prone to recall bias than a case-control study	• Nondiseased persons from whom the controls are selected may not be representative of the original cohort because of death or loss to follow-up among cases

be used for descriptive, exploratory purposes, as is often the case for ecologic and cross-sectional surveys, when a specific research hypothesis is formulated from an observed problem and research question, and data are collected under one of these study designs for the express purpose of testing the hypothesis, it is an analytic epidemiologic study.

CROSS-SECTIONAL STUDY DESIGN

A cross-sectional study involves a survey administered to a group of people at a specific point in time. There is no follow-up of participants of these surveys. There are a number of reasons for conducting cross-sectional surveys: they provide information about a disease or condition; they identify the extent (prevalence) of the public health problem; they identify attitudes, behaviors, and beliefs; they characterize a public health problem according to person, place, and time factors; they assist in planning and resource allocation; and they identify avenues for future research that can provide insights about an etiologic relationship between an exposure and health outcome. Because cross-sectional survey data are often used to determine prevalence data, they are also called *prevalence surveys*. For example, cross-sectional surveys have been used to estimate the prevalence of cancer and other chronic diseases.[1-5] Cross-sectional surveys that are routinely collected are called *serial surveys*, such as the United States census or the National Health Interview Survey.

ECOLOGIC STUDY DESIGN

An *ecologic study* is different than a cross-sectional study in that aggregated data are used for assessment rather than individual-level data. For example, suppose we are interested in obesity levels in the United States. National survey data from the Behavior Risk Factor Surveillance System provide state-level percentages of obesity among adults. These data are aggregated, representing state-level information. When a study involves ecologic data, we refer to it as an *ecologic study*.

Ecologic variables are often assessed to determine whether associations exist. For example, we may be interested in whether the state-level obesity data correlate with state-level dietary information. Ecologic studies are perhaps best suited for environmental settings. For instance, accidents and unintentional injuries are often associated with characteristics in the environment. In addition, modifications to physical, social, technological, political, economic, and organizational environments (i.e., group-focused interventions) may be more effective than trying to influence behaviors on an individual level.[6]

CASE-CONTROL STUDY DESIGN _____

The case-control study design originated in the 1920s and is particularly well suited for investigating chronic diseases where there is a long latency period.[7] This study design allows researchers to evaluate one or more exposures that may be associated with a given outcome. Other names for this study design that appear in the literature include *case-comparison study* and *case-referent study*.

A *case-control study* involves grouping people as cases (persons experiencing a health-related state or event) and controls and investigating whether the cases are more or less likely than the controls to have had past experiences, lifestyle behaviors, or exposures. In other words, what is it about their past that made them cases? We always consider the outcome status before the exposure status in a case-control study. Because this study design begins with the outcome and looks back at an antecedent variable or variables, it is retrospective in nature. *Retro spicere* means "to look back."

The first step in conducting a case-control study is to establish the diagnostic criteria and definition of disease. The aim is to ensure that the cases reflect as homogeneous a disease entity as possible. Cases may consist of new cases (incidence) that show selected characteristics during a specific time period in a specified population and a particular area. Cases may also consist of new and existing cases (prevalence). The timing of when the exposure was evaluated could have a large impact on the

---

History

Janet Lane-Claypon (1877–1967), an English physician, initially applied her skills in the research lab, investigating the biochemistry of milk and reproductive physiology, which later informed her thinking on the epidemiology of breast cancer. In 1912, she published a novel cohort study showing that babies fed breastmilk gained more weight than those fed cow's milk. Lane-Claypon used statistical methods to show that the difference in weight between the two groups was unlikely due to chance or confounding. In 1923, Lane-Claypon conducted a case-control study that involved 500 women with a history of breast cancer (cases) and 500 women without a history of breast cancer (controls). Then she investigated whether the cases differed from the controls with respect to occupation and infant mortality (proxies of social status), nationality, marital status, and age. In 1926, she conducted another groundbreaking cohort study that followed a large cohort of surgically treated women with pathologically confirmed breast cancer for up to 10 years. She showed statistically that stage at the time of diagnosis was directly related to survival, and she recognized the importance of accurate staging and potential biases that could influence the results. She also showed statistically that breast cancer risk was greater for women who did not have children, married at a later-than-average age, or did not breastfeed.[8,9]

association between exposure and health outcome. We typically prefer incidence cases because they can be more directly linked with potential causes; that is, for prevalence cases, it is often more difficult to link a specific cause with a disease outcome because both the development and duration of the disease influence prevalence. For example, assessing whether an association exists between exercise and the prevalence of breast cancer is difficult because it may be that exercise patterns before the development of the disease are much different than after the onset of symptoms.

Sources for cases can come from records from public health clinics, physician offices, health maintenance organizations, hospitals, and industrial and government organizations. Cases should be representative of all persons with the disease. In some situations, all persons with the disease may be included in the study. It is more common, however, that cases come from sampled data. In order for the sampled data to reflect the population of interest, random selection is required.

Controls in a case-control study should look like the cases, with the exception of not having the disease. Thus, controls should be selected from the same population from which the cases were drawn. An epidemiologic assumption is that controls are representative of the general population in terms of probability of exposure and that controls have the same possibility of being selected or exposed as the cases. Controls drawn from a population of the same area or populace as the cases should reflect the same gender, age, and other significant factors.

Controls can be randomly selected from a larger population when the entire population of eligible controls is known. Selection of controls can also be made systematically (i.e., every nth person listed), assuming that the order of potential controls is not related to factors such as age, gender, and education. It is often convenient to obtain controls from hospitals, or from family, friends, or relatives of the cases. Specific advantages and disadvantages of these types of controls are presented in **Table 10.2**.[10] In some situations, researchers select more than one control group in order to see whether the selection of controls influences the measured association between the exposure and outcome variables. In addition, in situations where there are a limited number of cases, statistical power can be increased by collecting more controls than cases, although the ratio of controls to cases should not exceed 4 to 1.

Once cases and controls have been identified, exposure status is determined. Exposure status is obtained through medical records, interviews, questionnaires, or surrogates such as spouses, siblings, or employers.

TABLE 10.2	**Advantages and Disadvantages of Controls from Hospitals, the General Population, and Special Groups**	
Controls	**Advantages**	**Disadvantages**
Hospital	• Easily identified, sufficient number, low cost • Subjects more likely aware of antecedent events or exposures • Selection factors that influence decision to come to a particular hospital similar to those for cases • More likely to cooperate, thereby minimizing potential bias from nonresponse	• Differ from the general population such that they do not accurately represent the exposure distribution in the population where cases were obtained
General population	• Represent the population from which cases were selected	• More costly and time consuming than hospital controls • Population lists may not be available • May be difficult to contact healthy people with busy work and leisure schedules • May have poorer recall than hospital controls • Less motivated to participate than controls from the hospital or special groups
Special groups (e.g., family, relatives, friends)	• Healthier than hospital controls • More likely to cooperate than people in the general population • Provide more control over possible confounding factors	• If the exposure is similar to the one experienced by cases, an underestimation of the true association would result

Data from: Hennekens CH, Buring JE. *Epidemiology in Medicine.* Boston, MA: Little, Brown and Company, 1987.

COHORT STUDY DESIGN

Cohort as a general term means a group or body of people. As time passes, the group moves through different and successive time periods of life; as the group ages, changes can be seen in the health and vital statistics of the group. Researchers track health-related states or events as well as deaths in cohorts. In epidemiology, a cohort study generally involves the study of persons over time to determine whether

Definitions

In a **prospective cohort study**, the investigator measures the predictor variable before the outcome has occurred.

In a **retrospective cohort study**, the investigator reconstructs a historical cohort with data on the predictor variable (measured in the past) and data on the outcome collected (measured in the past after some follow-up period).

people exposed to something are more likely to develop a particular health outcome than people not exposed. Cohorts of persons within a group can be studied as a group, either prospectively or retrospectively. The defining distinction between a prospective and retrospective cohort study is the time when the investigator initiates the study. In a retrospective cohort study the investigator collects data from existing records and does not follow patients up as in a prospective cohort study.

As the cohort advances through time, the researcher tracks the incidence rate of the outcome of interest and compares it between exposed and unexposed groups. An advantage of the cohort study over the case-control study is that the incidence rate of several outcome variables can be determined and associated with the exposure variable. As time passes, an increasing number of outcome variables may be considered.

SELECTING THE STUDY COHORT

Both inclusion and exclusion criteria should be considered when assembling the study cohort. Inclusion criteria focus on who should be in the study. For example, we need to identify those people or groups that are at risk of becoming cases. Individuals who already have a disease outcome of interest (prevalent cases) or who are not at risk should not be included in the study. Additionally, people should be excluded from the study if their presence is likely to bias the study results. Those who are not likely to be available for follow-up assessment should be excluded, such as terminally ill patients, those beyond a certain age, individuals moving out of state, or those suffering from dementia. In the interest of saving time and money and avoiding unnecessary testing and effort, appropriate inclusion and exclusion criteria for a cohort study must be given utmost attention.

Restriction is commonly used in cohort studies to improve the feasibility and focus of the study and lower the risk of bias. Restriction may involve just including only high-risk individuals into a study or people in a certain age range or racial group. For example, cohort studies focusing on respiratory disease may restrict the study to coke workers at steel mills or garment factory workers; cohort studies focusing on heart disease may restrict the study to men at least 40 years of age; cohort studies wishing to minimize confounding due to smoking or age may restrict the study to just smokers or just nonsmokers or to individuals in a certain age range. A limitation of restriction is that it narrows to whom the study results may be generalized.

When the cohort population of interest is large, a sample may be necessary. Adequate sample size should be considered in order to capture the outcome of interest. To obtain a sufficiently large sample size, researchers may restrict the cohort to high-risk individuals, such as middle-aged morbidly obese individuals. For some rare outcomes, it might not be feasible to conduct a prospective cohort study. In such cases, a retrospective cohort or case-control study should be employed.

DOUBLE-COHORT STUDY DESIGN

Distinct from the conventional cohort study design is the *double-cohort study design* wherein two separate populations are involved with different levels of an exposure of interest. In a double-cohort study, samples are taken from each of the two populations, unless the populations are small enough such that they are considered in their entirety. Both cohorts are followed and selected outcome information is obtained. The double-cohort design is useful when the exposure is rare and a relatively small number of people are affected.

Table 10.3 presents a number of strengths and weaknesses of cohort studies.[11]

NESTED CASE-CONTROL STUDY DESIGN

The *nested case-control study design* (sometimes called a *case-cohort study design*) involves a case-control study nested within a cohort study. A sample of cases and noncases are selected, and their exposure status is compared. The primary advantage of using a nested case-control study over a case-control study is that a nested case-control study is less prone to recall bias. The primary advantage to its use over a cohort study is that a smaller sample size is required.

CHANCE, BIAS, AND CONFOUNDING

In assessing the relationship between or among variables, we are interested in valid measures of association that are not explained by chance, bias, or confounding. Each of the study designs presented in this chapter may be influenced by these factors. This section will describe chance, bias, and confounding and present ways to minimize their effects.

CHANCE

In statistical inference, we assume the sample is representative of the population, which may be accomplished through random selection. Hypothesis tests incorporate the role of chance. Obtaining a result due to chance is a possibility whenever samples are involved.

TABLE 10.3	**Selected Strengths and Weaknesses of Prospective and Retrospective Cohort and Double-Cohort Studies**		
Study Design	**Description**	**Strengths**	**Weaknesses**
Prospective cohort	The investigator identifies participants, measures exposure status, and follows the cohort over time to monitor outcome events	• More control over selection of participants and exposure and outcome measures than the retrospective cohort	• More expensive • Longer duration than the retrospective cohort • Limited to one exposure variable
Retrospective cohort	The investigator identifies a cohort with already available exposure and outcome data	• Shorter duration • Less expensive • Fewer numbers required than the prospective cohort • More than one exposure can be identified and studied in the same data set	• Less control over selection of participants and exposure and outcome measures than the prospective cohort
Double-cohort	Two distinct populations with different levels of the exposure are followed	• Useful when distinct cohorts have different or rare exposures	• Potential confounding bias from sampling two populations

Data from: Adapted from Newman TB, Browner WS, Cummings SR, Hulley SB. Designing a new study: II: Cross-sectional and case-control studies. In: Hulley SB, Cummings SR, eds. *Designing Clinical Research: An Epidemiologic Approach.* Baltimore, MD: Williams & Williams; 1988:75–86.

Studies in epidemiology and medicine often rely on sampled data. However, when samples are involved, the characteristics of subjects in a sample may vary from sample to sample and an association between an exposure and outcome, or a lack thereof, might be the result of *chance* (i.e., the luck of the draw). Sample size is directly related to chance. Increasing the sample size decreases the probability that the result is due to chance. The *P* value

> **Definitions**
> **Chance** may explain a study finding if the investigation is based on sample data. The degree to which chance variability occurs can be monitored by the *P* value.

provides a means for evaluating the role of chance. However, although the *P* value is directly influenced by the sample size, it is also influenced by effect size. Consequently, a small *P* value may result from an extremely large sample size and a small effect size, or a strong effect size but a small or moderate sample size. For this reason, many journals prefer the confidence interval over the *P* value. Specifically, a confidence interval reveals more about the sample size because the width of the interval is directly related to the sample size. In addition, the confidence interval can be used to evaluate statistical significance.

BIAS

A study result may exist merely because of bias. There is usually very little that can be done to correct for bias once it is present in a study. For this reason, it is critical that the study be designed to minimize bias by identifying likely sources of bias, their direction, and the potential magnitude of their effect.

> **Definitions**
> **Bias** is deviation of the results from the truth; it can cause an observed association between exposure and outcome variables that is not real.

BIAS IN CROSS-SECTIONAL STUDIES

Response bias is a type of selection bias where those who respond to a questionnaire are systematically different from those who do not respond.[12] Responders to a survey may be more likely to be nonsmokers, be concerned about health matters, have a higher level of education, be more likely to be employed in professional positions, be more likely to be married and have children, be more active in the community, and so on. Consequently, the results will not be representative of the population of interest. Assuring a representative sample is a primary concern in survey sampling.

BIAS IN ECOLOGIC STUDIES

In ecologic studies, an error may occur when interpreting the association between variables by mistakenly assuming that because the majority of a group has a characteristic, the characteristic is definitively associated with those experiencing a health-related state or event in the group. This is called *ecologic fallacy*. It is possible that although higher levels of fruit and vegetable consumption, for example, may occur in states with lower levels of obesity, those eating five or more servings of fruit and vegetables per day may not be the ones with the lower weight. Perhaps those with the lower weight are more physically active or younger.

BIAS IN CASE-CONTROL STUDIES

Systematic error that arises from inaccurate measurements or misclassification of subjects according to exposure and outcome status in a case-control study is also referred to as *observation bias*. If exposure information is based on individual recall, there is a potential for bias. For example, suppose we are interested in assessing the association between chest radiographs during adolescence and female breast cancer later in life. If women with breast cancer had better recall of having had chest radiographs than women without breast cancer, bias would result. To avoid this bias, exposure information from medical records is always preferable, when available. Bias may be further minimized by blinding interviewers or those assessing medical records as to who the cases are and who the controls are, because such knowledge could influence how they probe or scan records for information.

Selection bias is a possibility whenever a factor associated with the outcome capable of influencing study participation exists in some participants at the beginning of the study. *Volunteer bias* is a type of selection bias. For example, in a study assessing the association between smoking and disease, family or friends of the cases may readily volunteer to participate as controls in the study, but they are likely to have higher levels of smoking than the general population from which the cases derive. If smoking is associated with the disease, the exposure-disease relationship will be underestimated. Two other types of selection bias common in case-control studies are called *Berkson's bias* and *Neyman's bias*. Berkson's bias is named

Definitions

Volunteer bias occurs when those who volunteer to participate in a study differ systematically with regard to either exposure or disease status from those who do not volunteer.

Berkson's bias is a type of selection bias that may occur in case-control studies when cases and controls are entirely selected from hospital patients.

Neyman's bias (also called prevalence-incidence bias) is a form of selection bias in case-control studies attributed to selective survival among the prevalent cases (i.e., mild, clinically resolved, or fatal cases being excluded from the case group).

after Dr. Joseph Berkson, who described this type of bias in the 1940s. The bias occurs when hospital patients are used as controls in case-control studies. If both cases and controls are selected from the hospital, the controls tend to be more likely exposed to the same thing under consideration than the general population from which the cases were obtained. In 1955, Jerzy Neyman identified a potential bias (now called Neyman's bias) that may result in case-control studies. This is a form of selection bias that occurs when less serious or more serious cases are not as likely to be represented among the cases.

BIAS IN COHORT STUDIES

Two common types of selection bias common in cohort studies are the *healthy worker effect* and *loss to follow-up*. With respect to the healthy worker effect, suppose the researcher is interested in measuring the association between employment at a steel mill and all-cause mortality. Although the workers may be exposed to certain harmful environmental factors, their jobs are often physically demanding, requiring a relatively high level of physical health. These workers may be in better health than a group of people from the same community where the steel workers reside. Consequently, a positive association between working at the steel mill and all-cause mortality is likely to be negatively biased. To avoid underestimation bias, a better comparison group would be workers at another manufacturing plant who are not exposed to the same environmental factors as those in the steel mill.

Loss to follow-up is a common problem in cohort studies, increasingly so in cohorts with longer follow-up times. Loss of participants eligible for follow-up may arise for a number of reasons. Some subjects may refuse to continue their participation, and some cannot be located or are unavailable for interview. Participant death is also always a possibility. Loss to follow-up can result in a biased estimate of an association if the extent of loss to follow-up is associated with both exposure and disease. For example, in a study assessing the association between childhood sexual abuse and psychosocial disorders, sexually abused individuals were more likely lost to follow-up if

Definitions

The **healthy worker effect** occurs in cohort studies when workers represent the exposed group and a sample from the general population represents the unexposed group. This is because workers tend to be healthier, on average, than the general population. In order to work and maintain a job, a certain level of health is required (e.g., some workers must pass a physical examination). On the other hand, the general population includes persons who are not able to get or keep a job because of health problems.

Definitions

Loss to follow-up is a circumstance in which researchers lose contact with study participants, resulting in unavailable outcome data on those people. If these individuals are systematically different from those who remain in the study, bias results.

they developed psychosocial disorders than if a person without a history of sexual abuse developed psychosocial disorders.

As a general rule, the validity of a study requires that loss to follow-up not exceed 20%. Excluding those not likely to remain in the study, making periodic contact with participants, and providing incentives are approaches frequently used to minimize the problem.

CONFOUNDING

Definition

A **confounder** is an extraneous variable that correlates with both the independent and the dependent variable to distort the relationship.

The word *confounding* means to cause surprise or confusion. In epidemiology and biostatistics, a *confounding variable* (also called a lurking variable or confounder) may affect (positively or negatively) the association between two variables you want to examine; that is, confounding occurs when the relationship between an exposure and a disease outcome is influenced by a third factor, which is related to the exposure and, independent of this relationship, is also related to the health outcome. Confounding should always be considered as a possible threat to validity in observational study designs involving assessment of associations among variables, particularly in ecologic and cross-sectional studies, but also in observational case-control and cohort studies. Only the randomized experimental study allows us to balance out anticipated and unanticipated confounding among groups. To illustrate, suppose smoking is a potential confounder and a large number of people are randomly assigned to either a treatment or control group. In this situation, we would expect that the distribution of smokers in terms of duration and intensity of smoking would be similar between the two groups. When randomization is not possible, approaches such as matching and restriction have been employed at the design level of study, and stratification and multiple regression have been employed at the analysis level of study to control for confounding. These methods may also be useful for controlling for confounding in observational studies.

The threat of confounding is typically greater in descriptive epidemiologic studies because there is not a control group. However, confounding can also bias measures of association in case-control, cohort, and experimental studies.

Controlling for Confounding at the Design Level of a Study
Case-control—matching
Cohort—restriction, matching
Experimental—randomization

Matching is most commonly used in case-control studies, although it may also be used in cohort studies; restriction involves selecting a cohort that reflects a single level of the potential confounding variable, as previously described; and randomization of participants to either the intervention or control arm of an experimental study balances out the effects of known or unknown confounding factors, if the sample size is sufficiently large. Matching is a method used to ensure that two study groups are similar with regard to an extrinsic factor or factors that might distort or confound a relationship between an exposure and outcome being studied. It is known that smoking increases the risk of heart disease and coffee drinkers are more likely to be smokers than non–coffee drinkers. Smoking, therefore, confuses or confounds the relationship between coffee drinking and heart disease. In order to eliminate the confounding effect of smoking in a case-control study, one could ensure that the diseased and control groups have equal proportions of smokers. There are two approaches—*pair (individual) matching* and *frequency matching*. Note that care must be given to matching in that there can be substantial loss of power if a case-control study matches on a factor that is not actually a confounder.

> **Definitions**
>
> **Pair (individual) matching** links each member of the case group to a member of the control group with respect to a potential confounding factor (e.g., age, sex, and smoking status).
>
> **Frequency matching** is more commonly used. The control subjects are chosen to ensure that the frequency of the matching factors is the same as found in the case group; that is, the distribution of a potential confounder is determined for the case group and controls are selected to match this frequency distribution.

If we have not adequately controlled for confounders at the design level of a study, it is not too late. Various methods are used to control for confounding in the analysis, including stratified analysis and multiple regression techniques. *Stratified analysis* involves an evaluation of the association between the exposure and outcome variables within homogeneous strata of the confounding variable. *Multiple regression* involves the simultaneous control of confounding factors. When the outcome variable is dichotomous, multiple logistic regression analysis is often used. Note that we can only control for confounding factors in the analysis if we have the foresight to collect data on these variables. Unfortunately, we often fail to anticipate all the potential confounders, such that controlling for effects in the analysis is impossible.

EXERCISES

1. Which descriptive study design is useful for identifying the prevalence (magnitude) of a public health problem?
2. Which descriptive study design is useful for identifying new, emerging health problems?

3. To compare the relationship between injury rates and education among various workplaces, which study design would be appropriate?

4. Match the descriptions in the left column with the appropriate study design in the right column?

___ Aggregate data involved (i.e., no information is available for specific individuals)	A. ecologic study
___ Takes advantage of preexisting data	B. case study
___ Produces prevalence	C. cross-sectional study
___ In-depth description	
___ Exposures and disease or injury outcomes not measured on the same individuals	
___ Potential bias from low response rate	
___ Potential measurement bias	
___ Higher proportion of long-term survivors	
___ Not feasible with rare exposures or outcomes	
___ Qualitative descriptive research of the facts in chronological order	

5. What is the primary distinction between an observational and an experimental analytic epidemiologic study?

6. Which study design is most appropriate for describing the incidence and natural history of a health-related state or event?

7. What is the distinction between prospective and retrospective cohort studies?

8. Describe key features of the case-control study design.

9. Describe key features of the cohort study design.

10. How is a double-cohort design distinct from a standard cohort design?

11. What are some strengths of the cohort study design?

12. List an advantage of using a nested case-control study over (1) a case-control study or (2) a cohort study.

13. Match the descriptions in the left column with the appropriate study design in the right column.

___ Best suited for generating hypotheses versus testing hypotheses	A. cross-sectional
___ Best suited for assessing an exposure–disease relationship when the outcome is rare	B. cohort
___ Best suited for determining the prevalence of a given health-related state or event	C. case-control
___ Best suited if the exposure is extremely rare	D. double-cohort
___ Best suited for generating incidence rates	

14. What is selection bias?
15. What is one important way to avoid selection bias?
16. What is observation bias?
17. Cohort studies are also prone to bias because of selection. Explain how the healthy worker effect is a type of selection bias.
18. When will loss to follow-up result in selection bias in a cohort study?
19. List some ways to minimize loss to follow-up.
20. Match the ways to control for confounding in the right column with the study designs in the left column. (You may use the letters more than once.)

___	Case-control	A. matching
___	Cohort	B. restriction
___	Experimental	C. randomization

REFERENCES

1. Byrne J, Kessler LG, Devesa SS. The prevalence of cancer among adults in the United States: 1987. *Cancer.* 1992;68:2,154–2,159.
2. Hewitt M, Breen N, Devesa S. Cancer prevalence and survivorship issues: analyses of the 1992 National Health Interview Survey. *J Natl Cancer Inst.* 1999;91(17):1,480–1,486.
3. Ahluwalia IB, Mack KA, Murphy W, Mokdad AH, Bales VS. State-specific prevalence of selected chronic disease-related characteristics—Behavioral Risk Factor Surveillance System, 2001. *MMWR.* 2003;52(8):1–80.
4. Harris MI, Flegal KM, Cowie CC, et al. Prevalence of diabetes, impaired fasting glucose, and impaired glucose tolerance in US adults. The Third National Health and Nutrition Examination Survey, 1988–1994. *Diabetes Care.* 1998;21(4):518–524.
5. Roy N, Merrill RM, Thibeault S, Parsa RA, Gray SD, Smith EM. Prevalence of voice disorders in teachers and the general population. *J Speech Lang Hear Res.* 2004;47(2):281–293.
6. Stevenson M, McClure R. Use of ecological study designs for injury prevention. *Injury Prev.* 2005;11:2–4.
7. Schlesselman JJ. *Case-Control Studies: Design, Conduct, Analysis.* New York: Oxford University Press; 1982.
8. Winkelstein W Jr. Vignettes of the history of epidemiology: three firsts by Janet Elizabeth Lane-Claypon. *Am J Epidemiol.* 2004;160(2):97–101.
9. Leopold E, Winkelstein W Jr. Unsung heroines: unveiling history. Janet Elizabeth Lane-Claypon. *BCA Newsletter.* May/June 2004;81. http://archive.bcaction.org/index.php?page=newsletter-81c. Accessed December 22, 2011.
10. Hennekens CH, Buring JE. *Epidemiology in Medicine.* Boston: Little, Brown and Company; 1987.
11. Newman TB, Browner WS, Cummings SR, Hulley SB. Designing a new study: II. cross-sectional and case-control studies. In: Hulley SB, Cummings SR, eds. *Designing Clinical Research: An Epidemiologic Approach.* Baltimore, MD: Williams & Williams; 1988:75–86.
12. Last JM, ed. *A Dictionary of Epidemiology.* New York: Oxford University Press; 1995.

CHAPTER 11

Statistical Measures of Association Among Variables

The study design used for addressing the research question describes the approach and type of data that will be employed. The type of exposure and outcome data obtained in the study dictates the kind of statistical measure to use when assessing associations between variables. The fourth general area of biostatistics involves statistical techniques. Three examples of statistical techniques include the contingency table, comparison of means, and analysis of variance, as introduced in Chapter 8. Selected techniques for measuring the association between variables and evaluating the association for statistical significance will be presented in this chapter.

CLASSIFICATION OF STATISTICAL TECHNIQUES AND TESTS BY VARIABLE TYPE

There are many approaches to evaluating data. Some of the statistical techniques and statistical tests for assessing types of exposure and outcome variables are presented in **Table 11.1**.[1] When measuring the association between two nominal or ordinal variables, data are entered into a contingency table, and the frequency distribution of one variable is compared with the frequency distribution of the other variable. If two numerical measures were taken on the same subjects, a scatter plot would be an appropriate way to display the data. This graph is a useful summary of the association between two numerical variables.

The *correlation coefficient* (also called the *Pearson correlation coefficient*) measures the strength of the linear association between two variables. The method assumes both variables are normally distributed and that a linear association exists between the variables. When the latter assumption is violated, the investigator may choose to apply the correlation measure over a subsection of the data where linearity holds. The correlation coefficient ranges between −1 and +1.

A related measure is the *coefficient of determination* (denoted by r^2), which is the square of the correlation coefficient, and represents the proportion of the total variation

TABLE 11.1   Classification of Selected Statistical Techniques (and Tests) by Types of Variables

Exposure Variable	Outcome Variable			
	Nominal with 2 categories (dichotomous)	Nominal with > 2 categories (multichotomous)	Continuous, not normally distributed, or ordinal with > 2 categories	Continuous, normally distributed
Continuous, normally distributed	Logistic regression (likelihood ratio test)	Analysis of variance (*F* test)	*Spearman rank correlation*	Correlation coefficient (*t* test) Linear regression (*t* test, *F* test)
Continuous, not normally distributed, or ordinal with > 2 categories	*Wilcoxon rank sum*	*Kruskall-Wallis*	*Spearman rank correlation*	*Spearman rank correlation*
Nominal with > 2 categories	Logistic regression (likelihood ratio test) Contingency table (chi-square)	Contingency table (chi-square)	*Kruskall-Wallis*	Analysis of variance (*F* test)
Nominal with 2 categories	Logistic regression (likelihood ratio test) Poisson regression (chi-square) Contingency table (chi-square)	Contingency table (chi-square)	*Wilcoxon rank sum*	Comparison of means (*t* test)

Note: Nonparametric tests (shown in italics) are distribution-free tests because they do not follow a specific distribution (e.g., normal). The Kruskal-Wallis test evaluates whether the population medians on a dependent variable are the same across all levels of an independent variable. The Wilcoxon rank-sum test is a nonparametric alternative to the two-sample *t* test that is based solely on the order in which the observations from the two samples fall.

Data from: Feigal D, Black D, Grady D, et al. Planning for data management and analysis. In: Hulley SB, Cummings SF. *Designing Clinical Research: An Epidemiologic Approach.* Baltimore, MD: Williams & Wilkins; 1988:159–171.

Calculating the Correlation Coefficient for a Sample

$$r = \frac{\sum (x - \bar{x})(y - \bar{y})}{\sqrt{\sum (x - \bar{x})^2 (y - \bar{y})^2}}$$

where x is the independent (or exposure) variable and y is the dependent (or outcome) variable. The population parameter is ρ (the lower case Greek letter rho). In a sample, ρ is estimated by r.

in the dependent variable that is determined by the independent variable. If a perfect positive or negative association exists, then all of the variation in the dependent variable would be explained by the independent variable. Generally, however, only part of the variation in the dependent variable can be explained by a single independent variable.

When the population parameter is hypothesized to be zero, the following mathematical expression involving the correlation coefficient, often called the t ratio, has a t distribution with $n - 2$ degrees of freedom:

$$t = \frac{r\sqrt{n-2}}{\sqrt{1-r^2}}$$

Spearman's rho or *rank correlation coefficient* is an alternative to the correlation coefficient when outlying data exist such that one or both of the distributions are skewed. This method is robust to outliers.

Calculating the Spearman's Rho

$$r = \frac{\sum (R_X - \bar{R}_X)(R_Y - \bar{R}_Y)}{\sqrt{\sum (R_X - \bar{R}_X)^2 (R_Y - \bar{R}_Y)^2}}$$

where R_X is the rank of the variable X, R_Y is the rank of the variable Y, $\bar{R}_X$ is the mean rank of the variable X, and $\bar{R}_Y$ is the mean rank of the variable Y.

Regression analysis provides an equation that estimates the change in the dependent variable (Y) per unit change in an independent variable (X). This method assumes (1) that for each value of X, Y is normally distributed, (2) that the standard deviation of the outcomes Y do not change over X, (3) that the outcomes Y are independent, and (4) that a linear relationship exists between X and Y. Data transformations and other methods are used to respond to violations of these assumptions. In some situations when outliers exist, the model is estimated after the outliers have been dropped. In situations where a linear relationship between variables does not hold, piecewise linear regression or polynomial regression is employed. Simple linear regression involves an equation with one independent variable. This method fits a linear line to the data that minimizes the squared deviations of each point from the straight line. The equation includes an intercept, slope, and error term, as follows:

$$Y = \beta_0 + \beta_1 X + \epsilon$$

If y_i is the observed outcome of Y_i for a particular value x_i, and $\hat{y}_i$ is the corresponding predicted value, then

$$e_i = y_i - \hat{y}_i$$

The distance e_i is known as the *residual*. When the regression equation is used to describe the relationship in the sample, it is often written as:

$$\hat{y} = b_0 + b_1 x$$

where b_0 represents the y-intercept of the linear fitted line, and b_1 represents the slope. The slope is a measure of association that indicates how much y changes when x changes by one unit. Linear regression finds the best fitting straight line, called the least squares regression line.

Calculating the Simple Regression Model

$$b_1 = \frac{\sum (x - \bar{x})(y - \bar{y})}{\sum (x - \bar{x})^2}$$

$$b_0 = \bar{y} - b_1 \bar{x}$$

The t statistic for evaluating the slope coefficient in the regression model is expressed as follows:

$$t = \frac{b_1 - \beta_1}{se_{b_1}}$$

This expression follows the t distribution with $n - 2$ degrees of freedom under the assumptions of the regression model and is used to test H_0: $\beta_1 = 0$ against H_a: $\beta_1 \neq 0$. Note that

$$se_{b_1} = \sqrt{\frac{\frac{1}{n-2}\sum(y_i - \hat{y}_i)^2}{\sum(x_i - \hat{x}_i)^2}}$$

EXAMPLE 11.1

Consider state and territory level data in the United States for 2010 that reflects the percentage of the adult population who are obese and the percentage with diabetes.[2] Suppose that, in a scatter plot, we observe that a linear relationship exists between the variables. Because the ecologic data are numerical, we can use the correlation coefficient, the coefficient of determination, and the regression line to further assess the relationship between obesity and diabetes. However, because there are 54 observations for each variable, computing these statistics by hand would be very tedious. Let us test the hypothesis that there is an association between obesity and diabetes. Applying the steps of hypothesis testing for this ecologic study gives the following:

1. H_0: $\rho = 0$
2. H_a: $\rho \neq 0$
3. $\alpha = 0.05$, $n = 54$
4. t ratio with $n - 2 = 52$ degrees of freedom
5. Using the PROC CORR procedure in SAS gives $r = 0.620$

$$t = \frac{0.620\sqrt{54 - 2}}{\sqrt{1 - 0.620^2}} = 5.70$$

6. Referring to Table 4 in Appendix B, the calculated t statistic corresponds with a $P < 0.001$.

Thus, we reject H_0 and conclude that the strength of the linear association between obesity and diabetes is significantly positive.

Confidence intervals define an upper limit and a lower limit with an associated probability. The general formula for the confidence interval is the point estimate, plus or minus the confidence coefficient multiplied by the standard error estimate. For the correlation coefficient, we use the following equation:

Fisher's z transformation of $r \pm 1.96 \times \sqrt{1/(n-3)}$

Fisher's z transformation is:

$$z(r) = \frac{1}{2}\ln\left(\frac{(1+r)}{(1-r)}\right) = \frac{1}{2}\ln\left(\frac{(1+0.620)}{(1-0.620)}\right) = 0.725$$

where ln is the natural logarithm. The 95% confidence interval is:

$$0.725 \pm 1.96 \times \sqrt{1/(54-3)}$$

$$\rightarrow 0.451 - 0.999$$

The coefficient of determination is merely r^2: 0.384. This means that 38.4% of the variation among states and territories in the percentage of adults with diabetes is explained by obesity. The Spearman correlation coefficient is employed by applying the ranked data. The SAS code for this example shows that the Spearman correlation coefficient can be obtained by typing in the word *Spearman* on the procedure line.

EXAMPLE 11.2

Using simple linear regression analysis is also a possibility for assessing the association between obesity and diabetes. A plot of the residuals is shown against the fitted values of diabetes mellitus in **Figure 11.1**. From this plot, the assumptions of normality, constant variance, independence, and linearity appear to be satisfied.

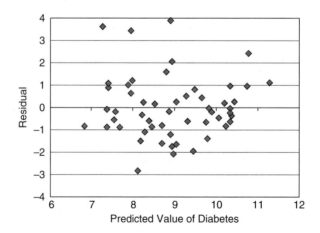

FIGURE 11.1 Residual plot—obesity and diabetes mellitus.
Data from: Centers for Disease Control and Prevention. Behavior Risk Factor Surveillance System. Prevalence and Trend Data. http://apps.nccd.cdc.gov/BRFSS/. Accessed July 1, 2011.

Applying the steps of hypothesis testing gives the following:

1. H_0: $\beta_1 = 0$
2. H_a: $\beta_1 \neq 0$
3. $\alpha = 0.05$, $n = 54$
4. t with $n - 2 = 52$ degrees of freedom
5. Using the PROC REG procedure in SAS gives the estimated linear regression line as:

$$Diabetes = -0.433 + 0.340 \times Obesity$$

Diabetes is treated as the dependent (outcome) variable and obesity as the independent (explanatory or predictor) variable. The researcher decides, which variable is to be the dependent or independent variable, based on observation and experience. To determine whether the estimates are statistically significant, the t statistic was used:

$$t_{b_1} = \frac{b_1}{se_{b_1}} = \frac{0.340}{0.060} = 5.69, P < 0.001$$

6. Thus we reject H_0 and conclude that for every percent increase in obesity among the adult population in the United States, diabetes increases, on average, by 0.34%.

For the regression coefficients, the standard errors are difficult to compute by hand. However, it is relatively easily obtained using statistical software. For example, the standard error for the estimated slope coefficient is 0.060. The formula for the 95% confidence intervals of the slope estimate is:

$$0.340 \pm 1.96 \times 0.060$$

$$\rightarrow 0.222 - 0.458$$

In addition, notice that if the percentage of obese people in the adult population were 0, the level of diabetes would be −0.433, according to the model. Of course this makes no sense. As a general rule, when interpreting the results from a regression analysis, estimating Y beyond the range of the values of X may result in misleading and nonsensical results.

The simple linear regression model can be expanded to include other potential explanatory variables. When more than one independent variable is included in the model, it is called *multiple regression*. Recall that obesity only explained 38.4% of the variation in diabetes. Other variables that may have been included in the model, which can explain additional variation in diabetes, include age, sex, race, diet, and family history of diabetes. Epidemiologist and medical researchers often employ multiple regression to evaluate the association between variables while adjusting for the potential confounding effects of other variables. For example, in a study assessing the association between a certain diet and blood pressure, age, sex, and race were considered to be potential confounders. By merely including these variables in the regression model, the researchers were able to assess the relationship between diet and blood pressure, adjusting for the potential confounding effects of age, sex, and race.

Definition

Multiple regression is an extension of simple regression analysis in which there are two or more independent variables. In multiple regression, the effects of multiple independent variables on the dependent variable can be simultaneously assessed. This type of model is useful for adjusting potential confounders.

The equation may be written as:

$$Y = \beta_0 + \beta_1 X_1 + \beta_2 X_2 + \cdots + \beta_k X_k + \epsilon$$

When the regression equation is used to describe the relationship in the sample, it is expressed as:

$$\hat{y} = b_0 + b_1 x_1 + b_2 x_2 + \cdots + b_k x_k$$

where b_0 represents the y-intercept of the linear fitted line, and b_1 represents the change in y mean value per unit change in x_1, adjusting for the other variables in the model.

Assumptions: (1) the errors are normally distributed, (2) the mean of the errors is zero, (3) the errors have a constant variance, and (4) the model errors are independent.

Interpretation: The slope (b_i) estimates the average value of y changes by b_i units for each 1 unit increase in x_i, holding all other variables constant.

EXAMPLE 11.3

In a study involving quality-of-life indicators in an older population, one of the quality-of-life indicators is general health (with the score ranging from 0 to 100, with a higher score reflecting better general health).[3] Suppose we are interested in assessing whether general health is associated with exercise (average days per week). However, we want to control for the potential confounding effects of BMI and age. A plot of the residuals is shown against the fitted values of general health in **Figure 11.2**. From

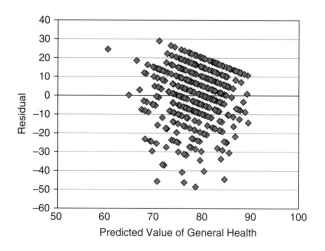

FIGURE 11.2 Residual plot—general health and exercise. *Data from:* Centers for Disease Control and Prevention. Behavior Risk Factor Surveillance System. Prevalence and Trend Data. http://apps.nccd.cdc.gov/BRFSS/. Accessed July 1, 2011.

this plot, the assumptions of normality, constant variance, independence, and linearity appear to be satisfied.

Applying the steps of hypothesis testing gives the following:

1. H_0: $\beta_1 = 0$
2. H_a: $\beta_1 \neq 0$
3. $\alpha = 0.05$, $n = 461$
4. t statistic with $n - 2 = 459$ degrees of freedom
5. Using the PROC REG procedure in SAS gives the estimated linear regression line as:

$$General\ Health = 89.171 + 2.207 \times Exercise_{Days/week} - 0.394 \times BMI - 0.126 \times Age$$

The t statistic and corresponding P value for the estimated exercise variable are 5.45 with $P < 0.001$.

6. There is a positive association between general health and exercise, after adjusting for BMI and age.

The standard error for the estimated regression coefficient for exercise, obtained from SAS, is 0.405. Thus, the 95% confidence interval for the regression coefficient for exercise is:

$$2.207 \pm 1.96 \times 0.405$$

$$\rightarrow 1.413 - 3.001$$

In this particular model, age was not significant at the 0.05 level. Generally, the researcher would drop this variable and reestimate the equation in order to provide greater power and more stable estimates.

If the dependent variable is not numerical but rather dichotomous (two levels), as is often the case in epidemiology and clinical medicine where the outcome variable reflects the presence (yes or no) of a health-related state or event, then an alternative regression model, called *logistic regression*, may be appropriate. Logistic regression is commonly used in epidemiology because many of the outcome measures considered involve nominal data (e.g., ill/not ill, injured/not injured, disabled/not disabled, dead/alive). We can define π as the probability of a success for a single trial and $1 - \pi$ as the probability of a failure for a single trial. It is inappropriate to evaluate the following model using standard regression:

$$\pi = \beta_0 + \beta_1 X + \epsilon$$

This is because π is a probability that ranges from 0 to 1. Hence, the assumption presented earlier for regression, that for each value of X, Y is normally distributed, is violated. It can be shown that

$$\ln(\text{odds}) = \ln\left[\frac{\pi}{1-\pi}\right] = \beta_0 + \beta_1 X + \epsilon$$

The expression on the left is called the *ln(odds)*—it is normal, and the relationship between it and X is linear. When the regression equation is used to describe the relationship in the sample, it is often written as:

$$\ln(\text{odds}) = \ln\left[\frac{f}{1-f}\right] = b_0 + b_1 x$$

where ln is the natural logarithm. The slope b_1 is the change in the ln(odds) of the outcome per unit change in x.

Consider b_1 in a logistic model when x_1 is a dichotomous variable such as "equal to 1 if exposed and 0 if unexposed," as follows:

> **Definition**
>
> **Logistic regression** is a type of regression in which the dependent variable is a dichotomous variable.

$$\textit{ln}(\textit{odds})_{Exposed} = b_0 + b_1 \times 1$$

$$\textit{ln}(\textit{odds})_{Unexposed} = b_0 + b_1 \times 0$$

$$b_1 = \textit{ln}(\textit{odds})_{Exposed} - \textit{ln}(\textit{odds})_{Unexposed} = \ln(\text{Odds Ratio})$$

$$\textit{Odds Ratio} = e^{b_1}$$

e^{b_1} is the odds ratio comparing exposed and unexposed groups. The odds ratio is further discussed later in this chapter as a primary measure of association in case-control studies involving exposure and outcome variables, each consisting of two levels.

EXAMPLE 11.4

Continuing with the same data set as in the last example, suppose we are interested in whether a history of voice disorders (dependent variable) is associated with a family history of voice disorders (independent variable). A voice disorder is defined as the voice not working, performing, or sounding as you feel it normally should so that it interferes with communication.

Applying the steps of hypothesis testing gives the following:

1. $H_0: \beta_1 = 0$
2. $H_a: \beta_1 \neq 0$

3. $\alpha = 0.05$, $n = 461$
4. Chi-square (χ^2) with 1 degrees of freedom
5. The estimated logistic regression model derived using PROC GENMOD in SAS is:

$$ln(odds) = -1.722 + 2.703 \times FH$$

$$e^{2.7031} = 14.93$$

6. The chi-square for the slope estimate in the regression model is 15.35, and the corresponding $P < 0.001$, so we reject H_0 and conclude that the odds of having a family history of voice disorders among those with a history of voice disorders is 14.93 times greater than among those without a history of voice disorders.

The 95% confidence interval for the slope coefficient, with the standard error of 0.690 obtained from SAS, is

$$2.703 \pm 1.96 \times 0.690$$

$$\rightarrow 1.351 - 4.055$$

The 95% confidence interval for the odds ratio is:

$$e^{2.703 \pm 1.96 \times 0.690} = e^{1.351} - e^{4.055}$$

$$\rightarrow 3.861 - 57.685$$

EXAMPLE 11.5

To extend the logistic regression model to the multiple logistic regression model in order to control for potential confounding variables that the researcher anticipates, we merely add these variables to the model. The multiple logistic regression model obtained using PROC GENMOD in SAS is:

$$ln(odds) = -0.960 + 2.338 \times FH - 0.008 \\ \times Age - 0.462 \times Gender_{M/F}$$

$$e^{2.338} = 10.39$$

Definition

Multiple logistic regression is an extension of logistic regression in which two or more independent variables are included in the model. It allows the researcher to look at the simultaneous effect of multiple independent variables on the dependent variable.

The equation may be written as:

$$\ln(odds) = \beta_0 + \beta_1 X_1 + \beta_2 X_2 \\ + \cdots + \beta_k X_k + \epsilon$$

When the regression equation is used to describe the relationship in the sample, it is expressed as:

$$\ln(odds) = b_0 + b_1 x_1 + b_2 x_2 \\ + \cdots + b_k x_k$$

where b_0 represents the y-intercept of the linear fitted line, and b_1 represents the change in log odds of the outcome per unit change in x_1, adjusting for the other variables in the model.

Assumptions: (1) The true conditional probabilities are a logistic function of the independent variables, (2) no important variables are omitted, (3) no extraneous variables are included, (4) the independent variables are measured without error, (5) the observations are independent, and (6) the independent variables are not linear combinations of each other.

Interpretation: The odds ratio is e^b, which means that if we increase x_i by one unit, the odds will change by e^b, holding all other variables constant.

The chi-square is 10.39 with 1 degree of freedom and $P < 0.005$. Hence, the significant association between a history of voice disorders and a family history of voice disorders remains significant after adjusting for age and gender.

The 95% confidence interval, with the standard error of 0.725 obtained from SAS, is:

$$2.338 \pm 1.96 \times 0.725$$

$$\rightarrow 0.917 - 3.759$$

The 95% confidence interval for the odds ratio is:

$$e^{2.338 \pm 1.96 \times 0.725} = e^{0.917} - e^{3.759}$$

$$\rightarrow 2.502 - 42.906$$

Another important regression model in epidemiology and clinical medicine is the *Poisson regression model*. Poisson regression is appropriate when the dependent events occur infrequently, the events occur independently, and the events occur over some continuous medium such as time or area. The probability of a single event occurring is influenced by the length of the interval. Counts or rates of rare diseases are well suited for modeling with Poisson regression.[4] To describe the meaning of b_1 in a Poisson model when x_1 is a dichotomous variable equal to 1 if exposed and 0 if unexposed,

$$ln\,(rate)_{Exposed} = b_0 + b_1 \times 1$$

$$ln\,(rate)_{Unexposed} = b_0 + b_1 \times 0$$

$$b_1 = ln\,(rate)_{Exposed} - ln\,(rate)_{Unexposed} = \ln(\text{Rate Ratio})$$

$$Rate\ Ratio = e^{b_1}$$

e^{b_1} is the rate ratio comparing exposed and unexposed groups. If additional variables are included in the model, then e^{b_1} is adjusted for those variables. The rate ratio is further discussed later in this chapter as a primary measure of association in cohort studies involving exposure and outcome variables, each consisting of two levels.

EXAMPLE 11.6

Consider the data in **Table 11.2**, obtained from a cohort study conducted by Iso and colleagues.[5]

TABLE 11.2	Total Cardiovascular Disease According to Smoking Status	
Current Smoker	**Disease Cases**	**Person-Years**
Yes	882	220,965
No	673	189,254

Suppose we are interested in testing the hypothesis that current smoking is associated with cardiovascular disease in this cohort study. Applying the steps of hypothesis testing gives the following:

1. H_0: $\beta_1 = 0$
2. H_a: $\beta_1 \neq 0$
3. $\alpha = 0.05$, $n = 1,555$
4. Chi-square (χ^2) with 1 degree of freedom
5. Using PROC GENMOD in SAS to compute a Poisson regression for this data resulted in the following:

   $$ln\,(rate) = -5.6391 + 0.1155 \times Smoker$$

   $$e^{0.1155} = 1.12$$

6. The chi-square is 5.10, with $P = 0.024$. Hence, we reject H_0 and conclude that smokers are 1.12 (or 12%) more likely than nonsmokers to develop cardiovascular disease.

The 95% confidence interval, with the standard error of 0.051 obtained from SAS, is:

$$0.116 \pm 1.96 \times 0.051$$

$$\rightarrow 0.015 - 0.216$$

The 95% confidence interval for the rate ratio is:

$$e^{0.116 \pm 1.96 \times 0.051} = e^{0.015} - e^{0.216}$$

$$\rightarrow 1.015 - 1.241$$

Note that additional variables could have been added to the Poisson model to adjust for potential confounding effects, in the same manner as the multiple regression models already discussed.

Deciding on the variables that best predict the dependent variable is a process called model building. Selecting the variables for regression models can be accomplished in various ways. In one approach, all independent variables thought to potentially predict the dependent variable are included in the model. Then, the variables that are not statistically significant are sequentially dropped from the model. The model is rerun after each insignificant variable is eliminated, beginning with the least significant variable. Computer programs contain routine approaches to select an optimal set of independent variables (see Appendix C).

In the remainder of this chapter, we will present measures of association that are commonly used in epidemiology and clinical medicine: the odds ratio, the risk ratio, the rate ratio, and the prevalence ratio. These measures involve nominal exposure and outcome variables, each with two levels. They are statistically assessed for significance using the chi-square test.

History

John Snow was an English physician who investigated a cholera outbreak in 1848. In 1854, a larger cholera outbreak occurred in London. At this time, much of London received its water supply from either the Lambeth Water Company or the Southwark and Vauxhall Water Company (S&V). The Lambeth Water Company's intake source was upriver on the Thames, above the sewage outlets. On the other hand, the Southwark and Vauxhall Water Company's intake source was on the Thames, below the sewage outlets. Throughout the south district of the city, both water companies had pipes down every street. The citizens were free to pick and choose which water company they wanted for their household water. Thus, by mere coincidence, John Snow encountered a populace using water randomly selected throughout the south district. Snow could not have arranged better sampling techniques than those that had occurred by chance.[6-8]

Vital statistics data and death rates compared according to water supplier presented conclusive evidence as to the source of contamination (**Table 11.3**). The death rate was greater for the districts supplied by S&V compared with Lambeth. Thus, Snow was finally able to prove his hypothesis that contaminated water passing down the sewers into the river, then being drawn from the river and distributed through miles of pipes into peoples' homes, produced cholera throughout the community. Snow showed that cholera was a water-borne disease that traveled in both surface and groundwater supplies.[6-8]

TABLE 11.3 Mortality from Cholera in the Districts of London Supplied by the Southwark and Vauxhall Company or the Lambeth Water Company, July 8–August 26, 1854

Group of districts with water supplied by:	Population in 1851	Deaths from Cholera	Death rate per 1,000 population
Southwark and Vauxhall Company	167,654	738	4.4
Lambeth Water Company	19,133	4	0.2
Areas served by both companies			
Southwark and Vauxhall Company	98,862	419	4.2
Lambeth Water Company	154,615	80	0.5
Rest of London	1,921,972	1,422	0.7

Data from: Snow J. *On the Mode of Communication of Cholera.* 2nd ed., 1855. New York, NY: Commonwealth Fund; 1936.

MEASURES OF ASSOCIATION FOR TWO-LEVEL NOMINAL EXPOSURE AND OUTCOME VARIABLES

To begin, we will refer to a 2×2 contingency table involving exposure and outcome variables, each with two levels (**Table 11.4**).

In a cohort study, the row totals are fixed, whereas in a case-control study, the column totals are fixed.

When person-time data is involved, the table is modified, where t_{ei} is the follow-up time for the ith person in the exposed group, and t_{uei} is the follow-up time for the ith person in the unexposed group (**Table 11.5**; see also **Table 11.2**). Time can be measured in different units (e.g., hours, days, weeks, months, years).

TABLE 11.4 2 × 2 Contingency Table

Exposed	Outcome		
	Yes	**No**	
Yes	a	b	$a + b$
No	c	d	$c + d$
	$a + c$	$b + d$	$n = a + b + c + d$

TABLE 11.5 2 × 2 Table Involving Cohort Person-Time Data			
	Disease		
Exposed	**Yes**	**No**	
Yes	a	—	Person Time (t_{ei})
No	c	—	Person Time (t_{oi})
	$a + c$	—	$T = \sum (t_{ei} + t_{oi})$

The formulas for measures of association using two-level nominal variables employed in case-control, cohort, and cross-sectional study designs employ rules of probability.

CASE-CONTROL STUDY

- Odds ratio (OR)

$$OR = \frac{P(exposed|disease)/P(unexposed|disease)}{P(exposed|no\ disease)/P(unexposed|no\ disease)} = \frac{a/c}{b/d} = \frac{a \times d}{b \times c}$$

The Mantel-Haenszel (MH) method is useful for estimating a pooled odds ratio across homogeneous strata, as follows:

$$OR_{MH} = \frac{\sum (a_i d_i / n_i)}{\sum (b_i c_i / n_i)}$$

COHORT STUDY

- Risk ratio (also called relative risk)

$$Risk\ Ratio = \frac{P(outcome|exposed)}{P(outcome|not\ exposed)} = \frac{a/(a+b)}{c/(c+d)}$$

$$= \frac{Attack\ rate\ for\ exposed}{Attack\ rate\ for\ not\ exposed}$$

$$RR_{MH} = \frac{\sum (a_i [c_i + d_i] / n_i)}{\sum (c_i [a_i + b_i] / n_i)}$$

- Rate ratio

$$Rate\ Ratio = \frac{P(outcome|exposed)}{P(outcome|not\ exposed)} = \frac{a/PT_e}{c/PT_o}$$

$$= \frac{Person-time\ rate\ for\ exposed}{Person-time\ rate\ for\ not\ exposed}$$

CROSS-SECTIONAL STUDY

- Prevalence ratio

$$PR = \frac{P(outcome|exposed)}{P(outcome|not\ exposed)} = \frac{a/(a+b)}{c/(c+d)}$$

The odds ratio, risk ratio, rate ratio, and prevalence ratio each range in values from 0 to infinity. A value greater than 1 indicates a positive association between the exposure and outcome; a value of 1 indicates no association between exposure and outcome variables; and a value less than 1 indicates a negative (or inverse) association between the exposure and outcome. The chi-square test is used to assess the hypothesis of independence between the variables (**Table 11.6**).

Confidence intervals for measures of association involving two-level nominal-scaled data indicate the level of precision in the estimate and can tell us whether a measured association is statistically significant. These are summarized in **Table 11.7**. [9-13]

EXAMPLE 11.7

Spasmodic dysphonia (SD) is an idiopathic, chronic, and disabling voice disorder. In a case-control study, investigators wanted to evaluate whether a statistical relationship exists between meningitis and spasmodic dysphonia. Applying the steps to hypothesis testing for this *case-unmatched control study* gives the following:

1. $H_0: OR = 1$
2. $H_a: OR \neq 1$
3. $\alpha = 0.05, n = 300$
4. Chi-square (χ^2) with 1 degree of freedom

TABLE 11.6   Selected Study Designs, Measures of Association, and Test Statistics

Study Design	Measure of Association	Tests of Significance
Case-control		
Unmatched	$Odds\ Ratio\ (OR) = \dfrac{a \times d}{b \times c}$	$\chi^2 = \dfrac{(\lvert ad - bc \rvert - n/2)^2\, n}{(a+b)(c+d)(a+c)(b+d)}$
Matched	$OR = \dfrac{b}{c}$	$\chi^2 = \dfrac{(\lvert b - c \rvert - 1)^2}{(b+c)}$
Summary odds ratio	$OR_{MH} = \dfrac{\sum (a_i d_i / n_i)}{\sum (b_i c_i / n_i)}$	$\chi^2_{MH} = \dfrac{\left\{ \sum a_i - \sum [(a_i + c_i)(a_i + b_i)/n_i] \right\}^2}{\sum (a_i + b_i)(c_i + d_i)(a_i + c_i)(b_i + d_i)/(n_i^2 [n_i - 1])}$
Cohort		
Attack rates	$Risk\ Ratio\ (RR) = \dfrac{a/(a+b)}{c/(c+d)}$	$\chi^2 = \dfrac{(\lvert ad - bc \rvert - n/2)^2\, n}{(a+b)(c+d)(a+c)(b+d)}$
Summary risk ratio	$RR_{MH} = \dfrac{\sum [a_i(c_i + d_i)/n_i]}{\sum [c_i(a_i + b_i)/n_i]}$	$\chi^2_{MH} = \dfrac{\left\{ \sum a_i - \sum [(a_i + c_i)(a_i + b_i)/n_i] \right\}^2}{\sum (a_i + b_i)(c_i + d_i)(a_i + c_i)(b_i + d_i)/(n_i^2 (n_i - 1))}$
Person-time rates	$Rate\ Ratio = \dfrac{a/T_e}{c/T_o}$	$\chi^2 = \dfrac{\{a - [T_e(a+c)]/T\}^2}{T_e[T_o(a+c)]/T^2}$
Cross-sectional	$Prevalence\ Ratio = \dfrac{a/(a+b)}{c/(c+d)}$	$\chi^2 = \dfrac{(\lvert ad - bc \rvert - n/2)^2\, n}{(a+b)(c+d)(a+c)(b+d)}$

MH = Mantel-Haenszel
a = number of exposed individuals with the outcome
b = number of exposed individuals without the outcome
c = number of unexposed individuals with the outcome
d = number of unexposed individuals without the outcome
n = total number of individuals in the sample
i = level of stratification
T = total time a cohort of exposed (e) and unexposed (o) people are followed

TABLE 11.7   Summary of Confidence Intervals for Evaluating Selected Hypotheses

For testing H_0: $OR = 1$ in an unmatched case-control study

$$95\%\ CI(OR) = \exp\left[\ln OR \pm \left(1.96 \times \sqrt{\frac{1}{a} + \frac{1}{b} + \frac{1}{c} + \frac{1}{d}}\right)\right]$$

For testing H_0: $OR = 1$ in a matched case-control study

$$95\%\ CI(OR) = \exp\left[\ln OR \pm \left(1.96 \times \sqrt{\frac{1}{b} + \frac{1}{c}}\right)\right]$$

For testing H_0: $OR = 1$ in a stratified case-control study

$$95\%\ CI(OR_{MH}) = OR_{MH}^{\left(1 \pm 1.96/\sqrt{\chi^2_{MH}}\right)}$$

For testing H_0: *risk ratio* $= 1$

$$95\%\ CI(RR) = \exp\left[\ln RR \pm \left(1.96 \times \sqrt{\frac{b/a}{a+b} + \frac{d/c}{c+d}}\right)\right]$$

For testing H_0: $RR = 1$ in a stratified cohort study

$$95\%\ CI(RR_{MH}) = RR_{MH}^{\left(1 \pm 1.96/\sqrt{\chi^2_{MH}}\right)}$$

For testing H_0: *rate ratio* $= 1$

$$95\%\ CI(Rate\ Ratio) = \exp\left[\ln(Rate\ Ratio) \pm 1.96 \times \sqrt{\frac{1}{a} + \frac{1}{c}}\right]$$

For testing H_0: Prevalence Ratio $= 1$ in a cross-sectional study

$$95\%\ CI(PR) = \exp\left[\ln PR \pm \left(1.96 \times \sqrt{\frac{b/a}{a+b} + \frac{d/c}{c+d}}\right)\right]$$

Data from: Katz D, Baptista J, Azen SP, Pike MC. Obtaining confidence intervals for the risk ratio in cohort studies. *Biometrics*. 1978;34:469–474. Ederer F, Mantel N. Confidence limits on the ratio for two Poisson variables. *Am J Epidemiol*. 1974;100:165–167. Ahlbom A. *Biostatistics for Epidemiologists*. Boca Raton, FL: Lewis Publishers; 1993. Woolf B. On estimating the relation between blood group and disease. *Ann Hum Genet*. 1955;19:251–253. Schlesselman JJ. *Case-Control Studies: Design, Conduct, Analysis*. New York: Oxford University Press; 1982.

5. In the study, 150 cases of SD were identified along with 150 controls. Of those with SD, 16 had previously experienced meningitis. Of the controls, 3 had previously experienced meningitis.

$$OR = \frac{16 \times 147}{3 \times 134} = 5.851$$

$$\chi^2_{df=1} = \frac{(|16 \times 147 - 3 \times 134| - 300/2)^2 \, 300}{(16+3)(134+147)(16+134)(3+147)} = 8.091$$

6. Referring to Table 5 in Appendix B, the calculated chi-square corresponds with a $P < 0.005$. Because the calculated value is in the rejection region, we reject H_0 and accept that there is an association between meningitis and spasmodic dysphonia.

$$95\% \; CI(5.851) = exp\left[\ln(5.851) \pm 1.96 \times \sqrt{\frac{1}{16} + \frac{1}{3} + \frac{1}{134} + \frac{1}{147}}\right]$$

$$\rightarrow 1.67 - 20.53$$

EXAMPLE 11.8

In a *matched case-control study* conducted in Morocco, investigators wanted to assess whether a relationship existed between lighting the home with candles and lung cancer.[14] Controls were matched to cases on smoking status, age, and gender. Applying the steps to hypothesis testing for this matched case-control study gives the following:

1. $H_0: OR = 1$
2. $H_a: OR \neq 1$
3. $\alpha = 0.05, n = 160$
4. Chi-square (χ^2) with 1 degree of freedom
5. The data appear in the following contingency table:

		Controls	
		Candle lighting	No candle lighting
Lung cancer	Candle lighting	25	25
	No candle lighting	10	100

$$OR = \frac{25}{10} = 2.5$$

$$\chi^2_{df=1} = \frac{(|25 - 10| - 1)^2}{(25 + 10)} = 5.6$$

6. Referring to Table 5 in Appendix B, the calculated chi-square corresponds with $0.025 < P < 0.010$. Because the calculated value is in the rejection region, we reject H_0 and accept that there is an association between candle lighting in the home and lung cancer in Morocco.

$$95\% \; CI(2.5) = exp\left[\ln(2.5) \pm 1.96 \times \sqrt{\frac{1}{25} + \frac{1}{10}} \right]$$

$$\rightarrow 1.20 - 5.21$$

EXAMPLE 11.9

Suppose a case-control study is conducted among a group of women aged 30 years and older to investigate the relationship between coffee drinking and osteoporosis. Smoking is believed to be a confounder, so data were collected on this variable so a stratified analysis could be performed. Applying the steps to hypothesis testing for this study gives the following:

1. $H_0: OR_{MH} = 1$
2. $H_a: OR_{MH} \neq 1$
3. $\alpha = 0.05$, $n = 400$
4. χ^2_{MH} with 1 degree of freedom
5. The data appear in the following contingency tables:

Coffee Drinking and Osteoporosis, Crude Data		
	Osteoporosis	
Coffee drinker	Yes	No
Yes	138	119
No	62	81

Coffee Drinking and Osteoporosis among Smokers		
	Osteoporosis	
Coffee drinker	Yes	No
Yes	96	62
No	24	18

Coffee Drinking and Osteoporosis among Nonsmokers		
	Osteoporosis	
Coffee drinker	Yes	No
Yes	42	57
No	38	63

$$OR_{Crude} = \frac{138 \times 81}{119 \times 62} = 1.52$$

$$OR_{Smokers} = \frac{96 \times 18}{62 \times 24} = 1.16$$

$$OR_{Nonsmokers} = \frac{42 \times 63}{57 \times 38} = 1.22$$

Before combining the information across strata, we must first verify that the odds ratios are constant across the different strata. If they are not, a single summary value for the overall relative odds is not beneficial. Rather, it is better to treat the data in the various tables as if they had been drawn from distinct populations and report a different odds ratio for each subgroup.

Because the stratified odds ratios are similar, we will apply the Mantel-Haenszel method for estimating a pooled odds ratio across the two homogeneous strata.

$$OR_{MH} = \frac{(96 \times 18)/200 + (42 \times 63)/200}{(62 \times 24)/200 + (57 \times 38)/200} = 1.197$$

$$\chi^2_{MH} = \frac{[(96+42) - (96+24)(96+62)/200 + (42+38)(42+57)/200]^2}{(96+62)(24+18)(96+24)(96+18)/200^2 \times (200-1)} = 0.646$$
$$+ (42+57)(38+63)(42+38)(57+63)/200^2 \times (200-1)$$

6. Referring to Table 5 in Appendix B, the calculated chi-square corresponds with $P > 0.100$.

$$95\% \; CI(1.197) = 1.197^{1 \pm 1.96/\sqrt{0.646}}$$

$$\rightarrow 0.772 - 1.856$$

EXAMPLE 11.10

A group of adults was randomly assigned to an intervention group or a control group. The intervention involved a dietary program. Each group had their BMI measured at baseline and after 6 months. Apply the steps of hypothesis testing to this *cohort study.*

1. $H_0: RR = 1$
2. $H_a: RR \neq 1$
3. $\alpha = 0.05, n = 348$
4. Chi-square (χ^2) with 1 degree of freedom
5. The data appear as in the following table.

	Lowered BMI	
Intervention	Yes	No
Yes	138	36
No	98	76

$$RR = \frac{138/(138+36)}{98/(98+76)} = 1.41$$

$$\chi^2_{df=1} = \frac{(|138 \times 76 - 36 \times 98| - 348/2)^2 \times 348}{(138+36)(98+76)(138+98)(36+76)} = 20.03$$

6. Referring to Table 7 in Appendix B, the calculated chi-square corresponds with $P < 0.001$. Thus, we reject H_0 and conclude that the intervention is efficacious at lowering BMI over 6 months of follow-up. Specifically, those who participated in the dietary program are 1.41 (or 41%) more likely to lower their BMI over the 6-month study period.

$$95\% \ CI(1.41) = exp\left[\ln(1.41) \pm \left(1.96 \times \sqrt{\frac{36/138}{138+36} + \frac{76/98}{98+76}} \right) \right]$$

$$\rightarrow 1.21, 1.64$$

EXAMPLE 11.11

Consider the BMI data again, but suppose we wanted to calculate a measure of association that adjusts for the potential confounding effect of gender. Application of the steps of hypothesis testing gives the following:

1. $H_0: RR_{MH} = 1$
2. $H_a: RR_{MH} \neq 1$
3. $\alpha = 0.05, n = 348$

4. Chi-square (χ^2) with 1 degree of freedom
5. The data presented in contingency tables for men and women are:

Men	Lowered BMI	
Intervention	Yes	No
Yes	40	7
No	35	16

Women	Lowered BMI	
Intervention	Yes	No
Yes	98	29
No	63	60

$$RR_{MH} = \frac{40(35+16)/98 + 98(63+60)/250}{35(40+7)/98 + 63(98+29)/250} = 1.41$$

$$\chi^2_{MH} = \frac{\{(40+98) - [(40+35)(40+7)/98 + (98+63)(98+29)/250]\}^2}{(40+7)(35+16)(40+35)(7+16)/(98^2(98-1))} = 21.77$$
$$+ (98+29)(63+60)(98+63)(29+60)/(250^2(250-1))$$

6. Referring to Table 5 in Appendix B, the calculated chi-square corresponds with $P < 0.001$. Hence, we reject H_0 and conclude that the intervention does significantly lower BMI through 6 months of follow-up, after controlling for gender.

$$95\% \; CI(1.41) = 1.41^{1 \pm 1.96/\sqrt{21.77}}$$

$$\rightarrow 1.22 - 1.63$$

EXAMPLE 11.12

In Example 11.6, we used Poisson regression to assess the association between current smoking and cardiovascular disease in a cohort study involving person-years. Another way to evaluate this data is shown here, using the steps of hypothesis testing.

1. H_0: *Rate Ratio = 1*
2. H_a: *Rate Ratio $\neq$ 1*
3. $\alpha = 0.05$, $n = 1,555$
4. Chi-square (χ^2) with 1 degree of freedom

5. $Rate\ Ratio = \dfrac{882/220,965}{673/189,254} = 1.123$

$$\chi^2_{df=1} = \dfrac{\{882 - (220,965[882+673])/410,219\}^2}{220,965(189,254[882+673])/410,219^2} = 5.120$$

6. Referring to Table 5 in Appendix B, the calculated chi-square corresponds with $0.010 < P < 0.025$. Hence, we reject H_0 and conclude that smokers are 1.12 (or 12%) more likely than nonsmokers to develop cardiovascular disease.

$$95\%\ CI(1.123) = \exp\left[\ln(1.123) \pm 1.96\sqrt{\dfrac{1}{882} + \dfrac{1}{673}}\right]$$

$$\rightarrow 1.016 - 1.241$$

EXAMPLE 11.13

In a cross-sectional survey, a group of 296 Latinos who immigrated to the United States were asked what their age was when they entered the United States and what language they usually spoke in the home. Researchers wanted to know whether there was an association between age at immigration to the United States and language usually spoken in the home. Applying the steps of hypothesis, they tested whether a younger age is associated with speaking English only in the home versus speaking Spanish only in the home.

1. H_0: *Prevalence Ratio = 1*
2. H_a: *Prevalence Ratio ≠ 1*
3. $\alpha = 0.05$, $n = 203$
4. Chi-square (χ^2) with 1 degree of freedom

	Language spoken at home		
Age entered the United States	English only	Spanish only	Both equally
< 18	7	18	21
≥ 18	16	162	72

$$Prevalence\ Ratio = \dfrac{7/(7+18)}{16/(16+162)} = 3.12$$

$$\chi^2_{df=1} = \dfrac{(|71 \times 62 - 18 \times 16| - 203/2)^2 \times 203}{(7+18)(16+162)(7+16)(18+162)} = 6.11$$

5. Referring to Table 5 in Appendix B, the calculated chi-square corresponds with $0.010 < P < 0.025$, so we reject H_0 and conclude that entering the United States prior to age 18 compared with 18 years or older is positively associated with speaking only English in the home.

$$95\% \ CI(3.12) = exp\left[\ln(3.12) \pm \left(1.96 \times \sqrt{\frac{18/7}{7+18} + \frac{162/16}{16+162}}\right)\right]$$

$$\rightarrow 1.43 - 6.83$$

A NOTE ON THE RISK AND ODDS RATIOS

There may be differences in the numerical values of the risk ratio and the odds ratio, but they will always point in the same direction. Unless there is no association between exposure and outcome variables, the odds ratio will always be farther from unity than the risk ratio. The odds ratio is a biased estimate of the risk ratio because it tends to overestimate the magnitude of the association. The *odds ratio* is the odds of exposure among cases relative to the odds of exposure among noncases. The *risk ratio* is the risk of the health-related state or event for those having the risk factor (exposed) compared with the risk of the health-related state or event for those not having the risk factor (unexposed).

The odds ratio can be interpreted in the same way as the risk ratio if the outcome is uncommon. Specifically, if the outcome is rare, then $(a + b) \approx b$ and $(c + d) \approx d$, such that:

$$RR = \frac{a/(a+b)}{c/(c+d)} \approx \frac{a/b}{c/d} = \frac{a \times d}{b \times c} = OR$$

In addition, if the controls reflect everyone in the population of interest that are not cases, rather than a subsample of the population of noncases, then even if a case-control study is being conducted, it is appropriate to use the risk ratio. This is because the entire exposed and unexposed populations are represented such that attack rates can be computed for both groups.

SOME COHORT-BASED MEASURES

There are several cohort-based measures that are used in epidemiology and clinical medicine that are useful for communicating health information. Selected measures are presented in **Table 11.8**. The formulas for these measures are defined in the context of data in the 2×2 contingency table (see Tables 11.4 and 11.5).

TABLE 11.8 Some Epidemiologic Measures for Describing Cohort Data		
	Measure	**Interpretation**
Cumulative incidence rate in the exposed group	$I_e = (a/[a+b]) \times 10^n$	Attack rate (risk) of the health-related state or event for those exposed
Cumulative incidence rate in the unexposed group	$I_t = ([a+c]/n) \times 10^n$	Attack rate (risk) of the health-related state or event for those unexposed
Cumulative incidence in the total group	$I_o = (c/[c+d]) \times 10^n$	Overall attack rate (risk) of the health-related state or event
Risk ratio	$RR = \dfrac{I_e}{I_o}$	Relative risk
Attributable risk	$AR = I_e - I_o$	Excess risk of disease among the exposed group attributed to the exposure, typically expressed per 10^n
Attributable-risk percent	$AR\% = \dfrac{I_e - I_o}{I_e} \times 100$ $= \left(\dfrac{[RR-1]}{RR}\right) \times 100$	For disease cases that are exposed, this statistic refers to the percentage of disease cases attributed to their exposure
Population-attributable risk	$PAR = I_t - I_o$	The excess risk of disease in the population attributed to the exposure, typically expressed per 10^n
Population attributable-risk percent	$PAR\% = \dfrac{I_t - I_o}{I_t} \times 100$	Percentage of the disease in the population that can be attributed to the exposure

EXAMPLE 11.14

A varicella (chicken pox) outbreak occurred in Nebraska in 2004.[15] In this area, a large number of children had been vaccinated. Researchers wanted to investigate the extent that the vaccination had a protective effect against the illness. On the basis of the data in the following table, we will illustrate the summary measures presented in the previous table.

	Varicella (chicken pox)		
Vaccinated	Yes	No	
No	18	9	27
Yes	15	100	115
	33	109	142

Attack rates for those not vaccinated (nv), vaccinated (v), and overall are:

$$I_{nv} = \frac{18}{27} \times 100 = 66.7$$

$$I_v = \frac{15}{115} \times 100 = 13.0$$

$$I_t = \frac{33}{142} \times 100 = 23.2$$

The risk ratio is:

$$RR = \frac{66.7}{13.0} = 5.13$$

Therefore, those who have not been vaccinated are 5.13 (or 413%) more likely to develop chicken pox. We could have inverted the rows in the table, in which case:

$$RR = \frac{13.0}{66.7} = 0.195$$

The *preventive fraction* (i.e., vaccine efficacy), based on this formulation of the risk ratio, is $1 - 0.195 = 0.805$ (or 80.5%). Therefore, the vaccine prevented about 80% of the cases that would have otherwise occurred.

To further illustrate the measures in the table, we will use the previous form of the risk ratio. The excess risk of chicken pox among those not vaccinated because of their failure to be vaccinated is:

$$AR = 66.7 - 13.0 = 53.7 \; per \; 100$$

Among the cases of chicken pox who were not vaccinated, the percentage of cases attributed to their not being vaccinated is:

$$AR\% = \frac{66.7 - 13.0}{66.7} \times 100 = \frac{53.7}{66.7} \times 100 = 80.5\%$$

The excess risk of chicken pox in the population attributed to not being vaccinated is:

$$PAR = 23.2 - 13.0 = 10.2 \; per \; 100$$

The percentage of chicken pox in the population that can be attributed to not being vaccinated is:

$$PAR\% = \frac{23.2 - 13.0}{23.2} = \frac{10.2}{23.2} \times 100 = 44.0\%$$

It is important to note that for each of these measures, we assume there is a causal association between the exposure and outcome variables.

Definitions

Immunity is a state of having sufficient biological defenses to avoid infection, disease, or other unwanted biological invasions.

Active immunity occurs when the body produces its own antibodies. This can occur through a vaccine or in response to having a specific disease pathogen invade the body.

Passive immunity is the transfer from one individual to another of active humoral immunity in the form of ready-made antibodies (e.g., transplacental transfer to the unborn child of a mother's immunity from diseases). **Acquired immunity** involves having had a dose of a disease that stimulates the natural immune system.

Antigen, a substance that prompts the immune system to produce antibodies when introduced into the body.

Herd immunity, which is the notion that if the herd (a population or group) is mostly protected from a disease by immunization, then the chance that a major epidemic will occur is limited.[16–21]

History

Jonas Edward Salk (1914–1995) is known for developing the first polio vaccine. From the Second World War until 1955, polio was considered the most frightening public health problem. Epidemics occurred annually and were becoming increasingly devastating. In 1952, nearly 58,000 cases were reported in the United States, of which 3,145 died and 21,269 were disabled. Most of the victims were children. News of a successful polio vaccine, developed by Salk, came on April 12, 1955. Many people deemed Salk a "miracle worker." Salk suggested that if a herd immunity level of 85% exists in a population, a polio epidemic will not occur.[22, 23] Today, herd immunity thresholds for polio and several other communicable diseases are available.[21] Salk's later years were devoted to searching for a vaccine against the human immunodeficiency virus.[22, 23]

EXAMPLE 11.15

On the basis of epidemiologic cohort studies, the following information has been obtained on cigarette smoking and two chronic diseases: lung cancer and coronary heart disease (**Table 11.9**).[24]

TABLE 11.9	Cigarette Smoking, Lung Cancer, and Coronary Heart Disease Population	
	Lung cancer incidence rate per 100,000	**Coronary heart disease incidence rate per 100,000**
Overall	$I_t = 60$	$I_t = 240$
Cigarette smokers	$I_e = 180$	$I_e = 420$
Nonsmokers	$I_o = 20$	$I_o = 180$

Data from: Oleckno WA. *Essential epidemiology: Principles and Applications.* Prospect Heights, IL: Waveland Press, Inc.; 2002.

The summary measures in Table 11.9 applied to this data are presented as follows:

	Lung cancer	Coronary heart disease
Risk ratio	9	2.3
Attributable risk	160	240
Attributable risk percent	89	57
Population attributable risk	40	60
Population attributable risk percent	67	25

Assuming a causal association exists between cigarette smoking and these chronic diseases, we can conclude that there is a much stronger association of risk between smoking and lung cancer than between smoking and coronary heart disease. However, the excess risk among the smokers attributed to their smoking is greater for coronary heart disease. In other words, the burden of smoking on coronary heart disease is greater than that of smoking on lung cancer because coronary heart disease is a much more prevalent disease. Further, among lung cancer cases who smoke, 89% of those cases are attributed to their smoking. The corresponding percent for coronary heart disease is 57. The lower attributable-risk percent for coronary heart disease is consistent with a weaker risk associated with smoking. Regarding the population-attributable risk, the greater value for coronary heart disease is consistent with this disease being more prevalent than lung cancer. Finally, if smoking were eliminated in the population, we could expect a 67% decrease in lung cancer and a 25% decrease in coronary heart disease.

SAMPLE SIZE ESTIMATION FOR THE CORRELATION COEFFICIENT

There are several formulas for calculating sample size in observational and experimental analytic studies. Despite there being variations in the approach for estimating sample size, certain steps are common to all the formulas. In addition to the sample size formulas presented in Chapter 9, which are useful in designing experimental studies, this section will show how to calculate the sample size using the correlation coefficient in a hypothesis-based cross-sectional or ecologic study. The sample size formula for determining whether a correlation coefficient differs from zero is presented in the following box.

Sample Size Formula for the Correlation Coefficient

$$n = \left(\left[z_\alpha + z_\beta\right] \div C\right)^2 + 3$$

where

$C = 0.5 \times \ln\left(\left[1 + r\right]/\left[1 - r\right]\right)$ and r is the correlation coefficient.

If we are interested in the sample size for testing whether the correlation, r_1, is different from r_2, the formula is modified as follows:

$$n = \left(\left[z_\alpha + z_\beta\right] \div \left[C_1 - C_2\right]\right)^2 + 3$$

where

$$C_1 = 0.5 \times \ln\left(\left[1 + r_1\right]/\left[1 - r_1\right]\right)$$
$$C_1 = 0.5 \times \ln\left(\left[1 + r_2\right]/\left[1 - r_2\right]\right)$$

EXAMPLE 11.16

The research question is whether the variables *percent body fat* and *bone density* are correlated in a group of women ages 40–59. The investigator believes that women with a high percentage of body fat have a higher level of bone density. A small preliminary study found a modest correlation ($r = 0.3$) among women in this age group. How many women will need to be enrolled?

1. H_0: $\rho \leq 0$
2. H_a: $\rho > 0$
3. The anticipated effect size (r) = 0.3
4. Variability is a function of r and is included in the formula
5. α (one-tailed) = 0.05 and $\beta = 0.1$
6. $C = 0.5 \times \ln\left(\dfrac{[1 + 0.3]}{[1 - 0.3]}\right) = 0.3095$

$$n = \left([1.645 + 1.282] \div 0.3095\right)^2 + 3 = 93$$

Thus, 93 women in the age range 40–59 will be required.

EXERCISES

1. Match the descriptions in the left column with the measures of linear association in the right column.

___ Alternative to the Pearson correlation coefficient that is used when outlying data exist such that one or both of the distributions are skewed. This method is robust to outliers.

___ Provides an equation that estimates the change in the dependent variable per unit change in an independent variable. This method assumes that for each value of x, y is normally distributed; that the standard deviation of the outcomes y do not change over x; that the outcomes y are independent; and that a linear relationship exists between x and y.

___ Measures the strength of the association between two variables (also called the Pearson correlation). The method assumes that both variables are normally distributed and that a linear association exists between the variables.

___ Is the correlation coefficient squared, and represents the proportion of the total variation in the dependent variable that is explained by the independent variable.

A. correlation coefficient

B. coefficient of determination

C. Spearman's rank correlation coefficient

D. regression analysis (slope coefficient)

2. Why is it important to create a scatter plot of the data when evaluating the relationship between two numerical random variables?

3. Referring to question 2, if a linear relationship does not hold, what is an alternative measure to the Pearson correlation coefficient?

4. In a study involving participants at the World Senior Games, 443 individuals completed questions about general health and emotional health.[3] The relationship between these two variables was approximately linear, and the Pearson correlation coefficient equaled 0.394. Use the t test with $\alpha = 0.05$ and evaluate the hypothesis H_0: $\rho = 0$ versus H_a: $\rho \neq 0$.

5. Referring to question 4, what is the coefficient of determination? Interpret your result.

6. Under what condition should we have used Spearman's rank correlation coefficient instead of the Pearson correlation coefficient?

7. Suppose we are interested in the association between the heights of fathers and the heights of their sons. Data were collected from 14 father-and-son pairs. Heights are presented in inches.

Father's height	Son's height	Father's height	Son's height
69	72	69	70
66	78	67	70
67	70	75	79
68	68	73	78
71	72	70	75
73	73	68	70
70	71	69	69

a. Construct a two-way scatter plot for these data.
b. Is there a linear relationship between the heights of the fathers and sons?
c. Compute r, the Pearson correlation coefficient.
d. At the 0.05 level of significance, test the null hypothesis that the population correlation ρ is equal to 0. What do you conclude?
e. Calculate r_s, the Spearman rank correlation coefficient.
f. How does the value of r_s compare with r?
g. Using r_s, test the null hypothesis that the population correlation is equal to 0. What do you conclude?

8. Referring to question 7, what should we do in order to perform a simple linear regression analysis?

9. How is correlation analysis distinct from simple linear regression?

10. What assumptions are made with the method of least squares to estimate a population regression line?

11. Why should we be careful when extrapolating an estimated linear regression line outside the range of the observed data used to estimate the line?

12. Why is the two-way scatter plot of the residuals versus the fitted values of the response useful in evaluating the fit of a least-squares regression line?

13. Refer to the data in question 7. Suppose the data for the second father-son combination had an error; that is, the son's height of 78-inches should have

been 68-inches. Fix this error. Plot the data and comment on the assumptions of constant variance, independence, and linearity.

14. Referring to question 13, what is the coefficient of determination? Interpret.

15. Referring to question 13, what is the slope coefficient? Interpret.

16. Referring to question 13, the standard error of the estimated slope is 0.235. Is the slope statistically significant?

17. What assumptions are made when the method of least squares is used to estimate a population regression line containing two or more independent variables?

18. Referring to question 4, we calculated the following regression model using SAS.

$$EH = 52.608 + 0.366 \times GH$$

The standard error for the slope was 0.043 and $r^2 = 0.143$. How well does general health explain emotional health, and is the association statistically significant?

19. The following residual plot accompanies this model. What can you conclude about the assumptions?

20. Referring to question 18, calculate the 95% confidence interval for the slope coefficient.

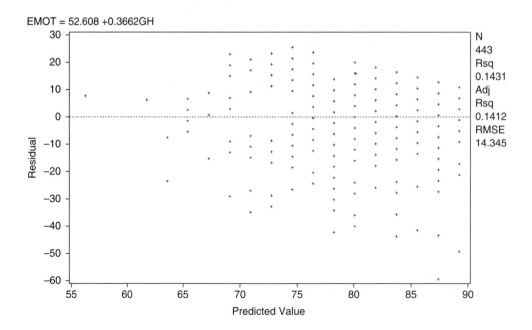

EMOT = 52.608 + 0.3662GH

N 443
Rsq 0.1431
Adj Rsq 0.1412
RMSE 14.345

21. Referring to question 18, we added age and gender to the model and calculated the following regression model using SAS:

$$EH = 62.413 + 0.348 \times GH - 0.150 \times Age + 3.526 \times Gender \ (M \ vs. \ F)$$

The standard errors were 0.042 for GH, 0.084 for age, and 1.363 for gender. In addition, the adjusted $r^2 = 0.160$. Comment on the significance of the model.

22. Which assumption in standard linear regression is violated if the dependent variable is dichotomous rather than continuous?

23. Suppose we are interested in whether the odds of disease change according to distance from a putative exposure. Five bands of distance from the exposure are from 1 to 5 kilometers. Now consider the following hypothetical case-control data:

Distance from putative exposure	Cases	Controls
1	40	100
2	35	100
3	30	100
4	15	100
5	12	100

With a dichotomous outcome variable (case versus control), use logistic regression to estimate the odds ratios and corresponding confidence intervals. Treat distance as a discrete variable.

24. The estimated logistic regression coefficient and standard error for the distance variable are −0.3045 and 0.0739, respectively. From these data, calculate the odds ratio and corresponding 95% confidence interval.

25. In a recent study, researchers evaluated the association of self-reported type 2 diabetes and primary open-angle glaucoma (POAG) among African American women.[25]

	POAG	
Type 2 diabetes	Cases	Person-years
Yes	57	23,488
No	308	389,470

Test the hypothesis of there being an association between type 2 diabetes and POAG.

26. Calculate the 95% confidence interval for the rate ratio estimated in the previous problem.

27. Consider the following data statements in SAS:

DATA CORONARY;
INPUT AGE $ SMOKE $ DEATH PYEARS;
LPYEARS = LOG(PYEARS);
DATALINES;

35–44	YES	32	52407
45–54	YES	104	43248
55–64	YES	206	28612
65–74	YES	186	12663
75–84	YES	102	5217
35–44	NO	2	18790
45–54	NO	12	10673
55–64	NO	28	5710
65–74	NO	28	2585
75–84	NO	31	1462

;

This data is from a study that Doll and Hill conducted (1966) in which they examined the relationship between death from coronary heart disease and smoking among male British doctors.[26] Use Poisson regression to assess the relationship between smoking and death, adjusting for age. What is the rate ratio and 95% confidence interval?

28. Researchers conducted a case-control study to investigate whether living near a high-hazard dump site compared with a low-hazard dump site increased the risk of having a low birth weight child.[27] Study results found that for women living near a high-hazard dump site while pregnant, 181 had a low birth weight child and 4,268 had a normal weight child. For women living near a low-hazard dump site while pregnant, 126 had a low birth weight child and 4,236 had a normal weight child. We can reformulate the hypotheses as: H_0: $OR = 1$ vs. H_a: $OR \neq 1$. Estimate the odds ratio and 95% confidence interval to evaluate your hypotheses.

29. Suppose you performed a case-control study to evaluate the association between voice disorders (VD) and the secondary teaching profession. Controls were matched to cases according to alcohol drinking status, smoking status, age, and gender. The following data were obtained:

		Controls	
		VD	No VD
Teacher	VD	24	35
	No VD	15	78

What are the odds ratio, the chi-square, the 95% confidence interval based on the matched data, and your conclusion about the association between teaching and voice disorders?

30. Using a case-control study design, researchers evaluated the association between oral contraceptive (OC) use and the risk of breast cancer in Chinese women.[28] The following data were obtained:

Use of oral contraceptives	Breast cancer	
	Yes	No
Ever	419	426
Never	1,654	1,657

Apply the steps of hypothesis testing to this data, using an appropriate measure of association.

31. In the United States, among a representative group of 6,006 white men and 1,126 black men aged 70–79 years at diagnosis with stage IV prostate cancer, 2,337 whites and 344 blacks were alive after 5 years of follow-up.[29] Compare the white and black patient survival at 5 years.

32. Now suppose that we want to adjust for age, and that for those aged 75–79, 856 out of 2,692 whites survive 5 years and 107 out of 470 blacks survive 5 years.[29] Redo the analysis, adjusting for age as a potential confounder.

33. A cohort study involving Swedish females born between 1952 and 1989 obtained data on mothers' education and whether their daughters had an eating disorder.[30] Calculate the rate ratio and 95% confidence interval for postsecondary compared with secondary (reference) maternal education. Use Poisson regression. Interpret your results and indicate whether the

relationship between mother's education and eating disorder is statistically significant.

Mother's education	Eating disorder Cases	Eating disorder Person-years
Secondary	21	80,468
Postsecondary	22	43,358

34. Consider the following prevalence data from the voice disorder study.[3]

Respiratory allergies	Voice disorder Yes	Voice disorder No
Yes	29	70
No	46	308

Evaluate the research hypothesis that there is an association between respiratory allergies and having a history of voice disorders.

35. Calculate the 95% confidence interval for the prevalence rate ratio found in the previous problem.

36. Under what condition will the odds ratio approximate the risk ratio?

37. For the data in question 33, calculate and interpret the *AR*, *AR%*, *PAR*, and *PAR%*. Treat postsecondary education as the exposure.

38. What is herd immunity?

39. The research question is whether the percentages of body fat and bone density are correlated. The investigator believes that those with a high percentage of body fat have a higher level of bone density. A previous study found a modest correlation ($r = 0.25$). How many will need to be enrolled, at α (one-sided) = 0.05 and $\beta = 0.2$?

REFERENCES

1. Adapted from Feigal D, Black D, Grady D, et al. Planning for data management and analysis. In: Hulley SB, Cummings SF. *Designing Clinical Research: An Epidemiologic Approach*. Baltimore, MD: Williams & Wilkins; 1988:159–171.

2. Centers for Disease Control and Prevention. Behavior risk factor surveillance system. Prevalence and trend data. http://apps.nccd.cdc.gov/BRFSS/. Published 2011. Accessed July 1, 2011.

3. Merrill RM, Anderson AE, Sloan A. Quality of life indicators according to voice disorders and voice-related conditions. *Laryngoscope*. 2011;121:2,004–2,011.

4. Frome EL, Checkoway H. Use of Poisson regression models in estimating incidence rates and ratios. *Am J Epidemiol*. 1985;212:309–323.

5. Iso H, Date C, Yamamoto A, et al. Smoking cessation and mortality from cardiovascular disease among Japanese men and women. The JACC study. *Am J Epidemiol*. 2005;161(2): 170–179.

6. Benenson AS, ed. *Control of Communicable Diseases in Man*. 15th ed. Washington, DC: American Public Health Association; 1990:367–373.

7. Snow J. *On the Mode of Communication of Cholera*. 2nd ed., 1855. New York, NY: Commonwealth Fund; 1936.

8. Snow J. *On the Mode of Communication of Cholera*. In: Buck C, Llopis A, Najera E, Terris M, eds. *The Challenge of Epidemiology: Issues and Selected Readings*. Washington, DC: World Health Organization; 1988:42–45.

9. Katz D, Baptista J, Azen SP, Pike MC. Obtaining confidence intervals for the risk ratio in cohort studies. *Biometrics*. 1978;34:469–474.

10. Ederer F, Mantel N. Confidence limits on the ratio for two Poisson variables. *Am J Epidemiol*. 1974;100:165–167.

11. Ahlbom A. *Biostatistics for Epidemiologists*. Boca Raton, FL: Lewis Publishers; 1993.

12. Woolf B. On estimating the relation between blood group and disease. *Ann Hum Genet*. 1955;19:251–253.

13. Schlesselman JJ. *Case-Control Studies: Design, Conduct, Analysis*. New York: Oxford University Press; 1982.

14. Sasco AJ, Merrill RM, Dari I, et al. A case-control study of lung cancer in Casablanca, Morocco. *Cancer Causes Control*. 2002;13(7):609–616.

15. Centers for Disease Control and Prevention. Varicella outbreak among vaccinated children— Nebraska, 2004. *MMWR*. 2006;55:749–752.

16. Evans AS, Brachman PS. *Bacterial Infections of Humans: Epidemiology and Control*. 2nd ed. New York, NY: Plenum Medical Book Company; 1991.

17. Bickley HC. *Practical Concepts in Human Disease*. 2nd ed. Baltimore, MD: Williams & Wilkins; 1977.

18. Sheldon H. *Boyd's Introduction to the Study of Disease*. Philadelphia, PA: Lea and Febiger; 1984.

19. Centers for Disease Control and Prevention. Summary of notifiable diseases, United States, 1997. *MMWR*. 1998;46(54):27.

20. Crowley LV. *Introduction to Human Disease*. 2nd ed. Sudbury, MA: Jones and Bartlett; 1988.

21. Merrill RM. *Introduction to Epidemiology*. 5th ed. Sudbury, MA: Jones and Bartlett; 2010.

22. Weiss RA. How does HIV cause AIDS? *Science*. 1993; 260(5112):1273–1279.

23. Douek DC, Roederer M, Koup RA. Emerging concepts in the immunopathogenesis of AIDS. *Annu Rev Med*. 2009;60:471–484.

24. Oleckno WA. *Essential Epidemiology: Principles and Applications*. Prospect Heights, IL: Waveland Press, Inc.; 2002.

25. Wise LA, Rosenberg L, Radin RG, et al. A prospective study of diabetes, lifestyle factors, and glaucoma among African-American women. *Ann Epidemiol*. 2011;21(6):430–439.

26. Doll R, Hill AB. Mortality in relation to smoking: 20 years' observations on male British doctors. *Br Med J.* 1976;2(6051):1525–1536.

27. Gilbreath S, Kass PH. Adverse birth outcomes associated with open dump sites in Alaska Native villages. *Am J Epidemiol.* 2006;164:518–528.

28. Xu WH, Shu XO, Long J, et al. Relation of FGFR2 genetic polymorphisms to the association between oral contraceptive use and the risk of breast cancer in Chinese women. *Am J Epidemiol.* 2011;173(8):923–931.

29. Surveillance, Epidemiology, and End Results (SEER) Program (www.seer.cancer.gov). SEER*Stat Database: Mortality—All COD, Aggregated with State, Total U.S. (1969–2007) <Katrina/Rita Population Adjustment>, National Cancer Institute, DCCPS, Surveillance Research Program, Cancer Statistics Branch. Underlying mortality data provided by NCHS. www.cdc.gov/nchs. Released June 2010. Accessed August 12, 2011.

30. Ahrén-Moonga J, Silverwood R, Klinteberg BA, Koupil I. Association of higher parental and grandparental education and higher school grades with risk of hospitalization for eating disorders in females: the Uppsala birth cohort multigenerational study. *Am J Epidemiol.* 2009;170(5): 566–575.

Experimental Studies

Observational study designs reflect the science of how information is assembled, described, and related. The investigators of observational studies observe diseases, events, behaviors, conditions, and associations without altering them. In contrast, in an *experimental study*, researchers evaluate the effects of an assigned intervention on an outcome. Thus, the researchers intervene in the study by influencing the exposure of the study participants. The purpose of this chapter is to present special types of experimental studies and ways to minimize bias and confounding in these research investigations.

History

James Lind (1716–1794), a Scottish naval surgeon, noticed that many sailors on long ocean voyages became sick with scurvy, a disease marked by spongy and bleeding gums, bleeding under the skin, and extreme weakness. He observed that scurvy began to occur after four to six weeks at sea. In 1747, while serving on the *HMS Salisbury,* he conducted an experimental study involving 12 ill patients with classic symptoms of scurvy. The sailors were put in six groups of two, all with a common diet of foods like water-gruel sweetened with sugar, fresh mutton broth, puddings, boiled biscuit with sugar, barley and raisins, rice and currents, and sago and wine. In addition, each of the groups received an additional dietary intervention. Two men received a quart of cider a day on an empty stomach; two men took two spoonfuls of vinegar three times a day on an empty stomach; two men were given a half-pint of sea water every day; two men were given lemons and oranges to eat on an empty stomach; two men received an elixir recommended by a hospital surgeon; and two men were fed a combination of garlic, mustard seed, and horseradish. Lind says that the men given the lemons and oranges ate them with "greediness." After six days, only the two sailors who supplemented their diet with lemons and oranges showed noticeable improvement. All the others had putrid gums, spots, lassitude, and weakness of the knees. In fact, the two receiving the supplementary diet of citrus fruit no longer had symptoms of scurvy and asked to nurse the others who were still sick. Thus, Lind discovered a remedy for scurvy occurring among sailors at sea.[1]

EXPERIMENTAL STUDY DESIGNS

The experimental study design resembles controlled experiments performed in scientific research. They are the most useful for establishing cause–effect relationships and for evaluating the efficacy of prevention and therapeutic interventions because the investigator has more control over the level of exposure, and they are best suited for controlling for bias and confounding. As will be discussed, when it is ethically acceptable to blind and randomize, blinding can be effective at minimizing bias and randomization can be effective at controlling for confounding.

The strongest methodological design is a *between-group design*, in which outcomes are compared between two or more groups of people receiving different levels of the intervention. Another study design that is commonly used and well suited for addressing certain research questions is the *within-group design*, in which the outcome in a single group is compared before and after an assigned intervention. The between-group design is more prone to individual type confounding factors (e.g., gender, race, genetic susceptibility). The within-group design is more susceptible to confounding from time-related factors (e.g., learning effects where participants do better on follow-up cognitive tests because they learned from the baseline test, influences from the media, or other external factors).

Experimental studies are defined according to the unit of measurement. The unit of measurement may be on the individual or community level. Sometimes experimental studies are referred to as *trials*, such as a clinical trial, if the experimental study is being performed in a clinical setting, or a community trial where the intervention is applied on a group level (e.g., school, classroom, or city). The types of trials, their descriptions, and selection issues according to the unit of measurement are presented in **Table 12.1**. For example, in an experimental study where the unit of measurement is the individual, researchers may conduct a clinical trial involving the investigation of a new drug in order to evaluate its efficacy and safety. Inclusion and exclusion criteria are used to improve the validity of the study.

Ideally, an experimental study will blind the patients and those assessing the outcome in order to minimize bias and also randomly assign participants to different levels of the intervention in order to eliminate confounding. However, blinding and randomization may pose ethical challenges, in which case alternative experimental designs may be needed. We will first describe the randomized, blinded trial, and then discuss alternative types of experimental studies.

RANDOM ASSIGNMENT

Randomly assigning participants to different levels of the intervention makes intervention and control groups look as similar as possible, thereby minimizing the potential influence of confounding factors. Assignment of participants to the different levels of the intervention is based on chance, such that the application of inferential statistical tests of probability and determination of the levels of significance are pos-

TABLE 12.1	Units of Measurement and Experimental Studies		
Unit of measurement	**Type of trial**	**Description**	**Selection of participants in relation to exposure and outcome**
Individuals	Clinical trial	Tests the efficacy and safety of a new drug or medical device.	Selected on the basis of outcome; usually inclusion and exclusion criteria.
	Prophylactic trial	Tests preventive measures.	Usually no selection; participants are typically healthy volunteers with a range of exposures and possible outcomes.
	Therapeutic trial	Tests new treatment methods.	Selected on basis of outcome; usually inclusion and exclusion criteria.
Community or group	Community trial	Tests a community intervention designed for the purpose of educational and behavioral changes at the population level. Community interventions generally use quasi-experimental designs (i.e., the investigators manipulate the study factors but do not assign individual participants to the intervention through random assignment).	The intervention is applied on a group level (e.g., school, classroom, neighborhood block). Initial screening may remove clinically diagnosed individuals at baseline. Community trials often focus on whether the intervention works in practice under day-to-day conditions that apply to the "real world."

sible. Randomization is typically used in clinical research trials. In clinical research, the efficacy of various levels of a treatment or combinations of treatments is investigated with inferential statistical tests of probability used and levels of significance determined.

Randomization is meant to balance out the effects of anticipated and unanticipated confounding factors among the assigned groups. Randomization of a sufficiently large number of participants will produce a similar distribution of participants among the assigned groups. Although it is possible to adjust for confounding factors at

Definition
Random assignment is the random allocation of participants to a given level of an intervention. Participants have an equal probability of being assigned to any of the groups. This process minimizes any confounding effects by balancing out the potential confounding factors among groups. The process requires a sufficiently large sample size.

the analysis phase of a study, this requires that data on the suspected confounders be collected at the outset of the study. However, although our best thinking might identify many possible confounding factors, there may be—and often are—some not considered. The great strength of randomization of a sufficiently large number of participants is that we can expect it to make the assigned groups look alike on average, and we do not need to be concerned that we have not considered all the potential confounders.

In a clinical setting, a physician may strongly believe in an intervention and place patients whom he or she perceives have the greatest amount to gain from the intervention in that group. Similarly, patients with more serious health problems may self-select the intervention. It is critical to design the random assignment procedure so that the investigators that have contact with the study participants are not able to influence their allocation. Treatment is often randomly assigned by computer programs, with rigorous precautions such that the assignments are tamper proof. Randomization has the advantage of eliminating conscious bias resulting from physician or patient selection and averages out unconscious bias from unknown factors. However, some may say that randomization jeopardizes the doctor–patient relationship and, in that sense, is not ethical, especially for studies involving certain health conditions.

NONRANDOM ASSIGNMENT

There are several possible reasons why researchers do not use random assignment, including feasibility and ethical issues. In experimental research, large populations are not always available, especially in clinical settings. The funds may simply not be available for conducting a large study involving treatment, follow-up assessment, testing of intervention, and control participants. There may also be a limited number of people with a given disease or condition under investigation or having a desire to participate in a randomized experimental study. Further, random assignment cannot occur if an entire population is to be affected or subjected to the treatment. For example, if fluoride is added to the water supply of a city, there is no way to include or exclude certain individuals. Similarly, if seat belt laws are implemented, we cannot randomly assign a group to not wear seat belts.

When randomization is not feasible, a concurrent comparison group in a nonrandom process (convenience sample) may be chosen. For example, if one city has fluoridated water, another city without fluoridated water could serve as a control, and dental outcomes from both groups could be used to evaluate the efficacy of fluoridation. In addition, if one state requires seat belt use and another does not, the death rate from motor vehicle accidents or some other seat belt–related outcome measure between the two states could be compared in order to determine the efficacy of seat belt use. A primary limitation of convenience samples is that they are more susceptible to unmeasured confounding factors.

> **Definition**
>
> **Convenience sampling** is a type of nonprobability sampling in which a sample population is selected because it is readily available and convenient.

BLINDING

Blinding is used in experimental studies to minimize potential bias. Bias may result because of the *placebo effect*. The placebo effect in a clinical trial is a response to a medical intervention that results from the intervention itself, not from the specific mechanism of action of the intervention.[2] In addition, just as a patient may respond to the intervention itself and not the specific therapeutic benefit of the intervention, an assessing investigator, despite trying to be honest in his/her assessment, may believe in a certain intervention to the extent that unconscious bias may arise, influencing the way the researcher evaluates those participants who receive the intervention.

> **Definition**
>
> The **placebo effect** is the influence on patient outcomes (improved or worsened) that may occur because of the expectation by a patient (or provider) that a particular intervention will have an effect. The placebo effect is independent of the true effect (pharmacologic, surgical, etc.) of a particular intervention.

Some studies are more amenable to the use of a placebo than others. Clinical trials involving the assessment of new drugs are particularly well suited for the use of a placebo because the placebos given to the control group are virtually indistinguishable (to blind the patients and providers, when possible) from the true intervention, providing a comparative basis for determining the effect of the treatment being investigated.[2] In a clinical trial involving the assessment of a new drug, a placebo is a pill of the same size, color, and shape as the treatment. However, it may be problematic to blind in drug studies where a treatment has characteristic side effects. Building side effects into a placebo may be unethical. For nondrug studies, such as those involving behavior changes or surgery, it is often impossible or unethical to blind.

History

The use of blinding to minimize the placebo effect in controlled clinical trials dates back about 100 years. In 1907, a double-blind placebo-controlled trial was conducted by W. H. R. Rivers to explore the association between alcohol and other substances and fatigue. Harry Gold advanced the double-blind placebo-controlled design in the 1940s and 1950s in several lectures and publications. In the 1950s, Henry Beecher estimated that in over two dozen studies that he assessed, the placebo effect was responsible for about one-third of those who showed improvement. The contributions of these and other researchers led the Food and Drug Administration to recommend but not require (in the 1970s) that new drug trials be double blinded.[3,4]

The need for blinding is related to whether the outcome is subjectively determined, such as when the outcome is a measurement of pain, fear, well-being, happiness, and so on. If the outcome measure is not based on a subjective response or assessment, such as a urine sample or blood test, blinding is unnecessary. In drug studies, compliance and retention in the study may be much better if a placebo is used, such that even those receiving no therapeutic benefit by being in the study are not aware of that fact.

There are three types of blinding: single, double, and triple. A *single-blind* placebo-controlled study blinds the participants so that they are not aware who received the active treatment; a *double-blind study* blinds both the participants and those doing the outcome assessment so that neither the participants nor the investigators know who is receiving the active treatment; and a *triple-blind study* involves blinding the participants, those doing the outcome assessment, and those analyzing the data are separate from the primary investigators.[5–9]

Some advantages of randomized, blinded experimental studies are that they are the best study design for demonstrating cause–effect relationships; they may produce a faster and cheaper answer than observational studies; they are the only appropriate approach for some research questions; and they allow the investigators to control the exposure levels, as needed.[10,11] On the other hand, they are often more costly in time and money. Many research questions are not suitable for experimental designs because of ethical barriers, and because of rare outcomes, many research questions are not suitable for blinding; standardized interventions may be different from common practice; and they may have a limited generalization because of the use of volunteers, eligibility criteria, and loss to follow-up.[10,11] A summary of these advantages and disadvantages of randomized, blinded studies is presented in **Table 12.2**.

TABLE 12.2	Selected Strengths and Weaknesses of Blinded Randomized Controlled Studies
Strengths	**Weaknesses**
• Can support cause–effect relationships with a high level of confidence because of the tightly controlled conditions not possible in observational studies • Sometimes produce a faster and cheaper answer to the research question than observational studies • Only appropriate approach for some research questions • Allow investigators to control the exposure levels as needed	• Often more costly in time and money • Many research questions are not suitable for experimental designs because of ethical barriers and because of rare outcomes • Many research questions are not suitable for blinding • Standardized interventions may be different from common practice • May have limited external validity because of the use of volunteers, eligibility criteria, and loss to follow-up

Data from: Hulley SB, Feigal D, Martin M, Cummings SR. Designing a new study: IV: experiments. In: Hulley SB, Cummings SR, eds. *Designing Clinical Research: An Epidemiologic Approach.* Baltimore, MD: Williams & Williams; 1988. Oleckno WA. *Essential Epidemiology: Principles and Applications.* Prospect Heights, IL: Waveland Press, Inc.; 2002.

DESIGNING A CLINICAL TRIAL

Prior to designing a clinical trial, a pilot study may be in order. A *pilot study* is a standard scientific approach that involves preliminary analysis, which can greatly improve the chance of obtaining funding for major clinical trials. Information from pilot studies can also markedly improve the chance that the trial will be successfully conducted. These studies require careful planning, with clear objectives and correct application of methods. Some of the primary reasons for conducting a pilot study are to:

- Determine the feasibility, required time, and cost of recruitment and randomization.
- Determine the feasibility and efficiency of planned measurements, data collection instruments, and data management systems; a phase I or phase II clinical trial (see Table 12.3) is a type of pilot study aimed at identifying an optimal intervention.
- Obtain information on the effect of the intervention on the main outcome; statistical variability allows for a more accurate sample size estimation.

There are six general steps to consider when designing a clinical trial, which are related to conducting experimental studies, in general. These steps are: (1) selecting the intervention, (2) selecting the outcome (also called the *end point*), (3) assembling the study cohort, (4) measuring baseline variables, (5) choosing a comparison group, and (6) ensuring compliance.[11,12] These steps are described in **Table 12.3**.

TABLE 12.3	Steps for Designing a Clinical Trial
Steps	**Description**
1. Selecting the intervention	• Interventions may involve prevention or treatment. • The choice and dose of an intervention should be based on its potential effectiveness and safety, relevance to clinical practice, simplicity, suitability for blinding, and feasibility of enrolling participants. • Stages of testing new therapies include: **Preclinical**—Study involving animals or cell cultures. **Phase I**—Unblinded, uncontrolled study with typically less than 30 volunteers. It is conducted to determine the safety of a treatment in humans. Patients go through intense monitoring. **Phase II**—Also relatively small (up to 50 people) and involves randomization and blinding. In this type of trial, the investigator explores test tolerability, safe dosage, side effects, and how the body copes with the drug. **Phase III**—Relatively large randomized blinded trial used to evaluate the efficacy of an intervention (see the following steps). **Phase IV**—Large study (it may or may not be a randomized trial) conducted after the therapy has been approved by the FDA to assess the rate of serious side effects and explore further therapeutic uses.
2. Selecting the outcome	• Clinical outcomes are best for providing evidence of whether/how to use treatment. • Clinically relevant outcome measures are best (e.g., pain, quality of life, cancer, and death). • Intermediate markers may be reasonable outcomes and should be considered.

3. Assembling the study cohort	• The primary objective in establishing inclusion and exclusion criteria is a valid result.
	• There is often a compromise between the population most efficient for answering the clinical question and the population best for generalizing the study findings.
	• Broad inclusion criteria may improve the extent to which we can generalize the study results, but this may not be feasible. However, choosing people at high risk for an uncommon outcome can improve the feasibility (i.e., decrease sample size and cost) of a study.
	• The primary reasons for excluding people from a clinical trial include the following:
	  • The person has high risk of adverse reaction to the treatment.
	  • The person would experience high risk if assigned a placebo.
	  • The person is at low risk of experiencing the outcome.
	  • The person has a medical condition and is unlikely to respond to treatment.
	  • The person is currently on a medication that would interact with the intervention.
	  • The person is unlikely to adhere to the intervention.
	  • The person is unlikely to complete the follow-up.
	  • The person has physical or mental limitations that make participation problematic.

TABLE 12.3   Steps for Designing a Clinical Trial *(continued)*

Steps	Description
4. Measuring baseline variables	• Personal identifying information (e.g., name, address, employer, family member) is collected and used to minimize loss to follow-up. • Demographic information (e.g., age, race, ethnicity, gender) and behavior information (e.g., smoking, exercise, diet) are useful for characterizing the study population and controlling for confounding. • Behavior and clinical information are required if the investigator wants to evaluate changes from before to after the intervention.
5. Choosing a comparison group	• The comparison group should be selected so that the control group is not contaminated by the intervention. • Placebo controlled is ideal in drug studies. • Often the comparison group is assigned the status quo rather than a placebo if withholding an efficacious treatment is unethical.
6. Ensuring compliance	• Contact the participant shortly before evaluation. • Provide reimbursement. • Minimize harm, stress, or complexity associated with the intervention.

The intervention is determined from the research objective, whether it is to treat or prevent disease. In studies investigating the efficacy of a treatment, the investigator must establish that the therapy is safe and active against the disease, provide evidence that the therapy is potentially better than another, and provide evidence that the therapy is likely to be implementable in the field. There are different phases for testing new therapies that are required before a drug is granted a license (see Table 12.3). Behavioral interventions usually begin with an identified problem. When a public health problem is observed in a population through descriptive epidemiologic methods, tailored programs can be developed. Identifying high-risk behaviors for disease, recognizing where these risk behaviors are most common, and understanding why these behaviors are more readily adopted by one group and not another are important for designing the intervention. Behavioral interventions are often developed from behavior theory and refined with focus groups. New interventions are often developed from existing interventions shown to be efficacious in other settings. Evaluation of behavioral interventions often requires pilot testing in order to provide evidence that a larger scale assessment is worth doing.

Selecting an outcome variable should be driven by whichever variable or variables are best for satisfying the research question. Clinically relevant outcome measures are most meaningful in clinical trials. For rare outcome measures, such as many forms of cancer, capturing them in a clinical trial generally requires a very large number of participants, followed for a long period of time. Hence, feasibility of the study is an issue. In other cases, the outcome may occur so far in the future that an *intermediate marker* (or *intermediate endpoint*) may be preferred. These are events that precede the outcome of interest, are associated with the outcome, and may predict the value of a given treatment with less time and money. For example, an AIDS-defining event (e.g., parasitic infection, fungal infection, bacterial infection, viral infection, neoplastic disease) may be used over death from AIDS when evaluating a treatment to slow the progression of AIDS. In a prevention program involving a certain dietary intervention aimed at lowering the risk of colon cancer among men and women in their 50s with a history of the disease, the development of polyps may be the outcome variable used instead of a diagnosis of colon cancer or death from colon cancer.

The power of a study is greater when the outcome variable is numerical rather than dichotomous (e.g., CD_4 counts versus the presence or absence of a bacterial infection in HIV/AIDS patients). For dichotomous outcome variables, power is influenced more by the number of occurrences of the outcome than by the number of subjects in the study.[13]

In clinical trials, there is a term called *intent-to-treat*. An intent-to-treat analysis consists of comparing outcomes between intervention and control groups, with each participant analyzed according to his or her random group assignment, regardless of whether the participant adhered to the assigned intervention. Although this approach may underestimate the treatment effect, it also minimizes bias.

In some cases, researchers include more than one outcome measure in their study in order to measure different aspects of a given phenomenon. For example, an intense diet and physical activity–modification program, designed to ultimately reduce the risk of chronic health problems, measured change in several health indicators between baseline and 6 weeks. Variables with improved scores included health knowledge, percent body fat, total steps per week, and most nutrition variables measured. Clinical improvements were seen in resting heart rate, total cholesterol, low-density lipoprotein cholesterol, and systolic and diastolic blood pressure.[14]

When planning the sample size and the length of the study, a single primary outcome should be selected. In other words, an experimental study may have more than one hypothesis about the effects of an intervention on selected outcome variables. In this case, the sample size calculation and length of the study should be based on what the researchers believe is the most important hypothesis.

Before assembling the study cohort, inclusion and exclusion criteria are established and an appropriate sample size is determined. Inclusion and exclusion criteria influence the extent to which the results can be generalized. Inclusion criteria focus on who should be included in the study, whereas exclusion criteria are employed to help control error. Exclusions should be limited because unnecessary exclusions reduce the extent to which the results can be generalized. Sample size calculations are employed to ensure that the number of participants is adequate to test the specific hypothesis or hypotheses motivating the study.

Measuring baseline variables is necessary for maintaining contact with the study subjects and for minimizing loss to follow-up. Demographic information is useful for characterizing the study cohort. The first table of reports and papers describing results from randomized controlled trials typically compares baseline characteristics, including demographics, in the study groups, which provides a quick assessment of how well the random assignment balanced out intervention and control participants. In nonrandomized studies, it is important to collect demographic and other information (e.g., smoking habits) so that their potential confounding effects can be adjusted for in the analysis. In addition, measuring baseline data provides information for comparison in within-group designs.

The comparison group makes it possible to assess hypotheses. The comparison group should look like the intervention group, which is accomplished through random assignment. In many instances where a proven intervention is available, it would not be ethical to give patients a placebo, but the comparison group would receive the current treatment. Comparing a new drug with nothing is rarely done, unless there is no efficacious treatment available for the disease. The aim is to identify whether improvements can be made over the status quo.

The validity of an experimental study is directly associated with compliance. Thus, several steps are often taken to minimize loss to follow-up, such as contacting patients by telephone or mail shortly before their appointments and providing reimbursement for time and travel. Compliance is better when the drug or behavioral intervention is well tolerated and not too demanding.

OTHER SELECTED TYPES OF EXPERIMENTAL STUDIES _____

There are a number of other types of study designs. In many situations, variations of the randomized, blinded experimental study may have some advantages. We saw earlier that in some situations, random assignment and/or blinding may not feasible or ethical. In **Table 12.4**, six additional study designs are described, along with their strengths and weakness.

TABLE 12.4 Selected Experimental Study Designs

Study type	Description	Strengths	Weaknesses
Run-in design	All eligible participants in the cohort are placed on placebo (or treatment). Those who remain in the study after some short period of time (e.g., days or weeks) are then randomly assigned to the different arms of the study.	This design is useful for minimizing bias due to loss of follow-up.	As some people are eliminated from the study, generalization of the results to a population of interest becomes limited.
2 × 2 factorial design	Eligible participants are randomly assigned to one of four groups. The groups represent the different combinations of two interventions.	This is an efficient design that allows us to test two hypotheses for the price of one.	Interactions between the effects of the intervention on the outcomes can produce misleading results.
Time-series design	Among the eligible participants, the outcome variables are measured, the intervention is applied to the whole cohort, the cohort is followed, and the outcome variables are again measured.	A single, non-randomized group minimizes the potential for confounding because each participant serves as his or her own control.	There is not a concurrent control group such that it is impossible to determine whether the intervention effect is attributed to a learning effect.
Crossover study design	A crossover design (also called a crossover trial) is a longitudinal study in which subjects receive a sequence of different treatments (or exposures).	This combines randomized and time-series designs to improve control over confounding, and fewer participants are required to obtain a given level of power.	A doubling of time for the study is required and there is an added level of complexity required in the analysis and interpretation.
Group randomization	The intervention is randomly assigned to naturally forming clusters (e.g., practices, schools, hospitals, communities).	Helps control for confounding factors.	Sample size estimation and data analysis are more complicated than for individual-level randomization. In addition, the sample size required to maintain adequate statistical power is larger than with individual level randomization.[15,16]
Randomized matched paired design	Eligible participants are matched in pairs according to some potential confounding factor (e.g., age, sex, race, ethnicity).	Improves balance among groups on potential confounding variables.	Matching complicates the study at the design and analysis level and is unnecessary to control for confounding when the sample size is sufficiently large.

For placebo-controlled studies, the *run-in design* can be useful for minimizing bias associated with loss to follow-up. A limitation of this design is that the participants in the cohort at the time of randomization may no longer reflect the population of interest. In a behavioral intervention study, it may be useful to place all participants on the intervention and then, after a short time period, randomly assign those compliant with the program to the different levels of the intervention. For example, recovering heart attack patients in a selected cohort could all be placed on a new dietary intervention, and after a run-in period, those who are compliant would be randomly assigned to remain on the program or change to a standard dietary program used for recovering heart attack patients. The efficacy of the new dietary intervention can be assessed, but depending on the extent of initial dropout, it may have limited generalization to the population of heart attack patients as a whole.

A *factorial design* allows investigators to address the efficacy of two or more interventions in a single cohort of participants. In Table 12.4, a description of a 2×2 factorial design is given. For example, suppose we are interested in testing the efficacy of two placebo-controlled drugs. Eligible participants would be randomly assigned to one of four groups: (1) drug A and drug B, (2) drug A and placebo B, (3) placebo A and drug B, and (4) placebo A and placebo B. Comparing the outcomes for groups 1 and 2 with groups 3 and 4 allows for an evaluation of the efficacy of drug A. Comparing the outcomes for groups 1 and 3 with groups 2 and 4 allows for an evaluation of the efficacy of drug B. Factorial designs also offer an efficient approach for studying combination effects of treatments on an outcome. They are further useful in studying primary prevention programs. In one study, investigators used the factorial design to evaluate low-dose aspirin (100 mg/day) and vitamin E (300 mg/day) as tools in the prevention of cardiovascular events (cardiovascular death, stroke, or myocardial infarction) in type 2 diabetic patients having at least one cardiovascular risk factor. Although low-dose aspirin was shown to lower the risk of cardiovascular events, no significant reduction in any of the end points occurred because of vitamin E.[17]

Time-series designs involve measurements on a cohort at two or more successive periods of time. The simple time-series design involves the collection of measurements made at regular intervals through repeated observations, such as the number of hospitalizations per day or the number of deaths per day. In an experimental study, measurements are taken before and after an intervention to assess change in the outcome of interest. Time-series analysis is also commonly used in monitoring and surveillance. Time-series analysis of cohort data allows researchers to study the pattern of illness or injury for a group of people who experienced an exposure at roughly the same time.

In a *crossover study*, the outcome variables are measured on the eligible participants, and the participants are randomized to an intervention or control arm of the study. Then the outcome variables are measured again after a follow-up period, a washout period occurs to reduce carryover effect, the former placebo group is assigned the intervention, the former intervention group is assigned the placebo, and the outcome variables are measured again at the end of the follow-up.

In *group randomization*, instead of individuals being randomly assigned the intervention, groups or naturally forming clusters are randomly assigned the intervention. Individuals or patients within a cluster are likely to be more similar to each other compared with those in other clusters according to selected variables. This study design may be more feasible for addressing the research question than a randomized experimental study, but it is more complex in terms of sample size, analysis, and interpretation.

Matching is a procedure that aims to make treatment and comparison groups similar with respect to extraneous (or confounding) factors.[18] After participants are matched on one or more extraneous factors, one subject is randomly assigned to the treatment group (e.g., a dietary program or a drug) in each matched pair, and the other is assigned to the control group. A randomized matched pair design is most useful for balancing confounding factors among groups when the number of study participants is small.

EXERCISES

1. Compare and contrast a between-group experimental study and a within-group experimental study.
2. What is a placebo?
3. Why is randomization important in experimental research?
4. Explain how blinding in the classic randomized clinical trial can help minimize bias.
5. Match the descriptions in the left column with the concepts in the right column.

   ___ Eliminates conscious bias due to physician or patient selection

   ___ Often impossible in nondrug studies

   ___ More subjective outcomes call for more serious consideration of this

   ___ Can improve compliance and follow-up

   ___ Interferes with the doctor–patient relationship

   ___ Effective at controlling for unmeasured confounding effects

   A. randomize
   B. blind
   C. placebo

6. What is the meaning of intent-to-treat in a trial, and why is it done?
7. Match the definitions in the left column with the stages of testing new therapies listed in the right column.

___ Studies involving animals or cell cultures	A. preclinical
___ Conducted to determine the safety of a treatment in humans; patients go through intense monitoring	B. phase I
	C. phase II
	D. phase III
___ Large studies (may or may not be a randomized trial) conducted after the therapy has been approved by the FDA to assess the rate of serious side effects and explore further therapeutic uses	E. phase IV
___ Relatively large randomized blinded trials used to evaluate the efficacy of an intervention	
___ Investigator explores test tolerability, safe dosage, side effects, and how the body copes with the drug	

8. Why might investigators choose to conduct a factorial design?
9. Which study design is particularly useful for increasing the proportion of study participants who adhere to the intervention and follow-up procedures?
10. Which study design is specifically meant to improve the balance of baseline variables in order to reduce confounding?
11. What is one advantage to selecting a high-risk population in a clinical trial?

REFERENCES

1. Lilienfeld AM, Lilienfeld DE. *Foundations of Epidemiology.* 2nd ed. New York, NY: Oxford; 1980:30–31.
2. U.S. National Library of Medicine. National Institutes of Health. HTA 101: glossary. http://www.nlm.nih.gov/nichsr/hta101/ta101014.html. Published September 8, 2008. Accessed January 25, 2012.
3. Shapiro AK, Shapiro E. *The Powerful Placebo: From Ancient Priest to Modern Physician.* Baltimore, MD: Johns Hopkins University Press; 1997:272.
4. Beecher HK. The powerful placebo. *JAMA.* 1955;159(17):1602–1606.
5. Alreck RL, Settle RB. *The Survey Research Handbook.* Homewood, IL: Irwin; 1985.
6. Kerlinger FN. *Foundations of Behavioral Research.* 3rd ed. New York: Holt, Rinehart and Winston; 1986.
7. Neale JM, Liebert RM. *Science and Behavior.* 3rd ed. Englewood Cliffs, NJ: Prentice Hall; 1986.

8. Timmreck TC, Braza G, Mitchell J. Growing older: a study of stress and transition periods. *Occup Health Saf.* 1984;53(9):39–48.

9. Rothman KJ. *Modern Epidemiology.* Boston: Little, Brown and Company; 1986.

10. Hulley SB, Feigal D, Martin M, Cummings SR. Designing a new study: IV: experiments. In: Hulley SB, Cummings SR, eds. *Designing Clinical Research: An Epidemiologic Approach.* Baltimore, MD: Williams & Williams; 1988:110-127.

11. Oleckno WA. *Essential Epidemiology: Principles and Applications.* Prospect Heights, IL: Waveland Press, Inc.; 2002.

12. ClinicalTrials.gov: a service of the U.S. National Institutes of Health. Understanding clinical trials. http://clinicaltrials.gov/ct2/info/understand. Published September 20, 2007. Accessed December 23, 2011.

13. Yusuf S, Collins R, Peto R. Why do we need some large, simple randomized trials? *Stat Med.* 1984;3:409–420.

14. Aldana SG, Greenlaw RL, Diehl HA, et al. Effects of an intensive diet and physical activity modification program on the health risks of adults. *J Am Diet Assoc.* 2005;105(3):371–381.

15. Cosby RH, Howard M, Kaczorowski J, Willan AR, Sellors JW. Randomizing patients by family practice: sample size estimation, intracluster correlation and data analysis. *Fam Pract.* 2003;20(1):77–82.

16. Underwood M, Barnett A, Hajioff S. Cluster randomization: a trap for the unwary. *Br J Gen Pract.* 1998;48(428):1089–1090.

17. Sacco M, Pellegrini F, Roncaglioni MC, et al. Primary prevention of cardiovascular events with low-dose aspirin and vitamin E in type 2 diabetic patients: results of the Primary Prevention Project (PPP) trial. *Diabetes Care.* 2003;26(12):3264–3272.

18. Greevy R, Lu B, Silber JH, Rosenbaum P. Optimal multivariate matching before randomization. *Biostatistics.* 2004;5(2):263–275.

CHAPTER 13

Survival Analysis

In many studies in epidemiology and medicine, the response variable of interest is the amount of time (e.g., days, weeks, months, or years) from an initial observation until a subsequent event (e.g., death, disease, relapse, or recovery). Some examples include time until death for heart transplant patients, time to pregnancy among women taking fertility medication, and time in remission for leukemia patients. The time from initial observation to a subsequent event is the survival time. We also often refer to the event as a failure, because the event of interest is usually negative, such as disease or death. However, it may also be positive, such as returning to work or recovery after an illness.

Survival time is a continuous variable, but it tends to be skewed to the right. When survival time is assessed, the focus is typically on the probability that an individual will survive for a specified period of time. Survival time data are generally characterized by not all patients experiencing the outcome of interest at the time of assessment or not all patients beginning the study at the same time. When survival times are long, the data may need to be analyzed prior to the follow-up event of interest occurring for all patients. Some patients may also be lost to follow-up. Incomplete time to failure is called *censoring*, wherein we do not know how long censored observations will go until the event of interest occurs.

Let capital T denote the random variable for a person's survival time, which includes all numbers equal to or greater than zero. Let lowercase t denote any specific value of interest for the random variable T. For example, if we are interested in whether a heart transplant patient survives at least 5 years after undergoing surgery, $t = 5$

> **Definitions**
>
> **Survival analysis** involves modeling time to failure or time to event. The outcome variable is time to failure or event. Survival analysis is able to account for censoring, compare survival between two or more groups, and assess the relationship between covariates and survival time.
>
> **Censoring** means that we do not know the exact survival time. This is generally because a person does not experience the event before the end of the study, is lost to follow-up, or withdraws from the study because of death (if death is not the event under consideration) or other reasons (e.g., adverse reaction to an intervention).

and we are interested in whether T exceeds 5. A distribution of survival times may be characterized by a *survival function* $S(t)$. The survival function is the probability that an individual survives beyond some specified time t. When T is a continuous random variable, then

$$S(t) = P(T > t)$$

A survival curve is shown graphically as $S(t)$ plotted against t. A theoretical survival curve is depicted in **Figure 13.1**. In practice, however, actual data usually gives a graph that has a step function rather than a smooth curve, as shown in **Figure 13.2**.

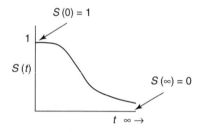

FIGURE 13.1 Theoretical $S(t)$.

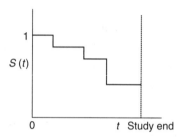

FIGURE 13.2 $S(t)$ in practice.

The purpose of this chapter is to describe two methods for evaluating survival data: the life table method (also called the actuarial method) and the product limit method (also called the Kaplan-Meier method). The log-rank test for evaluating differences in survival curves among two or more groups will also be presented.

THE LIFE TABLE METHOD

The life table method is the classic technique for estimating a survival curve. The computational ease in this approach made it the most commonly used method in medicine. It handles varying times of entry and varying times of withdrawal of individuals from the population. It calculates cumulative event-free probabilities and generates a survival curve.

In the life table method, survival times are grouped in intervals of fixed length, t to $t + n$; intervals should be mutually exclusive.

Life Table Notation for Survival Analysis

$q_x = \dfrac{d_x}{L_x + \frac{1}{2}d_x} = \dfrac{R_x}{1 + \frac{1}{2}R_x}$ is the probability of dying during the time interval t to $t + n$,

where $R_x = \dfrac{d_x}{L_x}$

$l_t = l_{t-1}(1 - q_{t-1}) =$ number alive at the beginning of the interval. l_0 is the radix and is an arbitrary value, typically 100,000

$d_t = l_t - l_{t+1} = q_t \times l_t =$ number of deaths during the time interval t to $t + n$

$p_t = 1 - q_t =$ probability of surviving in the time interval

$S(t) = \dfrac{l_t}{l_0} =$ proportion at time t that have not yet failed; cumulative probability of surviving at the beginning of the time interval or at the end of the previous interval

$S(t + 1) = p_{t+1} \times S(t)$

Additional Notation When Censoring Occurs

$w_t =$ number censored during the interval

$l' = l_t - w_t/2 =$ adjusted number at risk of the event in the interval

$q_t = \dfrac{d_t}{l'_t}$

In the life table method, we assume (1) there are no changes in survivorship over calendar time, (2) the experience of individuals who are lost to follow-up is the same as the experience of those who are followed, (3) withdrawal occurs uniformly within the interval, and (4) the event occurs uniformly within the interval.

EXAMPLE 13.1

A portion of the complete United States life table for 2006 is reproduced in **Table 13.1**.[1] The first column reflects the period of life between two exact ages stated in years. The second column is the proportion of persons dying during the interval. It is calculated from the age-specific death rates for the United States population in 2006. The third column begins with the radix equal to 100,000. To obtain the number of deaths in the next column, we multiply the proportion of persons dying during the interval by the radix to get 671. Then the number alive at the beginning of the next interval is:

$$l_2 = l_1 - d_1 = 100{,}000 - 671 = 99{,}329$$

TABLE 13.1   Life Table (Partial) for the Total Population in the United States, 2006

Age	Probability of dying during the time interval q_t	Number alive at the beginning of time t l_t	Number of deaths during the time interval d_t	Cumulative survival $S(t)$
0–<1	0.006713	100,000	671	1.00000
1–2	0.000444	99,329	44	0.99329
2–3	0.000300	99,285	30	0.99285
3–4	0.000216	99,255	21	0.99255
4–5	0.000179	99,233	18	0.99233
5–6	0.000168	99,216	17	0.99216
6–7	0.000156	99,199	15	0.99199
7–8	0.000143	99,184	14	0.99184
8–9	0.000125	99,169	12	0.99169
9–10	0.000103	99,157	10	0.99157
10–11	0.000086	99,147	9	0.99147
11–12	0.000088	99,138	9	0.99138
12–13	0.000125	99,130	12	0.99130
13–14	0.000206	99,117	20	0.99117
14–15	0.000317	99,097	31	0.99097
15–16	0.000438	99,065	43	0.99065
16–17	0.000552	99,022	55	0.99022
17–18	0.000657	98,967	65	0.98967
18–19	0.000747	98,902	74	0.98902
19–20	0.000825	98,828	82	0.98828
…				
98–99	0.282188	3,475	981	0.03475
99–100	0.303810	2,494	758	0.02494
100 and over	1.00000	1,737	1,737	0.01737

Data from: Arias E. United States life tables, 2006. *National vital statistics reports* 58(21). Hyattsville, MD: National Center for Health Statistics; 2010.

The fifth column is the survival function at time t, where

$$S(t) = \frac{l_t}{100,000}$$

The values of the third, fourth, and fifth columns are computed iteratively through the life table.

The survival curves for males and females in the United Sates, based on the life table approach, are presented in **Figure 13.3**. Females have greater survival than males across the age span. For our hypothetical cohort that we have aged through the life table, the proportion alive at age 70, for example, is 0.72 (or 72%) of males compared with 0.82 (or 82%) of females.

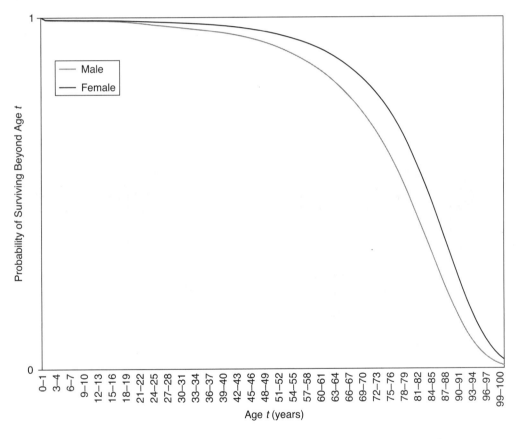

FIGURE 13.3 Survival curves for males and females in the United States population, 2006. *Data from:* Centers for Disease Control and Prevention. Behavior Risk Factor Surveillance System. Prevalence and Trend Data. Available at: http://apps.nccd.cdc.gov/BRFSS/. Accessed July 1, 2011.

The survival curves shown in Figure 13.3 reflect data from a *cross-sectional life table*. It was not practical to work with a *longitudinal life table*, which follows a cohort of individuals over their entire lifetimes, because this would take several decades. Hence, we apply current cross-sectional data to the life table. However, this approach assumes that current mortality rates will apply into the future, which may be unlikely. For smaller clinical studies in which patients are followed over a short period of time, a longitudinal life table is preferred.

EXAMPLE 13.2

Pancreatic cancer patients were diagnosed in 17 Surveillance, Epidemiology, and End Results (SEER) registries during 2003–2005 and followed up for survival status.[2] Cases were selected if they were actively followed with malignant pancreatic cancer. Cases were excluded if they were diagnosed at the time of autopsy and the cancer was a second or later primary. Initially, there were 19,109 patients. By monitoring the number of deaths among these patients each year and censoring and applying the equations for life table analysis, we obtained **Table 13.2**.

TABLE 13.2   Pancreatic Cancer Patients in 17 SEER Registries Diagnosed in 2003–2005, Followed through 3 Years after Diagnosis

Time since beginning of follow-up (years)	Number at beginning I_t	Deaths d_t	Number censored w_t	Adjusted number at risk I'	Probability of dying during the time interval $q_t = \dfrac{d_t}{I'}$	Probability of surviving the time interval $p_t = 1 - q_t$	Cumulative survival $\hat{S}(t)$
0	20,141	0	0	20,141	0.000	1.000	1.000
1	20,141	1,912	0	20,141	0.095	0.905	0.905
2	18,229	3,288	24	18,217	0.180	0.820	0.742
3	14,917	2,154	12	14,911	0.144	0.856	0.635
4	12,751	1,607	8	12,747	0.126	0.874	0.555
5	11,136	1,307	9	11,132	0.117	0.883	0.489
6	9,820	1,031	7	9,817	0.105	0.895	0.438

TABLE 13.2   Pancreatic Cancer Patients in 17 SEER Registries Diagnosed in 2003–2005, Followed through 3 Years after Diagnosis (*continued*)

Time since beginning of follow-up (years)	Number at beginning l_t	Deaths d_t	Number censored w_t	Adjusted number at risk l'	Probability of dying during the time interval $q_t = \dfrac{d_t}{l'}$	Probability of surviving the time interval $p_t = 1 - q_t$	Cumulative survival $\hat{S}(t)$
7	8,782	948	5	8,780	0.108	0.892	0.391
8	7,829	758	7	7,826	0.097	0.903	0.353
9	7,064	645	2	7,063	0.091	0.909	0.321
10	6,417	598	1	6,417	0.093	0.907	0.291
11	5,818	502	3	5,817	0.086	0.914	0.266
12	5,313	442	2	5,312	0.083	0.917	0.244
13	4,869	431	2	4,868	0.089	0.911	0.222
14	4,436	305	3	4,435	0.069	0.931	0.207
15	4,128	315	1	4,128	0.076	0.924	0.191
16	3,812	271	0	3,812	0.071	0.929	0.177
17	3,541	236	4	3,539	0.067	0.933	0.166
18	3,301	226	4	3,299	0.069	0.931	0.154
19	3,071	171	3	3,070	0.056	0.944	0.146
20	2,897	178	1	2,897	0.061	0.939	0.137
21	2,718	146	1	2,718	0.054	0.946	0.129
22	2,571	130	2	2,570	0.051	0.949	0.123
23	2,439	120	3	2,438	0.049	0.951	0.117
24	2,316	106	4	2,314	0.046	0.954	0.111
25	2,206	96	2	2,205	0.044	0.956	0.107
26	2,108	94	0	2,108	0.045	0.955	0.102
27	2,014	76	3	2,013	0.038	0.962	0.098
28	1,935	77	2	1,934	0.040	0.960	0.094

(continues)

TABLE 13.2   Pancreatic Cancer Patients in 17 SEER Registries Diagnosed in 2003–2005, Followed through 3 Years after Diagnosis (*continued*)

Time since beginning of follow-up (years)	Number at beginning l_t	Deaths d_t	Number censored w_t	Adjusted number at risk l'	Probability of dying during the time interval $q_t = \dfrac{d_t}{l'}$	Probability of surviving the time interval $p_t = 1 - q_t$	Cumulative survival $\hat{S}(t)$
29	1,856	66	1	1,856	0.036	0.964	0.091
30	1,789	61	1	1,789	0.034	0.966	0.088
31	1,727	62	2	1,726	0.036	0.964	0.084
32	1,663	49	3	1,662	0.029	0.971	0.082
33	1,611	51	3	1,610	0.032	0.968	0.079
34	1,557	43	4	1,555	0.028	0.972	0.077
35	1,510	50	1	1,510	0.033	0.967	0.075
36	1,459	44	0	1,459	0.030	0.970	0.072

Data from: Surveillance, Epidemiology, and End Results (SEER) Program (www.seer.cancer.gov). SEER*Stat Database: Mortality—All COD, Aggregated with State, Total U.S. (1969–2007) <Katrina/Rita Population Adjustment>, National Cancer Institute, DCCPS, Surveillance Research Program, Cancer Statistics Branch, released June 2010. Underlying mortality data provided by NCHS (www.cdc.gov/nchs).

The survival curve is plotted, using the life table method versus the point representing the start of each interval, and then the points were connected (**Figure 13.4**). Above 50% of the cohort died within 5 months of diagnosis.

EXAMPLE 13.3

To conclude this section on the life table method for estimating survival, consider 30 black pancreatic cancer patients diagnosed in Connecticut during 2000–2002 (**Table 13.3**). The number of deaths and censored cases each year are presented in the table. Iteratively calculating the probability of death and survival in each interval gives the results shown in the table. The small numbers and relatively good survival for this cancer show several intervals with no failures. Consequently, this data would be better assessed using the Product Limit method.

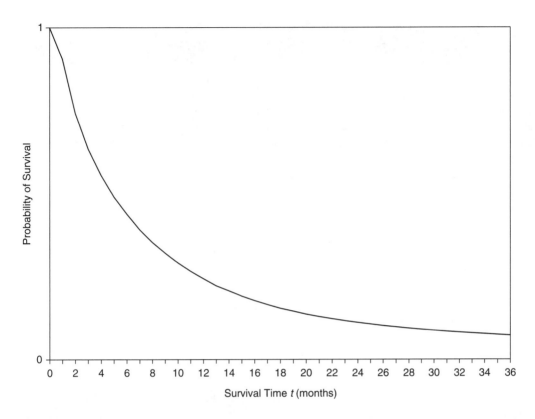

FIGURE 13.4 Survival curve for pancreatic cancer patients diagnosed in 2003–2005 and followed for 3 years.

Data from: Surveillance, Epidemiology, and End Results (SEER) Program (www.seer.cancer.gov). SEER*Stat Database: Mortality—All COD, Aggregated with State, Total U.S. (1969–2007) <Katrina/ Rita Population Adjustment>, National Cancer Institute, DCCPS, Surveillance Research Program, Cancer Statistics Branch, released June 2010. Underlying mortality data provided by NCHS (www.cdc .gov/nchs).

THE PRODUCT LIMIT METHOD

With the product limit method, instead of grouping survival times into intervals, as is done with the life table method, the exact survival time is used for each individual. Thus, it provides a more exact description of the pattern of survival seen in the cohort of patients; that is, this approach uses the exact times at which failures occur. This method generates the characteristic "stair step" survival curves. It is especially preferred with small data sets in which there can be intervals where failure does not occur.

TABLE 13.3   Liver Cancer in Black Patients in Connecticut, 2000–2002, Followed for 3 Years after Diagnosis

Time since beginning of follow-up (years)	Number at beginning l_t	Deaths d_t	Number censored w_t	Adjusted number at risk l'	Probability of dying during the time interval $q_t = \dfrac{d_t}{l'}$	Probability of surviving the time interval $p_t = 1 - q_t$	Cumulative survival $\hat{S}(t)$
0	30	0	0	30	0.000	1.000	1
1	30	1	0	30	0.033	0.967	0.967
2	29	4	0	29	0.138	0.862	0.833
3	25	1	0	25	0.040	0.960	0.800
4	24	2	0	24	0.083	0.917	0.733
5	22	0	0	22	0.000	1.000	0.733
6	22	2	0	22	0.091	0.909	0.667
7	20	0	0	20	0.000	1.000	0.667
8	20	0	0	20	0.000	1.000	0.667
9	20	2	0	20	0.100	0.900	0.600
10	18	0	0	18	0.000	1.000	0.600
11	18	0	0	18	0.000	1.000	0.600
12	18	0	0	18	0.000	1.000	0.600
13	18	0	1	18	0.000	1.000	0.600
14	17	0	0	17	0.000	1.000	0.600
15	17	0	0	17	0.000	1.000	0.600
16	17	0	0	17	0.000	1.000	0.600
17	17	0	1	17	0.000	1.000	0.600
18	16	0	0	16	0.000	1.000	0.600
19	16	1	0	16	0.063	0.938	0.563
20	15	0	0	15	0.000	1.000	0.563

TABLE 13.3   Liver Cancer in Black Patients in Connecticut, 2000–2002, Followed for 3 Years after Diagnosis (*continued*)

Time since beginning of follow-up (years)	Number at beginning l_t	Deaths d_t	Number censored w_t	Adjusted number at risk l'	Probability of dying during the time interval $q_t = \dfrac{d_t}{l'}$	Probability of surviving the time interval $p_t = 1 - q_t$	Cumulative survival $\hat{S}(t)$
21	15	0	0	15	0.000	1.000	0.563
22	15	1	0	15	0.067	0.933	0.525
23	14	0	0	14	0.000	1.000	0.525
24	14	0	0	14	0.000	1.000	0.525
25	14	0	0	14	0.000	1.000	0.525
26	14	0	0	14	0.000	1.000	0.525
27	14	0	0	14	0.000	1.000	0.525
28	14	0	0	14	0.000	1.000	0.525
29	14	0	0	14	0.000	1.000	0.525
30	14	0	0	14	0.000	1.000	0.525
31	14	0	0	14	0.000	1.000	0.525
32	14	0	0	14	0.000	1.000	0.525
33	14	0	0	14	0.000	1.000	0.525
34	14	0	0	14	0.000	1.000	0.525
35	14	0	0	14	0.000	1.000	0.525
36	14	0	0	14	0.000	1.000	0.525

Data from: Surveillance, Epidemiology, and End Results (SEER) Program (www.seer.cancer.gov). SEER*Stat Database: Mortality—All COD, Aggregated with State, Total U.S. (1969–2007) <Katrina/Rita Population Adjustment>, National Cancer Institute, DCCPS, Surveillance Research Program, Cancer Statistics Branch, released June 2010. Underlying mortality data provided by NCHS (www.cdc.gov/nchs).

The product limit method uses exact survival times, whereas the life table method groups survival times into intervals. With the computer, the product limit method is much more feasible with large data sets.

Features of the Product Limit Method[2]
1. The exact times events occur—rather than the intervals of follow-up.
2. The probability of the event is equal to the number of events at that time divided by the number at risk at that point in time (including those who had the events).
3. If there are withdrawals before the time of event, they are subtracted from the number at risk.

EXAMPLE 13.4

Table 13.4 shows the product limit estimate of the survival function based on the 30 patients presented in the previous example. With this method, survival at time t is assumed to remain the same over the time periods between deaths. In other words, it only changes when a subject fails. The left column of the table lists the months when a death or dropout occurred. Then, for each time a failure occurs, the probability of dying during the time interval, the probability of surviving in the time interval, and the cumulative probability of survival are presented. The survival curve corresponding to the function in Table 13.4 is presented in **Figure 13.5**. When the product limit method is used, $\hat{S}(t)$ is assumed to remain the same over the time periods between deaths, changing precisely when the subject fails.

TABLE 13.4   Product Limit Method of Estimating S(t) for 30 Liver Cancer Patients

Time (months)	q_t	p_t	$\hat{S}(t)$
0	0.000	1.000	1.000
1	0.033	0.967	0.967
2	0.138	0.862	0.833
3	0.040	0.960	0.800
4	0.083	0.917	0.733
6	0.091	0.909	0.667
9	0.100	0.900	0.600
19	0.063	0.938	0.563
22	0.067	0.933	0.525

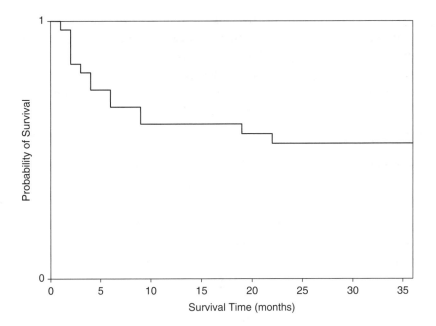

FIGURE 13.5 Survival curve for liver cancer among black patients diagnosed in 2000–2002 in Connecticut and followed for 3 years.
Data from: Surveillance, Epidemiology, and End Results (SEER) Program (www.seer.cancer.gov). SEER*Stat Database: Mortality–All COD, Aggregated with State, Total U.S. (1969–2007) <Katrina/ Rita Population Adjustment>, National Cancer Institute, DCCPS, Surveillance Research Program, Cancer Statistics Branch, released June 2010. Underlying mortality data provided by NCHS (www.cdc .gov/nchs).

LOG-RANK TEST

Investigators are often interested in comparing distributions of survival between two groups of patients. To compare whether survival curves significantly differ between groups, we need to apply a statistical test to the data. If no censored observations occur, then the *Wilcoxon rank-sum test* is appropriate for comparing the ranks of survival times between groups. This method is used to compare the median survival times. However, if some observations are censored, the nonparametric technique called the *log-rank test* is commonly used to evaluated whether the two distributions of survival times are identical or different. The Wilcoxon test places greater weights on events near time 0 than the log-rank test and, thus, is more likely to detect early differences.

The log-rank test involves a series of 2×2 contingency tables displaying the group versus survival status for each time t that a death occurred. After the entire sequence of tables is constructed, the data are assessed using the *Mantel-Haenszel chi-square* statistic, which compares the observed number of failures at each time to the expected number of failures given that the distributions of survival times for the two groups are identical. If the null hypothesis is true, the test statistic has an approximate chi-square distribution with a single degree of freedom. This approach is computationally tedious, so we will use the computer to calculate the log-rank test.

EXAMPLE 13.5

Pancreatic cancer patients who were black and diagnosed with localized disease in one of the 17 SEER registries in 2005 were followed up for survival status.[2] Cases were selected if they were actively followed and excluded if they were diagnosed at the time of autopsy or if the cancer was a second or later primary. The male and female cases included in the study are shown in **Table 13.5**. The log-rank test will be used to evaluate the hypotheses:

1. H_0: $S_M(t) = S_F(t)$
2. H_a: $S_M(t) \neq S_F(t)$

TABLE 13.5   Time to Death for Black Pancreatic Cancer Cases Diagnosed with Localized Disease in 2005 According to Sex

	Male			Female	
Patient number	Survival (months)	Censored*	Patient number	Survival (months)	Censored*
1	1	1	1	1	1
2	2	1	2	2	1
3	2	1	3	2	1
4	3	1	4	3	1
5	4	1	5	3	1
6	5	1	6	3	1
7	6	1	7	3	1
8	7	1	8	4	1
9	9	1	9	6	1
10	12	1	10	6	1
11	12	1	11	7	1
12	13	1	12	7	1
13	15	1	13	7	1

TABLE 13.5	Time to Death for Black Pancreatic Cancer Cases Diagnosed with Localized Disease in 2005 According to Sex *(continued)*				
Male			**Female**		
Patient number	**Survival (months)**	**Censored***	**Patient number**	**Survival (months)**	**Censored***
14	16	1	14	8	1
15	35	1	15	8	1
16	31	1	16	8	0
17	36	1	17	10	1
18	42	1	18	11	1
19	43	0	19	13	1
20	45	0	20	14	1
			21	17	1
			22	17	0
			23	18	1
			24	20	1
			25	22	1
			26	22	1
			27	23	1
			28	32	1
			29	35	1
			30	37	0
			31	39	0
			32	39	0
			33	39	0
			34	39	0
			35	39	0
			36	39	0
			37	46	0

*An event or failure is indicated by 1, and censoring is indicated by 0.

Data from: Surveillance, Epidemiology, and End Results (SEER) Program (www.seer.cancer.gov). SEER*Stat Database: Mortality—All COD, Aggregated with State, Total U.S. (1969–2007) <Katrina/Rita Population Adjustment>, National Cancer Institute, DCCPS, Surveillance Research Program, Cancer Statistics Branch, released June 2010. Underlying mortality data provided by NCHS (www.cdc.gov/nchs).

3. $\alpha = 0.05$, $n = 57$
4. Log-rank test with 1 degree of freedom
5. Using the PROC LIFETEST in SAS gives the following:

Test of Equality over Strata			
Test	**Chi-square**	**DF**	**Pr > Chi-square**
Log-rank	0.6916	1	0.4056
Wilcoxon	0.4693	1	0.4933

6. Because the P value is greater than 0.05, we fail to reject H_0 and conclude that the survival is similar between male and female patients. The SAS-generated graph for this data is shown in **Figure 13.6**.

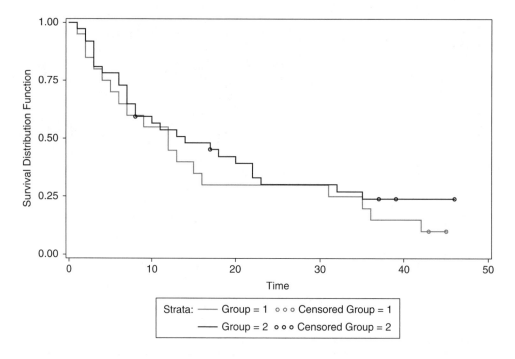

FIGURE 13.6 Kaplan-Meier survival curves for pancreatic cancer generated by SAS. (*Group = 1* refers to Males and *Group = 2* refers to females).

EXAMPLE 13.6

Gallbladder cancer patients who were diagnosed in New Mexico during 2005 were followed up for survival status.[2] Cases were selected if they were actively followed and were not diagnosed at the time of autopsy and if the cancer was a first primary. Cases are presented according to stage at diagnosis in **Table 13.6**. The steps of hypothesis testing give the following:

1. H_0: *No difference in survival curves*
2. H_a: *Difference in survival curves*

TABLE 13.6	Time to Death for Gallbladder Cancer Cases Diagnosed in New Mexico During 2005 According to Tumor Stage							
Local			Regional			Distant		
Patient number	Survival (months)	Censored*	Patient number	Survival (months)	Censored*	Patient number	Survival (months)	Censored*
1	1	1	1	3	1	1	4	1
2	6	1	2	4	1	2	4	1
3	8	1	3	5	1	3	4	1
4	9	1	4	6	1	4	6	1
5	9	1	5	7	1	5	14	1
6	20	1	6	10	1	6	20	1
7	21	1	7	14	1			
8	30	1	8	38	0			
9	35	0						
10	39	0						
11	44	0						
12	46	0						
13	48	0						

*An event or failure is indicated by 1, and censoring is indicated by 0.

Data from: Surveillance, Epidemiology, and End Results (SEER) Program (www.seer.cancer.gov). SEER*Stat Database: Mortality—All COD, Aggregated with State, Total U.S. (1969–2007) <Katrina/Rita Population Adjustment>, National Cancer Institute, DCCPS, Surveillance Research Program, Cancer Statistics Branch, released June 2010. Underlying mortality data provided by NCHS (www.cdc.gov/nchs).

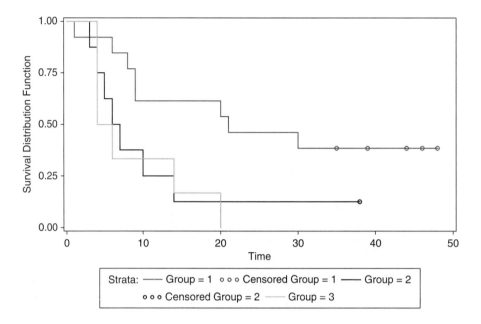

FIGURE 13.7 Kaplan-Meier survival curves for gallbladder cancer generated by SAS. (*Group = 1* refers to local stage, *Group = 2* refers to regional stage, and *Group 3* refers to distant stage).

3. $\alpha = 0.05$, $n = 27$
4. Log-rank test with 2 degrees of freedom
5. Using the PROC LIFETEST in SAS gives the following:

Test of Equality over Strata			
Test	**Chi-square**	**DF**	**Pr > Chi-square**
Log-rank	6.5908	2	0.0371
Wilcoxon	6.1435	2	0.0463

6. Because the *P* value is less than 0.05, we reject H_0 and conclude that the survival among the gallbladder cases is different among stage groups. The SAS-generated graph for this data is shown in **Figure 13.7**.

EXERCISES

1. What is survival analysis?
2. What are censored observations and how do they occur?
3. What is a survival function?

4. What is the primary difference between the life table method of estimating a survival curve and the product limit method?

5. Suppose you are interested in the survival times of 17 women, aged 70–79 years, diagnosed with ovarian cancer who were not recommended therapy because of other conditions.[2] Use the life table procedure to summarize the data for the 17 patients.

Patient number	Survival (months)	Patient number	Survival (months)
1	1	10	3
2	1	11	5
3	1	12	6
4	1	13	10
5	1	14	17
6	2	15	18
7	2	16	19
8	2	17	34
9	2		

6. Use the product limit method and display the estimate of the survival function using SAS.

7. What is the median survival?

8. What is the mean survival?

9. For the following abridged life table that reflects the total population in the United States, 2006, estimate and plot the survival curve.

Age	Probability of dying between ages x and x + n $_nq_x$	Number surviving to age x l_x	Number dying between ages x and x + n $_nd_x$	Person-years lived between ages x and x + n $_nL_x$	Total number of person-years lived about age x T_x	Expectation of life at age x e_x
0–<1	0.00671	100,000	671	99,409	7,769,651	77.7
1–4	0.00114	99,329	113	397,089	7,670,242	77.2
5–9	0.00069	99,216	69	495,906	7,273,153	73.3

(continues)

Age	Probability of dying between ages x and $x + n$ $_nq_x$	Number surviving to age x l_x	Number dying between ages x and $x + n$ $_nd_x$	Person-years lived between ages x and $x + n$ $_nL_x$	Total number of person-years lived about age x T_x	Expectation of life at age x e_x
10–14	0.00082	99,147	81	495,530	6,777,247	68.4
15–19	0.00321	99,065	318	494,531	6,281,717	63.4
20–24	0.00500	98,747	494	492,501	5,787,186	58.6
25–29	0.00503	98,253	495	490,031	5,294,686	53.9
30–34	0.00558	97,759	546	487,430	4,804,655	49.1
35–39	0.00739	97,213	718	484,270	4,317,225	44.4
40–44	0.01138	96,495	1,098	479,729	3,832,955	39.7
45–49	0.01726	95,397	1,647	472,866	3,353,227	35.2
50–54	0.02558	93,750	2,398	462,754	2,880,361	30.7
55–59	0.03606	91,352	3,295	448,523	2,417,607	26.5
60–64	0.05458	88,057	4,806	428,272	1,969,084	22.4
65–69	0.07917	83,251	6,591	399,781	1,540,811	18.5
70–74	0.12170	76,661	9,330	359,980	1,141,031	14.9
75–79	0.19501	67,331	13,130	303,831	781,051	11.6
80–84	0.30251	54,201	16,396	230,015	477,220	8.8
85–89	0.44721	37,805	16,907	146,757	247,205	6.5
90–94	0.61764	20,898	12,907	72,221	100,448	4.8
95–99	0.78268	7,991	6,254	24,318	28,227	3.5
100 and over	1.00000	1,737	1,737	3,909	3,909	2.3

10. Consider the following data. Treat the last two patients in the 60- to 69-year age group as censored. Test the hypothesis of difference in survival between the two age groups and plot the survival curves.

Patient number	Survival (months) Ages 60–69	Patient number	Survival (months) Ages 70–79
1	2	1	1
2	2	2	1
3	3	3	1
4	3	4	1
5	3	5	1
6	3	6	2
7	5	7	2
8	6	8	2
9	6	9	2
10	6	10	3
11	10	11	5
12	13	12	6
13	14	13	10
14	17	14	17
15	28	15	18
16	30	16	19
17	34	17	34
18	36		
19	36		
20	40		
21	41		

REFERENCES

1. Arias E. United States life tables, 2006. *National Vital Statistics Reports.* 58(21). Hyattsville, MD: National Center for Health Statistics; 2010.

2. Surveillance, Epidemiology, and End Results (SEER) Program (www.seer.cancer.gov). SEER*Stat Database: Mortality—All COD, Aggregated with State, Total U.S. (1969–2007) <Katrina/Rita Population Adjustment>, National Cancer Institute, DCCPS, Surveillance Research Program, Cancer Statistics Branch. Underlying mortality data provided by NCHS (www.cdc.gov/nchs). Released June 2010. Accessed September 3, 2011.

3. Diener-West M, Kanchanaraksa S. Life Tables. http://ocw.jhsph.edu/courses/FundEpi/PDFs/Lecture8.pdf. Published 2008. Accessed August 5, 2011.

CHAPTER 14

Cause and Effect

Throughout history, it has been observed that certain exposures, conditions, or behaviors tend to be associated with disease. Hippocrates, for example, observed that diseases like yellow fever and malaria were more common among people who lived near swampy areas.[1,2] However, it was not until 1900 that Walter Reed identified the mosquito as a vector for this disease.[3] More recently, the surgeon general of the United States concluded in 1964 that based on evidence from 29 case-control studies and 7 cohort studies, smoking is causally associated with lung cancer.[4]

History

Walter Reed (1851–1902) was a U.S. army physician. In May 1900, Reed was appointed head of the army board that the surgeon general charged with investigating tropical diseases, including yellow fever. While Reed was with the U.S. Army Yellow Fever Commission in Cuba, the board confirmed the transmission of yellow fever by mosquitoes. This finding dispelled the common belief that yellow fever could be transmitted by fomites such as clothing and bedding soiled by the body fluids and excrement of yellow fever sufferers. Many consider Reed's breakthrough in yellow fever research to be a milestone in biomedicine.[3]

Identifying the determinants (or causes) of health-related states or events is a central aim in epidemiology in order to prevent and control health problems. A cause produces an effect, result, or consequence. Without conclusions about cause-and-effect relationships, individuals and public health officials would not be able to make informed decisions; rather, they would be left to merely react to individual and public health crises. The connection between human health and physical, chemical, biological, social, and psychosocial factors is based on causal inference. The purpose of this chapter is to define causal inference, list selected criteria for establishing a cause-and-effect relationship, present selected causal models, and introduce webs of causation.

CAUSAL INFERENCE

Statistical inference involves reaching a conclusion about a population based on information from a sample, and using probability to indicate the level of reliability of that conclusion. Sample data are evaluated using statistical methods such as regression and survival analysis, and conclusions are drawn about the population. On the other hand, *causal inference* involves making conclusions about associations between variables based on lists of criteria or conditions applied to the results of scientific studies. Causal inference considers the totality of evidence in making a "judgment" about causality.[5] Causal inference provides a scientific basis for individual, medical, and public health action.

A valid statistical association does not necessarily mean that the association is causal. For example, in the 1700s, life expectancy in the United States was below 50 years. Today, life expectancy is about 80 years. Because people did not drive automobiles in the 1700s, but today most adults do, can we say that driving automobiles has extended life expectancy? No. The explanation is likely because in the earlier century, there were much higher rates of infant mortality, higher rates of women dying during childbirth, and higher rates of infectious disease.

Throughout our daily lives, each of us infers that something is true or highly probable based on our expectations and experiences. We may shower every day because we expect it will help our social relations, or we may eat a balanced diet because we expect it will help us maintain good physical and emotional health. Inference in epidemiology is similar to inference in daily life in that it also is based on expectations and experience; however, in science, expectations are referred to as *hypotheses, theories,* or *predictions,* and experiences are called *results, observations,* or *data.*[5] Inference in everyday life serves as a basis for action. In a similar manner, causal inference provides a scientific basis for medical and public health action.

The inferences we personally make are informal and based on expectations about a given event, reasons for its existence, and experience with similar situations. In contrast, scientists typically base their inferences on the application of formal methods. For instance, on the basis of sample data we may draw certain conclusions about the population. Probability is used to indicate the level of reliability in the conclusion. Sample techniques are used to obtain a representative sample, and data are evaluated using statistical methods.

In 1856, philosopher John Stuart Mill established three methods of hypothesis formulation in disease etiology: the method of difference, the method of agreement, and the method of concomitant variation.[6] These are described in **Table 14.1**.

Since Mill's postulates, others have developed criteria for causal inference (**Table 14.2**). Although criteria have been added over time, the evolutionary changes between 1959 and 1973 were minor. Causal methods used since are essentially the

TABLE 14.1 John Stuart Mill's Three Methods of Hypothesis Formulation in Disease Etiology

Method	Definition	Example
Method of difference	The frequency of disease occurrence is extremely different under different situations or conditions. If a risk factor can be identified in one condition and not in a second, it may be that factor, or the absence of it, that causes the disease.	Colon cancer is comparatively much lower in Japan than in the United States. The rate of colon cancer among Japanese immigrants to this country approaches the risk of people born in the United States, suggesting that lifestyle has a large influence on colon cancer risk.
Method of agreement	If a risk factor is common to a variety of different circumstances and the risk factor has been positively associated with a disease, then the probability of that factor being the cause is extremely high.	AIDS is relatively high in hemophiliacs, recipients of transfusions, and intravenous drug abusers, suggesting that the mode of transmission is the human immunodeficiency virus introduced into the blood.
Method of concomitant variation	The frequency or strength of a risk factor varies with the frequency of the disease.	Coronary heart disease rates are greater in areas with higher levels of fine particulate matter in the air.

Data from: Mills JS. *A System of Logic, Ratiocinative and Inductive.* 5th ed. London: Parker, Son and Bowin; 1862.

same. Definitions for selected criteria are summarized in **Table 14.3**. In general, the order in which epidemiologic study designs are effective at establishing causal associations is shown in **Figure 14.1**. The ranking involves the ability of the study design to establish a valid statistical association, a temporal sequence of events, and a biological gradient.

Although the randomized, blinded clinical trial provides the strongest evidence of a cause-and-effect association, it is often not appropriate or feasible to implement this study design. When randomization is not used, *propensity scoring* is a way to strengthen causal inferences. The propensity score is a conditional probability and is used to reduce selection bias by matching participants or patients on the probability

TABLE 14.2   Criteria for Causal Inference

Lilienfeld (1959)[7]	Sartwell (1960)[8]	Surgeon General (1964)[9] and Susser (1973)[10]	Hill (1965)[11]	MacMahon and Pugh (1970)[12]
• Consistency	• Replication	• Consistency	• Consistency	• Strength of association (including magnitude of association and dose-response)
• Magnitude of effect	• Strength of association	• Strength of association (including magnitude of effect and dose-response)	• Strength of association	
• Dose-response	• Dose-response		• Biological gradient	
• Biological mechanism	• Temporality		• Temporality	• Temporality
	• Biological reasonableness	• Temporality	• Experimental evidence	• Experimentation
		• Biological coherence	• Biological plausibility	• Consonance with existing knowledge
		• Specificity	• Biological coherence	• Biological mechanisms
			• Specificity	• Consistency
			• Analogy	• Exclusion of alternative explanations

Data from: Lilienfeld AM. On the methodology of investigations of etiologic factors in chronic diseases—some comments. *J Chronic Dis.* 1959;10:41–46. Sartwell PE. On the methodology of investigations of etiologic factors in chronic diseases—further comments. *J Chronic Dis.* 1960;11:61–63. Surgeon General's Advisory Committee on Smoking and Health. *Smoking and health: 1964.* Rockville, MD: U.S. Public Health Service, 1964 (DHEW publication no. (PHS) 1103). Susser M. *Causal Thinking in the Health Sciences.* New York, NY: Oxford University Press; 1973. Hill AB. The environment and disease: association or causation? *Proc R Soc Med.* 1965;58:295–300. MacMahon B, Pugh TF. *Epidemiology: Principles and Methods.* Boston, MA: Little, Brown, and Company; 1970.

that they would be assigned to a specific group. The interested reader may refer to other sources to learn more about propensity scores.[13–18]

To conclude this section, statistical methods alone are insufficient for establishing a cause-and-effect relationship. Conclusions about causality are based on the totality of evidence and involve judgment. Certainly, there is the possibility of error in causal inference, but it is a means to preventing and controlling health problems. The recommended systematic approach to causal inference is shown in **Figure 14.2**.

TABLE 14.3	**Description of Selected Causal Criteria**

Criterion	Definition
Strength of association	Following a research question, we formulate a hypothesis about the association between variables. A study design and an appropriate statistical test are then applied to the data. We either reject or fail to reject the null hypothesis. We then need to consider whether a measured association, or lack thereof, is real, because the measured relationship could be influenced by chance, bias, or confounding. A chance finding may result from nonrandom sampling or random sampling with small numbers, bias may influence the results if data are not correctly representative because of selection or observation, and confounding may cause a spurious result because it is not properly controlled for in the study design or analysis.
	In general, a stronger statistical association between an exposure and outcome provides greater evidence that the association is real.
Consistency of association	When measured associations are consistent in their direction among many different studies performed by various investigators in a range of settings with different methods, this strengthens the evidence of there being a causal association. If this criterion is satisfied, it further supports that a statistical association is real.
Specificity	Specificity of association means an exposure is associated with only one disease or that the disease is associated with only one exposure. If the biological response to the exposure varies, it is less likely to be causal. While this criterion can support a causal hypothesis, failure to satisfy it cannot rule out causality. For example, increased risk of lung cancer is associated with cigarette smoking, diet, radon gas, and asbestos. On the other hand, cigarette smoking has been associated with several cancers, heart disease, and stroke.
Temporal relationship of association	This is a very important criterion because in order for an exposure to cause a disease, the exposure must precede the disease. Temporality can be established in cohort and experimental studies, but it is often difficult or impossible to verify in other types of study designs.
Biological gradient	This exists if an increasing amount of exposure increases the risk of the outcome. However, a threshold value may exist and the biological gradient may not be linear.
Biological plausibility	Of interest is whether the association is biologically supported. Biological assessment often involves experiments in controlled laboratory environments involving animals.
Coherence	Causal inference is consistent with known epidemiologic patterns of disease.
Experimental evidence	The randomized, double-blind experimental study design is the best for establishing a cause-and-effect relationship. This is because the experimental aspect of the study design allows the researcher to have greater control over exposure levels and outcome measures, and randomization is effective at balancing out the effect of known and unknown confounders. In addition, blinding is an effective way to minimize bias. However, the use of randomization and blinding may be limited because of feasibility and ethical issues.

CAUSAL MODELS

A simple causal model for an outbreak of infectious disease that takes into account the interrelatedness of selected factors is the *epidemiology triangle*. This model involves the agent or disease-causing organism; the host; the environmental circumstances needed for a disease to thrive, survive, and spread; and time-related issues. The traditional triangle of epidemiology is shown in **Figure 14.3**.

An agent of infectious disease may be a pathogen (i.e., bacteria, virus, parasite, fungi, or mold). An agent for a noninfectious disease, disability, injury, or death may be a chemical from dietary foods, tobacco smoke, solvents, radiation or heat, rattlesnake poison, and so on. One or a combination of agents may contribute to an illness. A host offers subsistence and lodging for a pathogen and may or may not develop the disease. The level of immunity, genetic makeup, level of exposure, state of health, makeup of the host, and ability of the pathogen to accept the new environment can all influence the disease outcome. Environmental factors include the biological aspects as well as physical stresses (e.g., excessive heat, cold, and noise; radiation and vehicular collisions; workplace injuries), chemical influences (e.g., drugs, acids, alkali, heavy metals, poisons, and some enzymes), and psychosocial milieu (e.g., families and households, socioeconomic status, social networks and social support, neighborhoods and communities, formal institutions, and public health policy). The surroundings in which a pathogen lives and the effect the surroundings have on it are a part of the environment. An environment can be within a host or external to it in the community. Finally, time includes the severity of illness in relation to how long a person is infected or until the condition causes death or passes the threshold of danger toward recovery. Delays in time from infection to when symptoms develop, duration of illness, and threshold of an epidemic in a population are time elements with which the epidemiologist is concerned.

Definitions

The **agent** is the cause of the disease.

The **host** is an organism, usually a human or an animal, that harbors the disease.

The **environment** includes those surroundings and conditions external to the human or animal that cause or allow disease transmission.

Time accounts for incubation periods, life expectancy of the host or the pathogen, and duration of the course of the illness or condition.

Rank	Study Design
1	Randomized controlled trial
2	Community trial
3	Prospective cohort study
4	Retrospective cohort study
5	Case-control study
6	Cross-sectional study
7	Ecologic study
8	Case report or case series

FIGURE 14.1 Ranking of study designs for supporting causality.

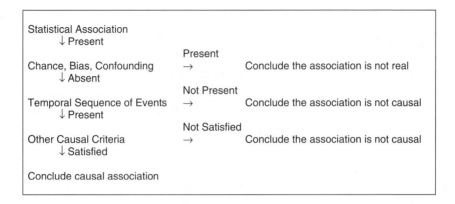

Statistical Association
↓ Present

Chance, Bias, Confounding   Present
↓ Absent   →   Conclude the association is not real

Temporal Sequence of Events   Not Present
↓ Present   →   Conclude the association is not causal

Other Causal Criteria   Not Satisfied
↓ Satisfied   →   Conclude the association is not causal

Conclude causal association

FIGURE 14.2 Systematic approach to causal inference.

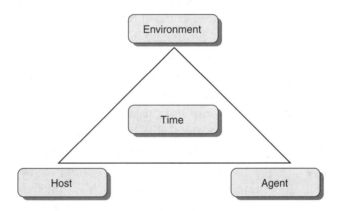

FIGURE 14.3 The triangle of epidemiology.
Source: Merrill R. *Introduction to Epidemiology. 5th ed.* Sudbury, MA: Jones & Bartlett Learning; 2010.

An epidemic can be stopped when one of the elements of the triangle is interfered with, altered, changed, or removed from existence so that the disease no longer continues along its mode of transmission.

MODES OF DISEASE TRANSMISSION

Disease transmission can be discussed in terms of communicability (vertical and horizontal) and disease transmission concepts. *Vertical transmission* is spread of an infectious agent from an individual to its offspring through sperm, placenta, milk, or vaginal fluids. *Horizontal transmission* is spread of an infectious agent from an infected individual to a

Definitions

Direct transmission is the direct and immediate transfer of an agent from a host/reservoir to a susceptible host. Direct transmission can occur through direct physical contact or direct person-to-person contact, such as touching with contaminated hands, skin-to-skin contact, kissing, or sexual intercourse.

Indirect transmission occurs when an agent is transferred or carried by some intermediate item, organism, means, or process to a susceptible host, resulting in disease (e.g., fomites, vectors, air currents, dust particles, water, food, oral–fecal contact, and other mechanisms that effectively transfer disease-causing organisms).

Mechanical transmission involves vector-borne disease transmission processes that are simply mechanical processes, such as when the pathogen, in order to spread, uses a host (e.g., a fly, flea, louse, or rat) as a mechanism for a ride, for nourishment, or as part of a physical transfer process.

Biological transmission is when the pathogen undergoes changes as part of its life cycle while within the host/vector and before being transmitted to the new host. For example, biological transmission occurs for malaria when the female Anopheles mosquito's blood meal is required for the Plasmodium protozoan parasite to complete its sexual development cycle. This can occur only with the ingested blood nutrients found in the intestine of the Anopheles mosquito.

susceptible contemporary. A *direct causal association* means that the cause and outcome relationship has no intermediate factor. For example, a trauma to the skin results in a bruise or infection while Salmonella results in enteritis. Eliminating the exposure will eliminate the adverse health outcome. On the other hand, an *indirect causal association* involves one or more intervening factors and is often much more complicated. For instance, poor diet and stress may cause high blood pressure, which in turn causes heart disease, wherein, diet and stress indirectly influence heart disease. It is also possible for there to be both direct and indirect causal associations. For example, a person may directly contract rabies by inhalation as she enters a cave where rabies-infected bats roost. He/she may also contract the disease by an infected skunk or fox living in the bat-infested cave.

Indirect transmission may involve *airborne transmission*, when droplets or dust particles carry the pathogen to the host and cause infection; *waterborne transmission*, when a pathogen such as cholera or shigellosis is carried in drinking water, swimming pools, streams, or lakes used for swimming; or *vehicle-borne transmission*, which involves transmission by a fomite such as eating utensils, clothing, washing items, combs, and shared drinking bottles.

The epidemiology triangle as used in a discussion of communicable disease is basic and foundational to all epidemiology. Another causal model that captures the fact that many health-related states or events result from the influence of multiple factors is Rothman's causal pies.[19] Rothman and other epidemiologists have stressed that the *one cause–one effect* understanding is overly simplistic because most health outcomes, whether illness or death, are caused by a chain or web consisting of many component causes. Causes can be distinguished as necessary, sufficient, or probabilistic conditions. If a necessary condition can be identified and controlled (e.g., antibodies to a disease agent), the harmful outcome can be avoided.

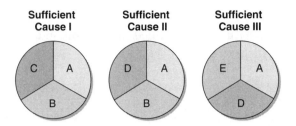

FIGURE 14.4 Three sufficient causes of an adverse health outcome.
Source: Merrill R. *Introduction to Epidemiology. 5th ed.* Sudbury, MA: Jones & Bartlett Learning; 2010.

Assume the factors that cause the adverse health outcome are pieces of a pie, with the whole pie being required to cause the health problem (**Figure 14.4**). The health-related state or event may have more than one sufficient cause, as illustrated in the figure, with each sufficient cause consisting of multiple contributing factors that are called component causes. The different component causes include the agent, host factors, and environmental factors. Where a given component cause is required in each of the different sufficient causes, it is referred to as a necessary cause.

Prevention and control measures do not require identifying every component of a sufficient cause because the health problem can be prevented by blocking any single component of a sufficient cause.

EXAMPLE 14.1

In Figure 14.4, the letter "A" represents a necessary cause because it is included in each of the three sufficient causes for the health problem. Exposure to the rubivirus is necessary for rubella-related birth defects to occur, but it is not sufficient to cause birth defects. Component causes that may be required to make a sufficient cause include a susceptible host who is not immune and illness during the first few months of pregnancy.

RISK FACTORS

A *risk factor* is a condition or behavior variable associated with the increased probability of a human health problem. It may be thought of as a component cause because it must be combined with other factors before an adverse health outcome occurs. It is not the same as a sufficient cause because not everyone who has the risk factor will experience the health problem. Risk factors are identified through analytic epidemiologic studies. After they have been identified, prevention and control measures can be taken.

> **History**
>
> The term *risk factor* was first introduced in 1961 by researchers involved in the Framingham Study, which showed that high blood pressure, high cholesterol, and smoking increase the risk of coronary heart disease.[20]

EXAMPLE 14.2

The component causes may be thought of as risk factors. Although smoking is a risk factor for lung cancer, the development of lung cancer may require smoking and other risk factors, such as the person's age, genetic predisposition (i.e., familial adenomatous polyposis), diet, and other environmental exposures.

A causal mechanism that requires the joint influence of multiple component causes includes factors that are predisposing, reinforcing, enabling, and precipitating.[21,22] These factors are described in **Table 14.4**. *Predisposing factors* influence the chance of developing a disease or condition. *Reinforcing factors* can help aggravate and perpetuate disease, conditions, disability, or death. These are called *negative reinforcing factors.* They may be repetitive patterns of behavior that recur, perpetuate, and support a disease that is spreading and running its course in a population. On the other hand, *positive reinforcing factors* are those that support, enhance, and improve the control and prevention of the causation of disease. *Enabling factors* include services, living conditions, programs, societal supports, skills, and resources that facilitate a health outcome's occurrence. *Precipitating factors* are essential to the development of the health problem, such as lead exposure, which is necessary for lead poisoning.

WEB OF CAUSATION

Although the epidemiologic triangle is useful for explaining how a single pathogen may cause an acute, infectious disease, chronic conditions caused by behavioral, occupational, or environmental factors require more sophisticated modeling. Rothman's pies expanded the epidemiologic triangle to illustrate that causes of disease often consist of combinations of risk factors such as predisposing, reinforcing, enabling, and precipitating factors.

TABLE 14.4   Predisposing, Reinforcing, Enabling, and Precipitating Factors

	Description	Examples
Predisposing factors	Factors already present that produce a susceptibility or disposition in a host to a disease or condition without actually causing it (e.g., age, immune status).	If the host is immunized against a disease or if the host has a natural resistance to the disease, he or she will respond by not developing the illness.
Reinforcing factors	Reinforcing factors have the ability to support the production and transmission of disease or conditions, and they have the ability to support and improve a population's health status and help control diseases and conditions.	A colleague encourages her friend to not drive after becoming intoxicated.
Enabling factors	Enabling factors can affect health through an environmental factor in either a positive or negative way.	Lack of public health services may enable a disease to spread, whereas the availability of and access to public health services can help prevent, control, intervene, treat, and facilitate recovery from diseases and conditions.
Precipitating factors	These are the factors essential to the development of diseases, conditions, injuries, disabilities, and death.	Lack of seat belt use in cars, drinking and driving, and lack of helmet use by motorcycle riders all precipitate a higher level of traffic deaths. The cause of a disease, condition, or injury may be fairly obvious, while in other cases it may not be so obvious. Several causal components may be present in the cause many times, especially in chronic diseases or those caused by lifestyle and behavior.

One way to model the complexity of causality for certain outcomes is a web of causation. A web of causation may be a graph, picture, or paradigmatic representation of complex sets of factors caused by an array of activities. The final outcome is the disease or condition. Webs can have many arms, branches, sources, inputs, and causes that are somehow interconnected or interrelated to the outcome. There may be a chain of events in which some events must occur before others can take place.

Steps for Constructing a Web of Causation

1. Identify the problem, affirm the condition, and obtain an accurate diagnosis of the disease.
2. Place the diagnosis at the center or bottom of the web.
3. Brainstorm and list all possible sources for the disease.
4. Brainstorm and list all risk factors and predisposing factors of the disease.
5. Develop subwebs and tertiary-level subwebs for the various branches of webs if needed.
6. Organize and arrange lists of sources and risk factors from general and most distant from the disease, in steps, being more specific and focused as the steps move closer toward the diagnosis of the disease.

Develop and work through causation decision trees for each element under consideration on the way toward the diagnosed disease.

EXAMPLE 14.3

A possible web of causation for lead poisoning is shown in **Figure 14.5**. Lead poisoning may result from a multitude of events and sources. Lead poisoning can occur by intake of lead by ingestion, inhalation, or absorption and can cause damage to the body's vital organs and nervous system. However, as illustrated in the figure, there are several factors that can influence the environment by which lead intake occurs, such as low education levels or low income. These factors often force people to live in older houses that may contain lead plumbing or lead-based paint. In turn, these housing conditions precipitate the ingestion of lead by individuals through drinking water or the accidental eating of lead paint. Because lead poisoning is a preventable disease, the key to controlling it is to understand its web of causation, especially the underlying contributors.

Although webs of causation are often complex, two concepts need emphasis. First, a complete understanding of the causal factors and mechanisms is not required or necessary for the development of effective prevention and control measures. Second, it is possible to interrupt the disease process by cutting the chains of occurrences of the various factors at strategic points.

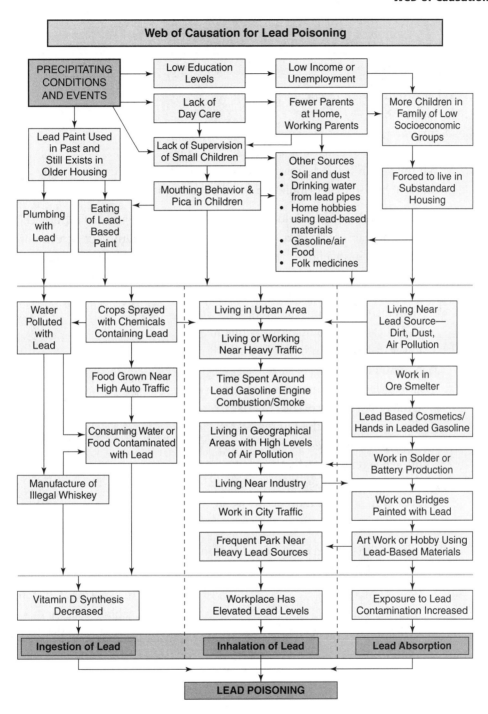

FIGURE 14.5 Example of a web of causation for lead poisoning.
Source: Merrill R. *Introduction to Epidemiology. 5th ed.* Sudbury, MA: Jones & Bartlett Learning; 2010.

EXERCISES

1. What is causal inference?
2. What is statistical inference?
3. Define *cause*.
4. Define *etiology*.
5. Is a risk factor the same thing as a cause? Explain.
6. Match the health-related situations described in the left column with the methods of hypothesis formulation listed in the right column.

    ___ AIDS is relatively high in hemophiliacs, recipients of transfusions, and intravenous drug abusers, suggesting that the mode of transmission is the human immunodeficiency virus introduced into the blood.

    ___ Colon cancer is comparatively much lower in Japan than in the United States. The rate of colon cancer among Japanese immigrants to the United States approaches the risk of people born in the United States, suggesting that lifestyle has a large influence on this cancer.

    ___ Coronary heart disease rates are greater in areas with higher levels of fine particulate matter in the air.

    A. Method of difference
    B. Method of agreement
    C. Method of concomitant variation

7. Match the health-related conditions listed in the left column with the types of risk factors in the right column.

    ___ Poor sanitation
    ___ Immunosuppressed
    ___ Li-Fraumeni syndrome
    ___ Peer influence
    ___ A toxin associated with the disease

    A. Predisposing risk factor
    B. Enabling risk factor
    C. Precipitating risk factor
    D. Reinforcing risk factor

8. Temporality is a criterion often used in causal inference. Explain why this is a critical element of causality.
9. Which study design is best suited for establishing temporality?

10. Underlying a valid statistical association is an accurate measure of both exposure and outcome data. Which is typically easier to measure, the exposure or the outcome? Why?

11. Consistency is a criterion often used in causal inference. Explain why this criterion may be supportive of causality.

12. Specificity is a criterion often used in causal inference. Explain why this criterion may be supportive or not supportive of causality.

13. Biological gradient is a criterion often used in causal inference. Explain why this criterion is important and how confounding can influence it.

14. Biological plausibility is a criterion often used in causal inference. What is biological plausibility and how useful do you think it is in causal inference?

15. Coherence is a criterion often used in causal inference. Critically assess this criterion.

16. Experimental evidence is a criterion often used in causal inference. Why is experimental evidence often considered the "gold standard," and what limitations does it have?

17. Order the following epidemiologic study designs (from 1 being the best, to 8 being the worst) in terms of their effectiveness in supporting causal inference.

    ____ Case report or case series
    ____ Cross-sectional study
    ____ Ecologic study
    ____ Case-control study
    ____ Prospective cohort study
    ____ Retrospective cohort study
    ____ Randomized, double-blind experimental study
    ____ Community experimental study

18. The aim of causal modeling is to present reasonable conjectures about underlying causal relationships between variables. The epidemiology triangle is a model that characterizes infectious disease causation. What are the interactive aspects of this model?

19. Although the epidemiologic triangle may work to explain how a pathogen leads to an acute, infectious disease, causal processes for behaviorally, occupationally, or environmentally caused chronic conditions or disorders require more sophisticated modeling. What is a web of causation?

20. Although webs of causation are often complex, two concepts universally apply with respect to prevention and control. Explain.

REFERENCES

1. Cumston CG. *An Introduction to the History of Medicine.* New York, NY: Alfred A. Knopf; 1926.
2. Garrison FH. *History of Medicine.* Philadelphia, PA: Saunders; 1926.
3. Pierce JR, Writer J. *Yellow Jack: How Yellow Fever Ravaged America and Walter Reed Discovered Its Deadly Secrets.* Hoboken, NJ: John Wiley and Sons; 2005.
4. U.S. Department of Health and Human Services. *Smoking and Health: Report of the Advisory Committee to the Surgeon General of the Public Health Service.* Publication PHS 1103. Washington, DC: U.S. Government Printing Office; 1964.
5. Weed DL. Causal and preventive inference. In: Greenwald P, Kramer BS, Weed DG, eds. *Cancer Prevention and Control.* New York: Mercel Dekker; 1995:285–302.
6. Mills JS. *A System of Logic, Ratiocinative and Inductive.* 5th ed. London: Parker, Son and Bowin; 1862.
7. Lilienfeld AM. On the methodology of investigations of etiologic factors in chronic diseases—some comments. *J Chronic Dis.* 1959;10:41–46.
8. Sartwell PE. On the methodology of investigations of etiologic factors in chronic diseases—further comments. *J Chronic Dis.* 1960;11:61–63.
9. Surgeon General's Advisory Committee on Smoking and Health. *Smoking and Health: 1964.* Rockville, MD: U.S. Public Health Service; 1964. DHEW publication no. (PHS) 1103.
10. Susser M. *Causal Thinking in the Health Sciences.* New York, NY: Oxford University Press; 1973.
11. Hill AB. The environment and disease: association or causation? *Proc R Soc Med.* 1965;58:295–300.
12. MacMahon B, Pugh TF. *Epidemiology: Principles and Methods.* Boston: Little, Brown, and Company; 1970.
13. Rosenbaum PR, Rubin DB. The central role of the propensity score in observational studies for causal effects. *Biometrica.* 1983;70:41–55.
14. Foster EM. Propensity score matching: an illustrated analysis of dose response. *Medical Care.* 2003;41(10)1183–1192.
15. Leslie RS, Ghomrawi H. *The Use of Propensity Scores and Instrument Variable Methods to Adjust for Treatment Selection Bias.* Proceedings of the SAS Global Forum 2008. San Antonio, Texas; 2008.
16. Parsons LS. Reducing bias in a propensity score matched-pair sample using greedy matching techniques. Proceedings of the 26th Annual SAS Users Group International Conference. Long Beach, California; 2001
17. Parsons LS. Performing a 1:N case-control match on propensity score. Proceedings of the 26th Annual SAS Users Group International Conference. Montreal, Canada; 2004
18. Patkar A, Fraeman KH. Economic impact of surgical site infection post-CABG surgery using multi-institutional hospitalization data. Presented at the 3rd Joint Meeting of the Surgical Infection Society–North America and the Surgical Infection Society of Europe. Chicago, IL; 2009.
19. Rothman KJ. Causes. *Am J Epidemiol.* 1976;104:587–592.
20. Kannel WB, Dawber TR, Kagan A, Revotski N, Stokes JI. Factors of risk in the development of coronary heart disease—six year follow-up experience; the Framingham Study. *Ann Intern Med.* 1961;55:33–50.
21. Evans AS. Causation and disease: the Henle-Koch postulates revisited. *Yale J Biol Med.* 1976;49:175–195.
22. Green L, Krueter M. *Health Promotion Planning.* 2nd ed. Mountain View, CA: Mayfield Publishing Company; 1991.

SAS Procedure Code

There are many computer packages available for assessing data. In this text, we have adopted the Statistical Analysis Software (SAS) system (Institute Inc., Cary, NC, USA, 2002–2010, version 9.3). There are three interactive windows in SAS: the Editor, Log, and Output, and each will be briefly described here.

SAS programs involve SAS statements. Each SAS statement ends with a semicolon; the semicolon completes the SAS statement. SAS statements are used to create SAS data sets and to run predefined statistical or other routines. A group of SAS statements used to define and create your SAS data set is called a Data Step. A Data Step tells SAS programs about the data. For example,

```
DATA EXAMPLE;
INPUT SUBJECT $ SEX $ AGE EXPOSED $ ILL $;
DATALINES;
1 Male 44 Yes Yes
2 Male 52 No No
3 Female 39 Yes No
.
.
.
;
```

The name of the data set is arbitrary but must begin with a letter. For categorical variables, follow the variable name on the INPUT line with "$". "DATALINES" comes prior to entering the data. Following the data set is a semicolon. It does not matter whether you choose to type words in upper- or lowercase.

PROC (meaning procedure) begins several predefined routines. Each PROC is followed by a specific option, such as PRINT, UNIVARIATE, MEAN, FREQ, REG, and so on. We finish the procedure statement with "RUN". For example, to obtain the mean age for males and females separately, we first sort the data according to sex.

```
PROC SORT DATA=EXAMPLE;
Title 'Sorted Data by Sex';
BY SEX;
RUN;
```

Then run PROC MEANS, using the following code:

```
PROC MEANS DATA=EXAMPLE;
Title 'Mean age by sex';
VAR AGE;
BY SEX;
RUN;
```

SAS programs are typed into the SAS Editor. Once the DATA STEP and procedure(s) are entered into the SAS EDITOR, they are submitted. When the procedure is submitted and executed, it produces a SAS LOG and a SAS OUTPUT. The SAS LOG is an annotated copy of the original program, with the data excluded. Any procedure coding errors and information about the data set (e.g., number of observations and variables) will be identified there. The SAS OUTPUT provides the results requested by the PROC statement.

SAS CODE FOR REFERENCE

The following consists of the SAS code typed in the SAS Editor for selected examples.

```
DATA EX2_1;
INPUT QUESTION AGREEMENT $ COUNT;
DATALINES;
 1 1-SA 185
 1 2-A 63
 1 3-D 3
 2 1-SA 137
 2 2-A 103
 2 3-D 11
```

```
DATA EX2_28;
INPUT AGE @@;
DATALINES;
 18 21 25 29 30 30 31
;

PROC MEANS DATA=EX2_28 RANGE;
VAR AGE;
RUN;
```

```
3 1-SA 65
3 2-A 88
3 3-D 98
;

PROC FREQ DATA=EX2_1;
WHERE QUESTION=1;
TABLE AGREEMENT;
WEIGHT COUNT;
RUN;


PROC FREQ DATA=EX2_1;
WHERE QUESTION=2;
TABLE AGREEMENT;
WEIGHT COUNT;
RUN;


PROC FREQ DATA=EX2_1;
WHERE QUESTION=3;
TABLE AGREEMENT;
WEIGHT COUNT;
RUN;
```

Examples 2.2–2.21 computed in Excel

```
DATA EX2_22;
INPUT AGE @@;
DATALINES;
 21 18 25 31 30 30 29
;

PROC MEANS DATA=EX2_22;
VAR AGE;
RUN;
```

```
DATA EX2_29;
INPUT AGE @@;
DATALINES;
 18 21 25 29 30 30 31
;

PROC MEANS DATA=EX2_29 Q1 Q3
QRANGE;
VAR AGE;
RUN;


DATA EX2_30;
INPUT AGE @@;
DATALINES;
 18 21 25 29 30 30 31
;

PROC MEANS DATA=EX2_30 STD VAR;
VAR AGE;
RUN;


DATA EX2_31;
INPUT AGE COUNT;
DATALINES;
 24 3
 25 7
 26 5
 27 2
;

PROC MEANS DATA=EX2_31 VAR;
VAR AGE;
FREQ COUNT;
RUN;
```

```
DATA EX2_23;
INPUT AGE COUNT;
DATALINES;
 24 3
 25 7
 26 5
 27 2
;

PROC MEANS DATA=EX2_23;
VAR AGE;
WEIGHT COUNT;
RUN;
```

Example 2.24 computed in Excel

```
DATA EX2_25A;
INPUT AGE @@;
DATALINES;
 21 18 25 31 30 30 29
;

PROC MEANS DATA=EX2_25A MEDIAN;
VAR AGE;
RUN;
```

```
DATA EX2_25B;
INPUT AGE @@;
DATALINES;
 21 18 25 31 30 30 29 32
;

PROC MEANS DATA=EX2_25B MEDIAN;
VAR AGE;
```

```
DATA EX2_32;
INPUT AGE @@;
DATALINES;
 18 21 25 29 30 30 31
;

PROC MEANS DATA=EX2_32 STD;
VAR AGE;
RUN;
```

```
DATA EX2_33;
INPUT AGE @@;
DATALINES;
 18 21 25 29 30 30 31
;

PROC MEANS DATA=EX2_33 STDERR;
VAR AGE;
RUN;
```

```
DATA EX2_34A;
INPUT AGE @@;
DATALINES;
 18 21 25 29 30 30 31
;

PROC MEANS DATA=EX2_34A CV;
VAR AGE;
RUN;
```

```
DATA EX2_34B;
INPUT AGE COUNT;
DATALINES;
 24 3
```

```
RUN;

Example 2.26 computed in Excel

Example 2.27 by inspection
```

```
25 7
26 5
27 2
;

PROC MEANS DATA=EX2_34B CV;
VAR AGE;
FREQ COUNT;
RUN;
```

```
DATA EX8_2;
INPUT AREA $ 1–16 POBESE 17–20;
DATALINES;
Maryland          27.9
Mississippi       34.5
North Dakota      27.9
Colorado          21.4
Nebraska          27.5
Wyoming           25.7
Rhode Island      26.0
Virgin Islands    30.0
Iowa              29.1
Arkansas          30.9
;

PROC MEANS DATA=EX8_2 LCLM UCLM;
VAR POBESE;
RUN;

PROC UNIVARIATE DATA=EX8_5;
WHERE GROUP='INTERVENTION';
VAR CBMI;
RUN;
```

```
DATA EX8_8;
INPUT SCREENING1 SCREENING2 COUNT;
TITLE "PUT TITLE HERE";
DATALINES;
1 1 13
1 2 2
2 1 8
2 2 27
;

PROC FREQ DATA=EX8_8;
TABLE SCREENING1*SCREENING2/AGREE;
WEIGHT COUNT;
RUN;

PROC TTEST DATA=EX8_9;
CLASS GROUP;
VAR AGE;
RUN;

PROC FREQ DATA=EX8_10;
TABLE SEX*GROUP/CHISQ CMH;
RUN;
```

```
PROC FORMAT;
VALUE $AGEFMT    '1' = '18–49'
                 '2' = '50–72';
RUN;

DATA EX8_7;
INPUT AGEGROUP $ SCREENING1
SCREENING2 COUNT;
FORMAT AGEGROUP AGEFMT.;
DATALINES;
  1 1 1 159
  1 1 2 18
  1 2 1 38
  1 2 2 26
  2 1 1 104
  2 1 2 14
  2 2 1 11
  2 2 2 15
;

PROC FREQ DATA=EX8_7;
TABLE AGEGROUP*SCREENING1*SCREENING2/
AGREE;
WEIGHT COUNT;
RUN;
```

```
PROC FORMAT;
VALUE $SITE    '1' = 'NEAR HIGH HAZARD DS'
               '2' = 'NEAR LOW HAZARD DS';
RUN;

DATA EX8_12;
INPUT RESIDENCE BIRTHWEIGHT COUNT;
DATALINES;
  1 1 181
  1 2 4268
  2 1 126
  2 2 4236
;

PROC FREQ DATA=EX8_12;
TABLE
RESIDENCE*BIRTHWEIGHT/CHISQ;
WEIGHT COUNT;
RUN;

PROC GLM DATA=EX8_13;
CLASS REPEAT;
MODEL SOCIAL_FUNCTIONING=REPEAT;
MEANS REPEAT/SNK;
RUN;
```

```
DATA EX11_1;
INPUT STATE $ 1–16 POBESE 17–24
PDIABETES 25–28;
DATALINES;
Alabama          33      13.2
Alaska           25.2    5.3
Arizona          24.7    11.4
Arkansas         30.9    9.6
California       24.7    8.6
Colorado         21.4    6
Connecticut      23      7.3
Delaware         28.7    8.7
District of Col  22.7    10.9
Florida          27.2    10.4
Georgia          30.4    9.7
Guam             27.6    11
Hawaii           23.1    8.3
Idaho            26.9    7.9
Illinois         28.7    8.7
Indiana          30.2    9.8
Iowa             29.1    7.5
Kansas           30.1    8.4
Kentucky         31.8    10
Louisiana        31.7    10.3
Maine            27.4    8.7
Maryland         27.9    9.3
Massachusetts    23.6    7.4
Michigan         31.7    10.1
Minnesota        25.4    6.7
Mississippi      34.5    12.4
Missouri         31.4    9.4
Montana          23.5    7
Nebraska         27.5    7.7
Nevada           23.1    8.5
New Hampshire    25.5    7.9
```

```
PROC GENMOD DATA=EX11_6;
CLASS EXPOSED;
MODEL CASES = EXPOSED/DIST = POISSON
LINK=LOG OFFSET = LPYEARS;
ESTIMATE 'SMOKER' EXPOSED 1-1/EXP;
RUN;


DATA EX11_7;
INPUT MENINGITIS SD COUNT;
DATALINES;
1 1 16
1 2 134
2 1 3
2 2 147
;


PROC FREQ DATA=EX11_7;
TABLE MENINGITIS*SD/CHISQ CMH;
WEIGHT COUNT;
RUN;


DATA EX11_9;
INPUT SMOKE CASE CONTROL COUNT;
DATALINES;
1 1 1 96
1 1 2 62
1 2 1 24
1 2 2 18
2 1 1 42
2 1 2 57
2 2 1 38
2 2 2 63
;
```

New Jersey	24.8	9.2
New Mexico	25.6	8.5
New York	24.5	8.9
North Carolina	28.6	9.8
North Dakota	27.9	7.4
Ohio	29.7	10.1
Oklahoma	31.3	10.4
Oregon	27.6	7.2
Pennsylvania	29.2	10.3
Puerto Rico	27.5	12.8
Rhode Island	26	7.8
South Carolina	32	10.7
South Dakota	27.7	6.9
Tennessee	31.7	11.3
Texas	31.7	9.7
Utah	23	6.5
Vermont	23.9	6.8
Virginia	26.4	8.7
Virgin Islands	30	9.1
Washington	26.2	7.6
West Virginia	32.9	11.7
Wisconsin	26.9	7.1
Wyoming	25.7	7.2

```
;

PROC CORR DATA=EX11_1
PEARSON SPEARMAN;
VAR POBESE PDIABETES;
RUN;

DATA EX11_2;
INPUT STATE $ 1–16 POBESE 17–24
PDIABETES 25–28;
DATALINES;
.
.
```

```
PROC FREQ DATA=EX11_9;
TABLE SMOKE*CASE*CONTROL/CMH;
WEIGHT COUNT;
RUN;


DATA EX11_10;
INPUT INTERVENTION BMISTATUS COUNT;
DATALINES;
1 1 138
1 2 36
2 1 98
2 2 76
;


PROC FREQ DATA=EX11_10;
TABLE INTERVENTION*BMISTATUS/CMH
CHISQ;
WEIGHT COUNT;
RUN;


DATA EX11_11;
INPUT SEX INTERVENTION BMISTATUS COUNT;
DATALINES;
1 1 1 40
1 1 2 7
1 2 1 35
1 2 2 16
2 1 1 98
2 1 2 29
2 2 1 63
2 2 2 60
;


PROC FREQ DATA=EX11_11;
TABLE SEX*INTERVENTION*BMISTATUS/CMH;
```

```
.
;

PROC REG DATA=EX11_2;
MODEL PDIABETES = POBESE;
PLOT R.*P.;
PRINT R P;
RUN;

PROC REG DATA=EX11_3;
MODEL GENHEALTH = EXERCISE BMI AGE;
RUN;

PROC GENMOD EX11_4;
CLASS FH;
MODEL VD = FH/DIST =
BINOMIAL LINK = LOGIT;
ESTIMATE 'FAMILY HISTORY'
FH 1-1/E EXP;
RUN;

PROC GENMOD EX11_5;
CLASS FH;
MODEL VD = FH AGE
SEX/DIST = BINOMIAL
LINK = LOGIT;
ESTIMATE 'FAMILY HISTORY'
FH 1-1/E EXP;
RUN;

DATA EX11_6;
INPUT EXPOSED $ CASES PYEARS;
LPYEARS=LOG(PYEARS);
DATALINES;
 1 882 220965
 2 673 189254
;
```

```
WEIGHT COUNT;
RUN;

DATA EX11_12;
INPUT SMOKE CVD COUNT;
DATALINES;
 1 1 882
 1 2 220083
 2 1 673
 2 2 188581
;

PROC FREQ DATA=EX11_12;
TABLE SMOKE*CVD/CMH;
WEIGHT COUNT;
RUN;

DATA EX11_13;
INPUT AGEGRP LANGUAGE COUNT;
DATALINES;
 1 1 7
 1 2 18
 1 3 21
 2 1 16
 2 2 162
 2 3 72
;

PROC FREQ DATA=EX11_13;
WHERE LANGUAGE IN (1 2);
TABLE AGEGRP*LANGUAGE/CMH CHISQ;
WEIGHT COUNT;
RUN;
```

```
DATA EX13_5;
INPUT GROUP PN TIME CENSOR;
DATALINES;
1    1    1    1
1    2    2    1
1    3    2    1
1    4    3    1
1    5    4    1
1    6    5    1
1    7    6    1
1    8    7    1
1    9    9    1
1    10   12   1
1    11   12   1
1    12   13   1
1    13   15   1
1    14   16   1
1    15   35   1
1    16   31   1
1    17   36   1
1    18   42   1
1    19   43   0
1    20   45   0
2    1    1    1
2    2    2    1
2    3    2    1
2    4    3    1
2    5    3    1
2    6    3    1
2    7    3    1
2    8    4    1
2    9    6    1
2    10   6    1
2    11   7    1
```

```
DATA EX13_6;
INPUT GROUP PN TIME CENSOR;
DATALINES;
1    1    1    1
1    2    6    1
1    3    8    1
1    4    9    1
1    5    9    1
1    6    20   1
1    7    21   1
1    8    30   1
1    9    35   0
1    10   39   0
1    11   44   0
1    12   46   0
1    13   48   0
2    1    3    1
2    2    4    1
2    3    5    1
2    4    6    1
2    5    7    1
2    6    10   1
2    7    14   1
2    8    38   0
3    1    4    1
3    2    4    1
3    3    4    1
3    4    6    1
3    5    14   1
3    6    20   1
;

PROC LIFETEST DATA=EX13_6 PLOTS=(S);
TIME TIME*CENSOR(0);
```

2	12	7	1
2	13	7	1
2	14	8	1
2	15	8	1
2	16	8	0
2	17	10	1
2	18	11	1
2	19	13	1
2	20	14	1
2	21	17	1
2	22	17	0
2	23	18	1
2	24	20	1
2	25	22	1
2	26	22	1
2	27	23	1
2	28	32	1
2	29	35	1
2	30	37	0
2	31	39	0
2	32	39	0
2	33	39	0
2	34	39	0
2	35	39	0
2	36	39	0
2	37	46	0

```
;

PROC LIFETEST DATA=EX13_5 PLOTS=(S);
TIME TIME*CENSOR(0);
STRATA GROUP;
RUN;
```

```
STRATA GROUP;
RUN;
```

Tables

TABLE 1. Cumulative Binomial Probabilities

n	x	0.01	0.05	0.1	0.15	0.2	0.25	0.3	0.35	0.4	0.45	0.5
2	0	0.9801	0.9025	0.8100	0.7225	0.6400	0.5625	0.4900	0.4225	0.3600	0.3025	0.2500
	1	0.9999	0.9975	0.9900	0.9775	0.9600	0.9375	0.9100	0.8775	0.8400	0.7975	0.7500
	2	1.0000	1.0000	1.0000	1.0000	1.0000	1.0000	1.0000	1.0000	1.0000	1.0000	1.0000
3	0	0.9703	0.8574	0.7290	0.6141	0.5120	0.4219	0.3430	0.2746	0.2160	0.1664	0.1250
	1	0.9997	0.9928	0.9720	0.9393	0.8960	0.8438	0.7840	0.7183	0.6480	0.5748	0.5000
	2	1.0000	0.9999	0.9990	0.9966	0.9920	0.9844	0.9730	0.9571	0.9360	0.9089	0.8750
	3	1.0000	1.0000	1.0000	1.0000	1.0000	1.0000	1.0000	1.0000	1.0000	1.0000	1.0000
4	0	0.9606	0.8145	0.6561	0.5220	0.4096	0.3164	0.2401	0.1785	0.1296	0.0915	0.0625
	1	0.9994	0.9860	0.9477	0.8905	0.8192	0.7383	0.6517	0.5630	0.4752	0.3910	0.3125
	2	1.0000	0.9995	0.9963	0.9880	0.9728	0.9492	0.9163	0.8735	0.8208	0.7585	0.6875
	3	1.0000	1.0000	0.9999	0.9995	0.9984	0.9961	0.9919	0.9850	0.9744	0.9590	0.9375
	4	1.0000	1.0000	1.0000	1.0000	1.0000	1.0000	1.0000	1.0000	1.0000	1.0000	1.0000
5	0	0.9510	0.7738	0.5905	0.4437	0.3277	0.2373	0.1681	0.1160	0.0778	0.0503	0.0313
	1	0.9990	0.9774	0.9185	0.8352	0.7373	0.6328	0.5282	0.4284	0.3370	0.2562	0.1875
	2	1.0000	0.9988	0.9914	0.9734	0.9421	0.8965	0.8369	0.7648	0.6826	0.5931	0.5000
	3	1.0000	1.0000	0.9995	0.9978	0.9933	0.9844	0.9692	0.9460	0.9130	0.8688	0.8125
	4	1.0000	1.0000	1.0000	0.9999	0.9997	0.9990	0.9976	0.9948	0.9898	0.9816	0.9688
	5	1.0000	1.0000	1.0000	1.0000	1.0000	1.0000	1.0000	1.0000	1.0000	1.0000	1.0000

(continues)

TABLE 1.   Cumulative Binomial Probabilities (*continued*)

n	x	0.01	0.05	0.1	0.15	0.2	0.25	0.3	0.35	0.4	0.45	0.5
6	0	0.9415	0.7351	0.5314	0.3772	0.2621	0.1780	0.1177	0.0754	0.0467	0.0277	0.0156
	1	0.9985	0.9672	0.8857	0.7765	0.6554	0.5339	0.4202	0.3191	0.2333	0.1636	0.1094
	2	1.0000	0.9978	0.9842	0.9527	0.9011	0.8306	0.7443	0.6471	0.5443	0.4415	0.3438
	3	1.0000	0.9999	0.9987	0.9941	0.9830	0.9624	0.9295	0.8826	0.8208	0.7447	0.6563
	4	1.0000	1.0000	0.9999	0.9996	0.9984	0.9954	0.9891	0.9777	0.9590	0.9308	0.8906
	5	1.0000	1.0000	1.0000	1.0000	0.9999	0.9998	0.9993	0.9982	0.9959	0.9917	0.9844
	6	1.0000	1.0000	1.0000	1.0000	1.0000	1.0000	1.0000	1.0000	1.0000	1.0000	1.0000
7	0	0.9321	0.6983	0.4783	0.3206	0.2097	0.1335	0.0824	0.0490	0.0280	0.0152	0.0078
	1	0.9980	0.9556	0.8503	0.7166	0.5767	0.4450	0.3294	0.2338	0.1586	0.1024	0.0625
	2	1.0000	0.9962	0.9743	0.9262	0.8520	0.7564	0.6471	0.5323	0.4199	0.3164	0.2266
	3	1.0000	0.9998	0.9973	0.9879	0.9667	0.9294	0.8740	0.8002	0.7102	0.6083	0.5000
	4	1.0000	1.0000	0.9998	0.9988	0.9953	0.9871	0.9712	0.9444	0.9037	0.8471	0.7734
	5	1.0000	1.0000	1.0000	0.9999	0.9996	0.9987	0.9962	0.9910	0.9812	0.9643	0.9375
	6	1.0000	1.0000	1.0000	1.0000	1.0000	0.9999	0.9998	0.9994	0.9984	0.9963	0.9922
	7	1.0000	1.0000	1.0000	1.0000	1.0000	1.0000	1.0000	1.0000	1.0000	1.0000	1.0000
8	0	0.9227	0.6634	0.4305	0.2725	0.1678	0.1001	0.0577	0.0319	0.0168	0.0084	0.0039
	1	0.9973	0.9428	0.8131	0.6572	0.5033	0.3671	0.2553	0.1691	0.1064	0.0632	0.0352
	2	1.0000	0.9942	0.9619	0.8948	0.7969	0.6785	0.5518	0.4278	0.3154	0.2201	0.1445
	3	1.0000	0.9996	0.9950	0.9787	0.9437	0.8862	0.8059	0.7064	0.5941	0.4770	0.3633
	4	1.0000	1.0000	0.9996	0.9972	0.9896	0.9727	0.9420	0.8939	0.8263	0.7396	0.6367
	5	1.0000	1.0000	1.0000	0.9998	0.9988	0.9958	0.9887	0.9747	0.9502	0.9115	0.8555
	6	1.0000	1.0000	1.0000	1.0000	0.9999	0.9996	0.9987	0.9964	0.9915	0.9819	0.9648
	7	1.0000	1.0000	1.0000	1.0000	1.0000	1.0000	0.9999	0.9998	0.9993	0.9983	0.9961
	8	1.0000	1.0000	1.0000	1.0000	1.0000	1.0000	1.0000	1.0000	1.0000	1.0000	1.0000
9	0	0.9135	0.6303	0.3874	0.2316	0.1342	0.0751	0.0404	0.0207	0.0101	0.0046	0.0020
	1	0.9966	0.9288	0.7748	0.5995	0.4362	0.3003	0.1960	0.1211	0.0705	0.0385	0.0195

Table 1   327

TABLE 1. Cumulative Binomial Probabilities (*continued*)

n	x	0.01	0.05	0.1	0.15	0.2	0.25	0.3	0.35	0.4	0.45	0.5
	2	0.9999	0.9916	0.9470	0.8592	0.7382	0.6007	0.4628	0.3373	0.2318	0.1495	0.0898
	3	1.0000	0.9994	0.9917	0.9661	0.9144	0.8343	0.7297	0.6089	0.4826	0.3614	0.2539
	4	1.0000	1.0000	0.9991	0.9944	0.9804	0.9511	0.9012	0.8283	0.7334	0.6214	0.5000
	5	1.0000	1.0000	0.9999	0.9994	0.9969	0.9900	0.9747	0.9464	0.9007	0.8342	0.7461
	6	1.0000	1.0000	1.0000	1.0000	0.9997	0.9987	0.9957	0.9888	0.9750	0.9502	0.9102
	7	1.0000	1.0000	1.0000	1.0000	1.0000	0.9999	0.9996	0.9986	0.9962	0.9909	0.9805
	8	1.0000	1.0000	1.0000	1.0000	1.0000	1.0000	1.0000	0.9999	0.9997	0.9992	0.9981
	9	1.0000	1.0000	1.0000	1.0000	1.0000	1.0000	1.0000	1.0000	1.0000	1.0000	1.0000
10	0	0.9044	0.5987	0.3487	0.1969	0.1074	0.0563	0.0283	0.0135	0.0061	0.0025	0.0010
	1	0.9957	0.9139	0.7361	0.5443	0.3758	0.2440	0.1493	0.0860	0.0464	0.0233	0.0107
	2	0.9999	0.9885	0.9298	0.8202	0.6778	0.5256	0.3828	0.2616	0.1673	0.0996	0.0547
	3	1.0000	0.9990	0.9872	0.9500	0.8791	0.7759	0.6496	0.5138	0.3823	0.2660	0.1719
	4	1.0000	0.9999	0.9984	0.9901	0.9672	0.9219	0.8497	0.7515	0.6331	0.5044	0.3770
	5	1.0000	1.0000	0.9999	0.9986	0.9936	0.9803	0.9527	0.9051	0.8338	0.7384	0.6231
	6	1.0000	1.0000	1.0000	0.9999	0.9991	0.9965	0.9894	0.9740	0.9452	0.8980	0.8281
	7	1.0000	1.0000	1.0000	1.0000	0.9999	0.9996	0.9984	0.9952	0.9877	0.9726	0.9453
	8	1.0000	1.0000	1.0000	1.0000	1.0000	1.0000	0.9999	0.9995	0.9983	0.9955	0.9893
	9	1.0000	1.0000	1.0000	1.0000	1.0000	1.0000	1.0000	1.0000	0.9999	0.9997	0.9990
	10	1.0000	1.0000	1.0000	1.0000	1.0000	1.0000	1.0000	1.0000	1.0000	1.0000	1.0000
11	0	0.8953	0.5688	0.3138	0.1673	0.0859	0.0422	0.0198	0.0088	0.0036	0.0014	0.0005
	1	0.9948	0.8981	0.6974	0.4922	0.3221	0.1971	0.1130	0.0606	0.0302	0.0139	0.0059
	2	0.9998	0.9848	0.9104	0.7788	0.6174	0.4552	0.3127	0.2001	0.1189	0.0652	0.0327
	3	1.0000	0.9985	0.9815	0.9306	0.8389	0.7133	0.5696	0.4256	0.2963	0.1911	0.1133
	4	1.0000	0.9999	0.9973	0.9841	0.9496	0.8854	0.7897	0.6683	0.5328	0.3971	0.2744
	5	1.0000	1.0000	0.9997	0.9973	0.9884	0.9657	0.9218	0.8513	0.7535	0.6331	0.5000
	6	1.0000	1.0000	1.0000	0.9997	0.9980	0.9924	0.9784	0.9499	0.9007	0.8262	0.7256

(continues)

TABLE 1.   Cumulative Binomial Probabilities (*continued*)

n	x	0.01	0.05	0.1	0.15	0.2	0.25	0.3	0.35	0.4	0.45	0.5
11	7	1.0000	1.0000	1.0000	1.0000	0.9998	0.9988	0.9957	0.9878	0.9707	0.9390	0.8867
	8	1.0000	1.0000	1.0000	1.0000	1.0000	0.9999	0.9994	0.9980	0.9941	0.9852	0.9673
	9	1.0000	1.0000	1.0000	1.0000	1.0000	1.0000	1.0000	0.9998	0.9993	0.9978	0.9941
	10	1.0000	1.0000	1.0000	1.0000	1.0000	1.0000	1.0000	1.0000	1.0000	0.9999	0.9995
	11	1.0000	1.0000	1.0000	1.0000	1.0000	1.0000	1.0000	1.0000	1.0000	1.0000	1.0000
12	0	0.8864	0.5404	0.2824	0.1422	0.0687	0.0317	0.0138	0.0057	0.0022	0.0008	0.0002
	1	0.9938	0.8816	0.6590	0.4435	0.2749	0.1584	0.0850	0.0424	0.0196	0.0083	0.0032
	2	0.9998	0.9804	0.8891	0.7358	0.5584	0.3907	0.2528	0.1513	0.0834	0.0421	0.0193
	3	1.0000	0.9978	0.9744	0.9078	0.7946	0.6488	0.4925	0.3467	0.2253	0.1345	0.0730
	4	1.0000	0.9998	0.9957	0.9761	0.9274	0.8424	0.7237	0.5834	0.4382	0.3044	0.1939
	5	1.0000	1.0000	0.9995	0.9954	0.9806	0.9456	0.8822	0.7873	0.6652	0.5269	0.3872
	6	1.0000	1.0000	1.0000	0.9993	0.9961	0.9858	0.9614	0.9154	0.8418	0.7393	0.6128
	7	1.0000	1.0000	1.0000	0.9999	0.9994	0.9972	0.9905	0.9745	0.9427	0.8883	0.8062
	8	1.0000	1.0000	1.0000	1.0000	0.9999	0.9996	0.9983	0.9944	0.9847	0.9644	0.9270
	9	1.0000	1.0000	1.0000	1.0000	1.0000	1.0000	0.9998	0.9992	0.9972	0.9921	0.9807
	10	1.0000	1.0000	1.0000	1.0000	1.0000	1.0000	1.0000	0.9999	0.9997	0.9989	0.9968
	11	1.0000	1.0000	1.0000	1.0000	1.0000	1.0000	1.0000	1.0000	1.0000	0.9999	0.9998
	12	1.0000	1.0000	1.0000	1.0000	1.0000	1.0000	1.0000	1.0000	1.0000	1.0000	1.0000
13	0	0.8775	0.5133	0.2542	0.1209	0.0550	0.0238	0.0097	0.0037	0.0013	0.0004	0.0001
	1	0.9928	0.8646	0.6213	0.3983	0.2337	0.1267	0.0637	0.0296	0.0126	0.0049	0.0017
	2	0.9997	0.9755	0.8661	0.6920	0.5017	0.3326	0.2025	0.1132	0.0579	0.0269	0.0112
	3	1.0000	0.9969	0.9658	0.8820	0.7473	0.5843	0.4206	0.2783	0.1686	0.0929	0.0461
	4	1.0000	0.9997	0.9935	0.9658	0.9009	0.7940	0.6543	0.5005	0.3530	0.2280	0.1334
	5	1.0000	1.0000	0.9991	0.9925	0.9700	0.9198	0.8346	0.7159	0.5744	0.4268	0.2905
	6	1.0000	1.0000	0.9999	0.9987	0.9930	0.9757	0.9376	0.8705	0.7712	0.6437	0.5000
	7	1.0000	1.0000	1.0000	0.9998	0.9988	0.9944	0.9818	0.9538	0.9023	0.8212	0.7095

Table 1   329

n	x	0.01	0.05	0.1	0.15	0.2	0.25	0.3	0.35	0.4	0.45	0.5
	8	1.0000	1.0000	1.0000	1.0000	0.9998	0.9990	0.9960	0.9874	0.9679	0.9302	0.8666
	9	1.0000	1.0000	1.0000	1.0000	1.0000	0.9999	0.9994	0.9975	0.9922	0.9797	0.9539
	10	1.0000	1.0000	1.0000	1.0000	1.0000	1.0000	0.9999	0.9997	0.9987	0.9959	0.9888
	11	1.0000	1.0000	1.0000	1.0000	1.0000	1.0000	1.0000	1.0000	0.9999	0.9995	0.9983
	12	1.0000	1.0000	1.0000	1.0000	1.0000	1.0000	1.0000	1.0000	1.0000	1.0000	0.9999
	13	1.0000	1.0000	1.0000	1.0000	1.0000	1.0000	1.0000	1.0000	1.0000	1.0000	1.0000
14	0	0.8688	0.4877	0.2288	0.1028	0.0440	0.0178	0.0068	0.0024	0.0008	0.0002	0.0001
	1	0.9916	0.8470	0.5846	0.3567	0.1979	0.1010	0.0475	0.0205	0.0081	0.0029	0.0009
	2	0.9997	0.9700	0.8416	0.6479	0.4481	0.2811	0.1608	0.0839	0.0398	0.0170	0.0065
	3	1.0000	0.9958	0.9559	0.8535	0.6982	0.5213	0.3552	0.2205	0.1243	0.0632	0.0287
	4	1.0000	0.9996	0.9908	0.9533	0.8702	0.7415	0.5842	0.4227	0.2793	0.1672	0.0898
	5	1.0000	1.0000	0.9985	0.9885	0.9562	0.8883	0.7805	0.6405	0.4859	0.3373	0.2120
	6	1.0000	1.0000	0.9998	0.9978	0.9884	0.9617	0.9067	0.8164	0.6925	0.5461	0.3953
	7	1.0000	1.0000	1.0000	0.9997	0.9976	0.9897	0.9685	0.9247	0.8499	0.7414	0.6047
	8	1.0000	1.0000	1.0000	1.0000	0.9996	0.9979	0.9917	0.9757	0.9417	0.8811	0.7880
	9	1.0000	1.0000	1.0000	1.0000	1.0000	0.9997	0.9983	0.9940	0.9825	0.9574	0.9102
	10	1.0000	1.0000	1.0000	1.0000	1.0000	1.0000	0.9998	0.9989	0.9961	0.9886	0.9713
	11	1.0000	1.0000	1.0000	1.0000	1.0000	1.0000	0.9999	0.9994	0.9979	0.9935
	12	1.0000	1.0000	1.0000	1.0000	1.0000	1.0000	1.0000	1.0000	0.9999	0.9998	0.9991
	13	1.0000	1.0000	1.0000	1.0000	1.0000	1.0000	1.0000	1.0000	1.0000	1.0000	0.9999
	14	1.0000	1.0000	1.0000	1.0000	1.0000	1.0000	1.0000	1.0000	1.0000	1.0000	1.0000
15	0	0.8601	0.4633	0.2059	0.0874	0.0352	0.0134	0.0048	0.0016	0.0005	0.0001	0.0000
	1	0.9904	0.8291	0.5490	0.3186	0.1671	0.0802	0.0353	0.0142	0.0052	0.0017	0.0005
	2	0.9996	0.9638	0.8159	0.6042	0.3980	0.2361	0.1268	0.0617	0.0271	0.0107	0.0037
	3	1.0000	0.9945	0.9444	0.8227	0.6482	0.4613	0.2969	0.1727	0.0905	0.0424	0.0176
	4	1.0000	0.9994	0.9873	0.9383	0.8358	0.6865	0.5155	0.3519	0.2173	0.1204	0.0592

(continues)

TABLE 1. Cumulative Binomial Probabilities (*continued*)

n	x	0.01	0.05	0.1	0.15	0.2	0.25	0.3	0.35	0.4	0.45	0.5
15	5	1.0000	1.0000	0.9978	0.9832	0.9390	0.8516	0.7216	0.5643	0.4032	0.2608	0.1509
	6	1.0000	1.0000	0.9997	0.9964	0.9819	0.9434	0.8689	0.7548	0.6098	0.4522	0.3036
	7	1.0000	1.0000	1.0000	0.9994	0.9958	0.9827	0.9500	0.8868	0.7869	0.6535	0.5000
	8	1.0000	1.0000	1.0000	0.9999	0.9992	0.9958	0.9848	0.9578	0.9050	0.8182	0.6964
	9	1.0000	1.0000	1.0000	1.0000	0.9999	0.9992	0.9964	0.9876	0.9662	0.9231	0.8491
	10	1.0000	1.0000	1.0000	1.0000	1.0000	0.9999	0.9993	0.9972	0.9907	0.9745	0.9408
	11	1.0000	1.0000	1.0000	1.0000	1.0000	1.0000	0.9999	0.9995	0.9981	0.9937	0.9824
	12	1.0000	1.0000	1.0000	1.0000	1.0000	1.0000	1.0000	0.9999	0.9997	0.9989	0.9963
	13	1.0000	1.0000	1.0000	1.0000	1.0000	1.0000	1.0000	1.0000	1.0000	0.9999	0.9995
	14	1.0000	1.0000	1.0000	1.0000	1.0000	1.0000	1.0000	1.0000	1.0000	1.0000	1.0000
	15	1.0000	1.0000	1.0000	1.0000	1.0000	1.0000	1.0000	1.0000	1.0000	1.0000	1.0000
20	0	0.8179	0.3585	0.1216	0.0388	0.0115	0.0032	0.0008	0.0002	0.0000	0.0000	0.0000
	1	0.9831	0.7358	0.3918	0.1756	0.0692	0.0243	0.0076	0.0021	0.0005	0.0001	0.0000
	2	0.9990	0.9245	0.6769	0.4049	0.2061	0.0913	0.0355	0.0121	0.0036	0.0009	0.0002
	3	1.0000	0.9841	0.8671	0.6477	0.4115	0.2252	0.1071	0.0444	0.0160	0.0049	0.0013
	4	1.0000	0.9974	0.9568	0.8299	0.6297	0.4148	0.2375	0.1182	0.0510	0.0189	0.0059
	5	1.0000	0.9997	0.9888	0.9327	0.8042	0.6172	0.4164	0.2454	0.1256	0.0553	0.0207
	6	1.0000	1.0000	0.9976	0.9781	0.9133	0.7858	0.6080	0.4166	0.2500	0.1299	0.0577
	7	1.0000	1.0000	0.9996	0.9941	0.9679	0.8982	0.7723	0.6010	0.4159	0.2520	0.1316
	8	1.0000	1.0000	0.9999	0.9987	0.9900	0.9591	0.8867	0.7624	0.5956	0.4143	0.2517
	9	1.0000	1.0000	1.0000	0.9998	0.9974	0.9861	0.9520	0.8782	0.7553	0.5914	0.4119
	10	1.0000	1.0000	1.0000	1.0000	0.9994	0.9961	0.9829	0.9468	0.8725	0.7507	0.5881
	11	1.0000	1.0000	1.0000	1.0000	0.9999	0.9991	0.9949	0.9804	0.9435	0.8692	0.7483
	12	1.0000	1.0000	1.0000	1.0000	1.0000	0.9998	0.9987	0.9940	0.9790	0.9420	0.8684
	13	1.0000	1.0000	1.0000	1.0000	1.0000	1.0000	0.9997	0.9985	0.9935	0.9786	0.9423
	14	1.0000	1.0000	1.0000	1.0000	1.0000	1.0000	1.0000	0.9997	0.9984	0.9936	0.9793

Table 2   331

TABLE 1. Cumulative Binomial Probabilities (*continued*)

n	x	0.01	0.05	0.1	0.15	0.2	0.25	0.3	0.35	0.4	0.45	0.5
	15	1.0000	1.0000	1.0000	1.0000	1.0000	1.0000	1.0000	1.0000	0.9997	0.9985	0.9941
	16	1.0000	1.0000	1.0000	1.0000	1.0000	1.0000	1.0000	1.0000	1.0000	0.9997	0.9987
	17	1.0000	1.0000	1.0000	1.0000	1.0000	1.0000	1.0000	1.0000	1.0000	1.0000	0.9998
	18	1.0000	1.0000	1.0000	1.0000	1.0000	1.0000	1.0000	1.0000	1.0000	1.0000	1.0000
	19	1.0000	1.0000	1.0000	1.0000	1.0000	1.0000	1.0000	1.0000	1.0000	1.0000	1.0000
	20	1.0000	1.0000	1.0000	1.0000	1.0000	1.0000	1.0000	1.0000	1.0000	1.0000	1.0000

TABLE 2. Cumulative Poisson Probabilities

λ

x	0.01	0.01	0.02	0.03	0.04	0.05	0.06	0.07	0.08	0.09
0	0.9950	0.9900	0.9802	0.9704	0.9608	0.9512	0.9418	0.9324	0.9231	0.9139
1	1.0000	1.0000	0.9998	0.9996	0.9992	0.9988	0.9983	0.9977	0.9970	0.9962
2	1.0000	1.0000	1.0000	1.0000	1.0000	1.0000	1.0000	0.9999	0.9999	0.9999
3	1.0000	1.0000	1.0000	1.0000	1.0000	1.0000	1.0000	1.0000	1.0000	1.0000

λ

x	0.1	0.2	0.3	0.4	0.5	0.6	0.7	0.8	0.9	1
0	0.9048	0.8187	0.7408	0.6703	0.6065	0.5488	0.4966	0.4493	0.4066	0.3679
1	0.9953	0.9825	0.9631	0.9384	0.9098	0.8781	0.8442	0.8088	0.7725	0.7358
2	0.9998	0.9989	0.9964	0.9921	0.9856	0.9769	0.9659	0.9526	0.9371	0.9197
3	1.0000	0.9999	0.9997	0.9992	0.9982	0.9966	0.9942	0.9909	0.9865	0.9810
4	1.0000	1.0000	1.0000	0.9999	0.9998	0.9996	0.9992	0.9986	0.9977	0.9963
5	1.0000	1.0000	1.0000	1.0000	1.0000	1.0000	0.9999	0.9998	0.9997	0.9994
6	1.0000	1.0000	1.0000	1.0000	1.0000	1.0000	1.0000	1.0000	1.0000	0.9999
7	1.0000	1.0000	1.0000	1.0000	1.0000	1.0000	1.0000	1.0000	1.0000	1.0000

(continues)

TABLE 2.   Cumulative Poisson Probabilities (*continued*)

					λ					
x	1.1	1.2	1.3	1.4	1.5	1.6	1.7	1.8	1.9	2
0	0.3329	0.3012	0.2725	0.2466	0.2231	0.2019	0.1827	0.1653	0.1496	0.1353
1	0.6990	0.6626	0.6268	0.5918	0.5578	0.5249	0.4932	0.4628	0.4337	0.4060
2	0.9004	0.8795	0.8571	0.8335	0.8088	0.7834	0.7572	0.7306	0.7037	0.6767
3	0.9743	0.9662	0.9569	0.9463	0.9344	0.9212	0.9068	0.8913	0.8747	0.8571
4	0.9946	0.9923	0.9893	0.9857	0.9814	0.9763	0.9704	0.9636	0.9559	0.9473
5	0.9990	0.9985	0.9978	0.9968	0.9955	0.9940	0.9920	0.9896	0.9868	0.9834
6	0.9999	0.9997	0.9996	0.9994	0.9991	0.9987	0.9981	0.9974	0.9966	0.9955
7	1.0000	1.0000	0.9999	0.9999	0.9998	0.9997	0.9996	0.9994	0.9992	0.9989
8	1.0000	1.0000	1.0000	1.0000	1.0000	1.0000	0.9999	0.9999	0.9998	0.9998
9	1.0000	1.0000	1.0000	1.0000	1.0000	1.0000	1.0000	1.0000	1.0000	1.0000

					λ					
x	2.1	2.2	2.3	2.4	2.5	2.6	2.7	2.8	2.9	3
0	0.1225	0.1108	0.1003	0.0907	0.0821	0.0743	0.0672	0.0608	0.0550	0.0498
1	0.3796	0.3546	0.3309	0.3084	0.2873	0.2674	0.2487	0.2311	0.2146	0.1991
2	0.6496	0.6227	0.5960	0.5697	0.5438	0.5184	0.4936	0.4695	0.4460	0.4232
3	0.8386	0.8194	0.7993	0.7787	0.7576	0.7360	0.7141	0.6919	0.6696	0.6472
4	0.9379	0.9275	0.9162	0.9041	0.8912	0.8774	0.8629	0.8477	0.8318	0.8153
5	0.9796	0.9751	0.9700	0.9643	0.9580	0.9510	0.9433	0.9349	0.9258	0.9161
6	0.9941	0.9925	0.9906	0.9884	0.9858	0.9828	0.9794	0.9756	0.9713	0.9665
7	0.9985	0.9980	0.9974	0.9967	0.9958	0.9947	0.9934	0.9919	0.9901	0.9881
8	0.9997	0.9995	0.9994	0.9991	0.9989	0.9985	0.9981	0.9976	0.9969	0.9962
9	0.9999	0.9999	0.9999	0.9998	0.9997	0.9996	0.9995	0.9993	0.9991	0.9989
10	1.0000	1.0000	1.0000	1.0000	0.9999	0.9999	0.9999	0.9998	0.9998	0.9997
11	1.0000	1.0000	1.0000	1.0000	1.0000	1.0000	1.0000	1.0000	0.9999	0.9999
12	1.0000	1.0000	1.0000	1.0000	1.0000	1.0000	1.0000	1.0000	1.0000	1.0000

Table 2   333

| TABLE 2. | Cumulative Poisson Probabilities *(continued)* | | | | | | | | | |

					λ					
x	3.1	3.2	3.3	3.4	3.5	3.6	3.7	3.8	3.9	4
0	0.0450	0.0408	0.0369	0.0334	0.0302	0.0273	0.0247	0.0224	0.0202	0.0183
1	0.1847	0.1712	0.1586	0.1468	0.1359	0.1257	0.1162	0.1074	0.0992	0.0916
2	0.4012	0.3799	0.3594	0.3397	0.3208	0.3027	0.2854	0.2689	0.2531	0.2381
3	0.6248	0.6025	0.5803	0.5584	0.5366	0.5152	0.4942	0.4735	0.4532	0.4335
4	0.7982	0.7806	0.7626	0.7442	0.7254	0.7064	0.6872	0.6678	0.6484	0.6288
5	0.9057	0.8946	0.8829	0.8705	0.8576	0.8441	0.8301	0.8156	0.8006	0.7851
6	0.9612	0.9554	0.9490	0.9421	0.9347	0.9267	0.9182	0.9091	0.8995	0.8893
7	0.9858	0.9832	0.9802	0.9769	0.9733	0.9692	0.9648	0.9599	0.9546	0.9489
8	0.9953	0.9943	0.9931	0.9917	0.9901	0.9883	0.9863	0.9840	0.9815	0.9786
9	0.9986	0.9982	0.9978	0.9973	0.9967	0.9960	0.9952	0.9942	0.9931	0.9919
10	0.9996	0.9995	0.9994	0.9992	0.9990	0.9987	0.9984	0.9981	0.9977	0.9972
11	0.9999	0.9999	0.9998	0.9998	0.9997	0.9996	0.9995	0.9994	0.9993	0.9991
12	1.0000	1.0000	1.0000	0.9999	0.9999	0.9999	0.9999	0.9998	0.9998	0.9997
13	1.0000	1.0000	1.0000	1.0000	1.0000	1.0000	1.0000	1.0000	0.9999	0.9999
14	1.0000	1.0000	1.0000	1.0000	1.0000	1.0000	1.0000	1.0000	1.0000	1.0000

					λ					
x	4.1	4.2	4.3	4.4	4.5	4.6	4.7	4.8	4.9	5
0	0.0166	0.0150	0.0136	0.0123	0.0111	0.0101	0.0091	0.0082	0.0074	0.0067
1	0.0845	0.0780	0.0719	0.0663	0.0611	0.0563	0.0518	0.0477	0.0439	0.0404
2	0.2238	0.2102	0.1974	0.1851	0.1736	0.1626	0.1523	0.1425	0.1333	0.1247
3	0.4142	0.3954	0.3772	0.3594	0.3423	0.3257	0.3097	0.2942	0.2793	0.2650
4	0.6093	0.5898	0.5704	0.5512	0.5321	0.5132	0.4946	0.4763	0.4582	0.4405
5	0.7693	0.7531	0.7367	0.7199	0.7029	0.6858	0.6684	0.6510	0.6335	0.6160
6	0.8786	0.8675	0.8558	0.8436	0.8311	0.8180	0.8046	0.7908	0.7767	0.7622
7	0.9427	0.9361	0.9290	0.9214	0.9134	0.9049	0.8960	0.8867	0.8769	0.8666

(continues)

TABLE 2.   Cumulative Poisson Probabilities (*continued*)

					λ					
x	4.1	4.2	4.3	4.4	4.5	4.6	4.7	4.8	4.9	5
8	0.9755	0.9721	0.9683	0.9642	0.9597	0.9549	0.9497	0.9442	0.9382	0.9319
9	0.9905	0.9889	0.9871	0.9851	0.9829	0.9805	0.9778	0.9749	0.9717	0.9682
10	0.9966	0.9959	0.9952	0.9943	0.9933	0.9922	0.9910	0.9896	0.9880	0.9863
11	0.9989	0.9986	0.9983	0.9980	0.9976	0.9971	0.9966	0.9960	0.9953	0.9945
12	0.9997	0.9996	0.9995	0.9993	0.9992	0.9990	0.9988	0.9986	0.9983	0.9980
13	0.9999	0.9999	0.9998	0.9998	0.9997	0.9997	0.9996	0.9995	0.9994	0.9993
14	1.0000	1.0000	1.0000	0.9999	0.9999	0.9999	0.9999	0.9999	0.9998	0.9998
15	1.0000	1.0000	1.0000	1.0000	1.0000	1.0000	1.0000	1.0000	0.9999	0.9999
16	1.0000	1.0000	1.0000	1.0000	1.0000	1.0000	1.0000	1.0000	1.0000	1.0000

					λ					
x	5.1	5.2	5.3	5.4	5.5	5.6	5.7	5.8	5.9	6
0	0.0061	0.0055	0.0050	0.0045	0.0041	0.0037	0.0033	0.0030	0.0027	0.0025
1	0.0372	0.0342	0.0314	0.0289	0.0266	0.0244	0.0224	0.0206	0.0189	0.0174
2	0.1165	0.1088	0.1016	0.0948	0.0884	0.0824	0.0768	0.0715	0.0666	0.0620
3	0.2513	0.2381	0.2254	0.2133	0.2017	0.1906	0.1800	0.1700	0.1604	0.1512
4	0.4231	0.4061	0.3895	0.3733	0.3575	0.3422	0.3272	0.3127	0.2987	0.2851
5	0.5984	0.5809	0.5635	0.5461	0.5289	0.5119	0.4950	0.4783	0.4619	0.4457
6	0.7474	0.7324	0.7171	0.7017	0.6860	0.6703	0.6544	0.6384	0.6224	0.6063
7	0.8560	0.8449	0.8335	0.8217	0.8095	0.7970	0.7841	0.7710	0.7576	0.7440
8	0.9252	0.9181	0.9106	0.9027	0.8944	0.8857	0.8766	0.8672	0.8574	0.8472
9	0.9644	0.9603	0.9559	0.9512	0.9462	0.9409	0.9352	0.9292	0.9228	0.9161
10	0.9844	0.9823	0.9800	0.9775	0.9747	0.9718	0.9686	0.9651	0.9614	0.9574
11	0.9937	0.9927	0.9916	0.9904	0.9890	0.9875	0.9859	0.9841	0.9821	0.9799
12	0.9976	0.9972	0.9967	0.9962	0.9955	0.9949	0.9941	0.9932	0.9922	0.9912
13	0.9992	0.9990	0.9988	0.9986	0.9983	0.9980	0.9977	0.9973	0.9969	0.9964
14	0.9997	0.9997	0.9996	0.9995	0.9994	0.9993	0.9991	0.9990	0.9988	0.9986

Table 2   335

TABLE 2.	Cumulative Poisson Probabilities	(continued)

					λ					
x	5.1	5.2	5.3	5.4	5.5	5.6	5.7	5.8	5.9	6
15	0.9999	0.9999	0.9999	0.9998	0.9998	0.9998	0.9997	0.9996	0.9996	0.9995
16	1.0000	1.0000	1.0000	0.9999	0.9999	0.9999	0.9999	0.9999	0.9999	0.9998
17	1.0000	1.0000	1.0000	1.0000	1.0000	1.0000	1.0000	1.0000	1.0000	0.9999
18	1.0000	1.0000	1.0000	1.0000	1.0000	1.0000	1.0000	1.0000	1.0000	1.0000

					λ					
x	6.1	6.2	6.3	6.4	6.5	6.6	6.7	6.8	6.9	7
0	0.0022	0.0020	0.0018	0.0017	0.0015	0.0014	0.0012	0.0011	0.0010	0.0009
1	0.0159	0.0146	0.0134	0.0123	0.0113	0.0103	0.0095	0.0087	0.0080	0.0073
2	0.0577	0.0536	0.0498	0.0463	0.0430	0.0400	0.0371	0.0344	0.0320	0.0296
3	0.1425	0.1342	0.1264	0.1189	0.1118	0.1052	0.0988	0.0928	0.0871	0.0818
4	0.2719	0.2592	0.2469	0.2351	0.2237	0.2127	0.2022	0.1920	0.1823	0.1730
5	0.4298	0.4141	0.3988	0.3837	0.3690	0.3547	0.3406	0.3270	0.3137	0.3007
6	0.5902	0.5742	0.5582	0.5423	0.5265	0.5108	0.4953	0.4799	0.4647	0.4497
7	0.7301	0.7160	0.7017	0.6873	0.6728	0.6581	0.6433	0.6285	0.6136	0.5987
8	0.8367	0.8259	0.8148	0.8033	0.7916	0.7796	0.7673	0.7548	0.7420	0.7291
9	0.9090	0.9016	0.8939	0.8858	0.8774	0.8686	0.8596	0.8502	0.8405	0.8305
10	0.9531	0.9486	0.9437	0.9386	0.9332	0.9274	0.9214	0.9151	0.9084	0.9015
11	0.9776	0.9750	0.9723	0.9693	0.9661	0.9627	0.9591	0.9552	0.9510	0.9467
12	0.9900	0.9887	0.9873	0.9857	0.9840	0.9821	0.9801	0.9779	0.9755	0.9730
13	0.9958	0.9952	0.9945	0.9937	0.9929	0.9920	0.9909	0.9898	0.9885	0.9872
14	0.9984	0.9981	0.9978	0.9974	0.9970	0.9966	0.9961	0.9956	0.9950	0.9943
15	0.9994	0.9993	0.9992	0.9990	0.9988	0.9986	0.9984	0.9982	0.9979	0.9976
16	0.9998	0.9997	0.9997	0.9996	0.9996	0.9995	0.9994	0.9993	0.9992	0.9990
17	0.9999	0.9999	0.9999	0.9999	0.9998	0.9998	0.9998	0.9997	0.9997	0.9996
18	1.0000	1.0000	1.0000	1.0000	0.9999	0.9999	0.9999	0.9999	0.9999	0.9999
19	1.0000	1.0000	1.0000	1.0000	1.0000	1.0000	1.0000	1.0000	1.0000	1.0000
20	1.0000	1.0000	1.0000	1.0000	1.0000	1.0000	1.0000	1.0000	1.0000	1.0000

(continues)

TABLE 2. Cumulative Poisson Probabilities *(continued)*

λ

x	7.1	7.2	7.3	7.4	7.5	7.6	7.7	7.8	7.9	8
0	0.0008	0.0007	0.0007	0.0006	0.0006	0.0005	0.0005	0.0004	0.0004	0.0003
1	0.0067	0.0061	0.0056	0.0051	0.0047	0.0043	0.0039	0.0036	0.0033	0.0030
2	0.0275	0.0255	0.0236	0.0219	0.0203	0.0188	0.0174	0.0161	0.0149	0.0138
3	0.0767	0.0719	0.0674	0.0632	0.0591	0.0554	0.0518	0.0485	0.0453	0.0424
4	0.1641	0.1555	0.1473	0.1395	0.1321	0.1249	0.1181	0.1117	0.1055	0.0996
5	0.2881	0.2759	0.2640	0.2526	0.2414	0.2307	0.2203	0.2103	0.2006	0.1912
6	0.4349	0.4204	0.4060	0.3920	0.3782	0.3646	0.3514	0.3384	0.3257	0.3134
7	0.5838	0.5689	0.5541	0.5393	0.5246	0.5100	0.4956	0.4812	0.4670	0.4530
8	0.7160	0.7027	0.6892	0.6757	0.6620	0.6482	0.6343	0.6204	0.6065	0.5925
9	0.8202	0.8096	0.7988	0.7877	0.7764	0.7649	0.7531	0.7411	0.7290	0.7166
10	0.8942	0.8867	0.8788	0.8707	0.8622	0.8535	0.8445	0.8352	0.8257	0.8159
11	0.9420	0.9371	0.9319	0.9265	0.9208	0.9148	0.9085	0.9020	0.8952	0.8881
12	0.9703	0.9673	0.9642	0.9609	0.9573	0.9536	0.9496	0.9454	0.9409	0.9362
13	0.9857	0.9841	0.9824	0.9805	0.9784	0.9762	0.9739	0.9714	0.9687	0.9658
14	0.9935	0.9927	0.9918	0.9908	0.9897	0.9886	0.9873	0.9859	0.9844	0.9827
15	0.9972	0.9969	0.9964	0.9959	0.9954	0.9948	0.9941	0.9934	0.9926	0.9918
16	0.9989	0.9987	0.9985	0.9983	0.9980	0.9978	0.9974	0.9971	0.9967	0.9963
17	0.9996	0.9995	0.9994	0.9993	0.9992	0.9991	0.9989	0.9988	0.9986	0.9984
18	0.9998	0.9998	0.9998	0.9997	0.9997	0.9996	0.9996	0.9995	0.9994	0.9993
19	0.9999	0.9999	0.9999	0.9999	0.9999	0.9999	0.9998	0.9998	0.9998	0.9997
20	1.0000	1.0000	1.0000	1.0000	1.0000	1.0000	0.9999	0.9999	0.9999	0.9999
21	1.0000	1.0000	1.0000	1.0000	1.0000	1.0000	1.0000	1.0000	1.0000	1.0000

λ

x	8.1	8.2	8.3	8.4	8.5	8.6	8.7	8.8	8.9	9
0	0.0003	0.0003	0.0002	0.0002	0.0002	0.0002	0.0002	0.0002	0.0001	0.0001
1	0.0028	0.0025	0.0023	0.0021	0.0019	0.0018	0.0016	0.0015	0.0014	0.0012

Table 2   337

TABLE 2.	Cumulative Poisson Probabilities *(continued)*								

					λ					
x	8.1	8.2	8.3	8.4	8.5	8.6	8.7	8.8	8.9	9
2	0.0127	0.0118	0.0109	0.0100	0.0093	0.0086	0.0079	0.0073	0.0068	0.0062
3	0.0396	0.0370	0.0346	0.0323	0.0301	0.0281	0.0262	0.0244	0.0228	0.0212
4	0.0940	0.0887	0.0837	0.0789	0.0744	0.0701	0.0660	0.0621	0.0584	0.0550
5	0.1822	0.1736	0.1653	0.1573	0.1496	0.1422	0.1352	0.1284	0.1219	0.1157
6	0.3013	0.2896	0.2781	0.2670	0.2562	0.2457	0.2355	0.2256	0.2160	0.2068
7	0.4391	0.4254	0.4119	0.3987	0.3856	0.3728	0.3602	0.3478	0.3357	0.3239
8	0.5786	0.5647	0.5507	0.5369	0.5231	0.5094	0.4958	0.4823	0.4689	0.4557
9	0.7041	0.6915	0.6788	0.6659	0.6530	0.6400	0.6269	0.6137	0.6006	0.5874
10	0.8058	0.7955	0.7850	0.7743	0.7634	0.7522	0.7409	0.7294	0.7178	0.7060
11	0.8807	0.8731	0.8652	0.8571	0.8487	0.8400	0.8311	0.8220	0.8126	0.8030
12	0.9313	0.9261	0.9207	0.9150	0.9091	0.9029	0.8965	0.8898	0.8829	0.8758
13	0.9628	0.9595	0.9561	0.9524	0.9486	0.9445	0.9403	0.9358	0.9311	0.9261
14	0.9810	0.9791	0.9771	0.9749	0.9726	0.9701	0.9675	0.9647	0.9617	0.9585
15	0.9908	0.9898	0.9887	0.9875	0.9862	0.9848	0.9832	0.9816	0.9798	0.9780
16	0.9958	0.9953	0.9947	0.9941	0.9934	0.9926	0.9918	0.9909	0.9899	0.9889
17	0.9982	0.9979	0.9977	0.9973	0.9970	0.9966	0.9962	0.9957	0.9952	0.9947
18	0.9992	0.9991	0.9990	0.9989	0.9987	0.9985	0.9983	0.9981	0.9978	0.9976
19	0.9997	0.9997	0.9996	0.9995	0.9995	0.9994	0.9993	0.9992	0.9991	0.9989
20	0.9999	0.9999	0.9998	0.9998	0.9998	0.9998	0.9997	0.9997	0.9996	0.9996
21	1.0000	1.0000	0.9999	0.9999	0.9999	0.9999	0.9999	0.9999	0.9998	0.9998
22	1.0000	1.0000	1.0000	1.0000	1.0000	1.0000	1.0000	1.0000	0.9999	0.9999
23	1.0000	1.0000	1.0000	1.0000	1.0000	1.0000	1.0000	1.0000	1.0000	1.0000

					λ					
x	9.1	9.2	9.3	9.4	9.5	9.6	9.7	9.8	9.9	10
0	0.0001	0.0001	0.0001	0.0001	0.0001	0.0001	0.0001	0.0001	0.0001	0.0000
1	0.0011	0.0010	0.0009	0.0009	0.0008	0.0007	0.0007	0.0006	0.0005	0.0005

(continues)

TABLE 2.   Cumulative Poisson Probabilities   (*continued*)

					λ					
x	9.1	9.2	9.3	9.4	9.5	9.6	9.7	9.8	9.9	10
2	0.0058	0.0053	0.0049	0.0045	0.0042	0.0038	0.0035	0.0033	0.0030	0.0028
3	0.0198	0.0184	0.0172	0.0160	0.0149	0.0138	0.0129	0.0120	0.0111	0.0103
4	0.0517	0.0486	0.0456	0.0429	0.0403	0.0378	0.0355	0.0333	0.0312	0.0293
5	0.1098	0.1041	0.0986	0.0935	0.0885	0.0838	0.0793	0.0750	0.0710	0.0671
6	0.1978	0.1892	0.1808	0.1727	0.1649	0.1574	0.1502	0.1433	0.1366	0.1301
7	0.3123	0.3010	0.2900	0.2792	0.2687	0.2584	0.2485	0.2388	0.2294	0.2202
8	0.4426	0.4296	0.4168	0.4042	0.3918	0.3796	0.3676	0.3558	0.3442	0.3328
9	0.5742	0.5611	0.5479	0.5349	0.5218	0.5089	0.4960	0.4832	0.4705	0.4579
10	0.6941	0.6820	0.6699	0.6576	0.6453	0.6329	0.6205	0.6080	0.5955	0.5830
11	0.7932	0.7832	0.7730	0.7626	0.7520	0.7412	0.7303	0.7193	0.7081	0.6968
12	0.8684	0.8607	0.8529	0.8448	0.8364	0.8279	0.8191	0.8101	0.8009	0.7916
13	0.9210	0.9156	0.9100	0.9042	0.8981	0.8919	0.8853	0.8786	0.8716	0.8645
14	0.9552	0.9517	0.9480	0.9441	0.9400	0.9357	0.9312	0.9265	0.9216	0.9165
15	0.9760	0.9738	0.9715	0.9691	0.9665	0.9638	0.9609	0.9579	0.9546	0.9513
16	0.9878	0.9865	0.9852	0.9838	0.9823	0.9806	0.9789	0.9770	0.9751	0.9730
17	0.9941	0.9934	0.9927	0.9919	0.9911	0.9902	0.9892	0.9881	0.9870	0.9857
18	0.9973	0.9969	0.9966	0.9962	0.9957	0.9952	0.9947	0.9941	0.9935	0.9928
19	0.9988	0.9986	0.9985	0.9983	0.9980	0.9978	0.9975	0.9972	0.9969	0.9965
20	0.9995	0.9994	0.9993	0.9992	0.9991	0.9990	0.9989	0.9987	0.9986	0.9984
21	0.9998	0.9998	0.9997	0.9997	0.9996	0.9996	0.9995	0.9995	0.9994	0.9993
22	0.9999	0.9999	0.9999	0.9999	0.9999	0.9998	0.9998	0.9998	0.9997	0.9997
23	1.0000	1.0000	1.0000	1.0000	0.9999	0.9999	0.9999	0.9999	0.9999	0.9999
24	1.0000	1.0000	1.0000	1.0000	1.0000	1.0000	1.0000	1.0000	1.0000	1.0000

					λ					
x	11	12	13	14	15	16	17	18	19	20
0	0.0000	0.0000	0.0000	0.0000	0.0000	0.0000	0.0000	0.0000	0.0000	0.0000
1	0.0002	0.0001	0.0000	0.0000	0.0000	0.0000	0.0000	0.0000	0.0000	0.0000

Table 2   339

TABLE 2. Cumulative Poisson Probabilities *(continued)*

x	11	12	13	14	15	16	17	18	19	20
2	0.0012	0.0005	0.0002	0.0001	0.0000	0.0000	0.0000	0.0000	0.0000	0.0000
3	0.0049	0.0023	0.0011	0.0005	0.0002	0.0001	0.0000	0.0000	0.0000	0.0000
4	0.0151	0.0076	0.0037	0.0018	0.0009	0.0004	0.0002	0.0001	0.0000	0.0000
5	0.0375	0.0203	0.0107	0.0055	0.0028	0.0014	0.0007	0.0003	0.0002	0.0001
6	0.0786	0.0458	0.0259	0.0142	0.0076	0.0040	0.0021	0.0010	0.0005	0.0003
7	0.1432	0.0895	0.0540	0.0316	0.0180	0.0100	0.0054	0.0029	0.0015	0.0008
8	0.2320	0.1550	0.0998	0.0621	0.0374	0.0220	0.0126	0.0071	0.0039	0.0021
9	0.3405	0.2424	0.1658	0.1094	0.0699	0.0433	0.0261	0.0154	0.0089	0.0050
10	0.4599	0.3472	0.2517	0.1757	0.1185	0.0774	0.0491	0.0304	0.0183	0.0108
11	0.5793	0.4616	0.3532	0.2600	0.1848	0.1270	0.0847	0.0549	0.0347	0.0214
12	0.6887	0.5760	0.4631	0.3585	0.2676	0.1931	0.1350	0.0917	0.0606	0.0390
13	0.7813	0.6815	0.5730	0.4644	0.3632	0.2745	0.2009	0.1426	0.0984	0.0661
14	0.8540	0.7720	0.6751	0.5704	0.4657	0.3675	0.2808	0.2081	0.1497	0.1049
15	0.9074	0.8444	0.7636	0.6694	0.5681	0.4667	0.3715	0.2867	0.2148	0.1565
16	0.9441	0.8987	0.8355	0.7559	0.6641	0.5660	0.4677	0.3751	0.2920	0.2211
17	0.9678	0.9370	0.8905	0.8272	0.7489	0.6593	0.5640	0.4686	0.3784	0.2970
18	0.9823	0.9626	0.9302	0.8826	0.8195	0.7423	0.6550	0.5622	0.4695	0.3814
19	0.9907	0.9787	0.9573	0.9235	0.8752	0.8122	0.7363	0.6509	0.5606	0.4703
20	0.9953	0.9884	0.9750	0.9521	0.9170	0.8682	0.8055	0.7307	0.6472	0.5591
21	0.9977	0.9939	0.9859	0.9712	0.9469	0.9108	0.8615	0.7991	0.7255	0.6437
22	0.9990	0.9970	0.9924	0.9833	0.9673	0.9418	0.9047	0.8551	0.7931	0.7206
23	0.9995	0.9985	0.9960	0.9907	0.9805	0.9633	0.9367	0.8989	0.8490	0.7875
24	0.9998	0.9993	0.9980	0.9950	0.9888	0.9777	0.9594	0.9317	0.8933	0.8432
25	0.9999	0.9997	0.9990	0.9974	0.9938	0.9869	0.9748	0.9554	0.9269	0.8878
26	1.0000	0.9999	0.9995	0.9987	0.9967	0.9925	0.9848	0.9718	0.9514	0.9221
27	1.0000	0.9999	0.9998	0.9994	0.9983	0.9959	0.9912	0.9827	0.9687	0.9475

(continues)

TABLE 2. Cumulative Poisson Probabilities (*continued*)

x	\(\lambda \) 11	12	13	14	15	16	17	18	19	20
28	1.0000	1.0000	0.9999	0.9997	0.9991	0.9978	0.9950	0.9897	0.9805	0.9657
29	1.0000	1.0000	1.0000	0.9999	0.9996	0.9989	0.9973	0.9941	0.9882	0.9782
30	1.0000	1.0000	1.0000	0.9999	0.9998	0.9994	0.9986	0.9967	0.9930	0.9865
31	1.0000	1.0000	1.0000	1.0000	0.9999	0.9997	0.9993	0.9982	0.9960	0.9919
32	1.0000	1.0000	1.0000	1.0000	1.0000	0.9999	0.9996	0.9990	0.9978	0.9953
33	1.0000	1.0000	1.0000	1.0000	1.0000	0.9999	0.9998	0.9995	0.9988	0.9973
34	1.0000	1.0000	1.0000	1.0000	1.0000	1.0000	0.9999	0.9998	0.9994	0.9985
35	1.0000	1.0000	1.0000	1.0000	1.0000	1.0000	1.0000	0.9999	0.9997	0.9992
36	1.0000	1.0000	1.0000	1.0000	1.0000	1.0000	1.0000	0.9999	0.9998	0.9996
37	1.0000	1.0000	1.0000	1.0000	1.0000	1.0000	1.0000	1.0000	0.9999	0.9998
38	1.0000	1.0000	1.0000	1.0000	1.0000	1.0000	1.0000	1.0000	1.0000	0.9999
39	1.0000	1.0000	1.0000	1.0000	1.0000	1.0000	1.0000	1.0000	1.0000	0.9999
40	1.0000	1.0000	1.0000	1.0000	1.0000	1.0000	1.0000	1.0000	1.0000	1.0000

TABLE 3. Normal Probabilities

The values in the body of the table are the areas between the mean and the value of Z.

Z	0	0.01	0.02	0.03	0.04	0.05	0.06	0.07	0.08	0.09
0	0	0.004	0.008	0.012	0.016	0.0199	0.0239	0.0279	0.0319	0.0359
0.1	0.0398	0.0438	0.0478	0.0517	0.0557	0.0596	0.0636	0.0675	0.0714	0.0753
0.2	0.0793	0.0832	0.0871	0.091	0.0948	0.0987	0.1026	0.1064	0.1103	0.1141
0.3	0.1179	0.1217	0.1255	0.1293	0.1331	0.1368	0.1406	0.1443	0.148	0.1517
0.4	0.1554	0.1591	0.1628	0.1664	0.17	0.1736	0.1772	0.1808	0.1844	0.1879
0.5	0.1915	0.195	0.1985	0.2019	0.2054	0.2088	0.2123	0.2157	0.219	0.2224
0.6	0.2257	0.2291	0.2324	0.2357	0.2389	0.2422	0.2454	0.2486	0.2517	0.2549
0.7	0.258	0.2611	0.2642	0.2673	0.2704	0.2734	0.2764	0.2794	0.2823	0.2852

Table 3   341

Z	0	0.01	0.02	0.03	0.04	0.05	0.06	0.07	0.08	0.09
0.8	0.2881	0.291	0.2939	0.2967	0.2995	0.3023	0.3051	0.3078	0.3106	0.3133
0.9	0.3159	0.3186	0.3212	0.3238	0.3264	0.3289	0.3315	0.3304	0.3365	0.3389
1	0.3413	0.3438	0.3461	0.3485	0.3508	0.3531	0.3554	0.3577	0.3599	0.3621
1.1	0.3643	0.3665	0.3686	0.3708	0.3729	0.3749	0.377	0.379	0.381	0.383
1.2	0.3849	0.3869	0.3888	0.3907	0.3925	0.3944	0.3962	0.398	0.3997	0.4015
1.3	0.4032	0.4049	0.4066	0.4082	0.4099	0.4115	0.4131	0.4147	0.4162	0.4177
1.4	0.4192	0.4207	0.4222	0.4236	0.4251	0.4265	0.4279	0.4292	0.4306	0.4319
1.5	0.4332	0.4345	0.4357	0.437	0.4382	0.4394	0.4406	0.4418	0.4429	0.4441
1.6	0.4452	0.4463	0.4474	0.4484	0.4495	0.4505	0.4515	0.4525	0.4535	0.4545
1.7	0.4554	0.4564	0.4573	0.4582	0.4591	0.4599	0.4608	0.4616	0.4625	0.4633
1.8	0.4641	0.4649	0.4656	0.4664	0.4671	0.4678	0.4686	0.4693	0.4699	0.4706
1.9	0.4713	0.4719	0.4726	0.4732	0.4738	0.4744	0.475	0.4756	0.4761	0.4767
2	0.4772	0.4778	0.4783	0.4788	0.4793	0.4798	0.4803	0.4808	0.4812	0.4817
2.1	0.4821	0.4826	0.483	0.4834	0.4838	0.4842	0.4846	0.485	0.4854	0.4857
2.2	0.4861	0.4864	0.4868	0.4871	0.4875	0.4878	0.4881	0.4884	0.4887	0.489
2.3	0.4893	0.4896	0.4898	0.4901	0.4904	0.4906	0.4909	0.4911	0.4913	0.4916
2.4	0.4918	0.492	0.4922	0.4925	0.4927	0.4929	0.4931	0.4932	0.4934	0.4936
2.5	0.4938	0.494	0.4941	0.4943	0.4945	0.4946	0.4948	0.4949	0.4951	0.4952
2.6	0.4953	0.4955	0.4956	0.4957	0.4959	0.496	0.4961	0.4962	0.4963	0.4964
2.7	0.4965	0.4966	0.4967	0.4968	0.4969	0.497	0.4971	0.4972	0.4973	0.4974
2.8	0.4974	0.4975	0.4976	0.4977	0.4977	0.4978	0.4979	0.4979	0.498	0.4981
2.9	0.4981	0.4982	0.4982	0.4983	0.4984	0.4984	0.4985	0.4985	0.4986	0.4986
3	0.4987	0.4987	0.4987	0.4988	0.4988	0.4989	0.4989	0.4989	0.499	0.499
3.1	0.499	0.4991	0.4991	0.4991	0.4992	0.4992	0.4992	0.4992	0.4993	0.4993
3.2	0.4993	0.4993	0.4994	0.4994	0.4994	0.4994	0.4994	0.4995	0.4995	0.4995
3.3	0.4995	0.4995	0.4995	0.4996	0.4996	0.4996	0.4996	0.4996	0.4996	0.4997
3.4	0.4997	0.4997	0.4997	0.4997	0.4997	0.4997	0.4997	0.4997	0.4997	0.4998

(continues)

TABLE 3.   Normal Probabilities (*continued*)

Z	0	0.01	0.02	0.03	0.04	0.05	0.06	0.07	0.08	0.09
3.5	0.4998	0.4998	0.4998	0.4998	0.4998	0.4998	0.4998	0.4998	0.4998	0.4998
3.6	0.4998	0.4998	0.4999	0.4999	0.4999	0.4999	0.4999	0.4999	0.4999	0.4999
3.7	0.4999	0.4999	0.4999	0.4999	0.4999	0.4999	0.4999	0.4999	0.4999	0.4999
3.8	0.4999	0.4999	0.4999	0.4999	0.4999	0.4999	0.4999	0.4999	0.4999	0.4999

TABLE 4.   Percentiles of the *t* Distribution

One Sided	75%	80%	85%	90%	95%	97.50%	99%	99.50%	99.75%	99.90%	99.95%
Two Sided	50%	60%	70%	80%	90%	95%	98%	99%	99.50%	99.80%	99.90%
df											
1	1	1.376	1.963	3.078	6.314	12.71	31.82	63.66	127.3	318.3	636.6
2	0.816	1.061	1.386	1.886	2.92	4.303	6.965	9.925	14.09	22.33	31.6
3	0.765	0.978	1.25	1.638	2.353	3.182	4.541	5.841	7.453	10.21	12.92
4	0.741	0.941	1.19	1.533	2.132	2.776	3.747	4.604	5.598	7.173	8.61
5	0.727	0.92	1.156	1.476	2.015	2.571	3.365	4.032	4.773	5.893	6.869
6	0.718	0.906	1.134	1.44	1.943	2.447	3.143	3.707	4.317	5.208	5.959
7	0.711	0.896	1.119	1.415	1.895	2.365	2.998	3.499	4.029	4.785	5.408
8	0.706	0.889	1.108	1.397	1.86	2.306	2.896	3.355	3.833	4.501	5.041
9	0.703	0.883	1.1	1.383	1.833	2.262	2.821	3.25	3.69	4.297	4.781
10	0.7	0.879	1.093	1.372	1.812	2.228	2.764	3.169	3.581	4.144	4.587
11	0.697	0.876	1.088	1.363	1.796	2.201	2.718	3.106	3.497	4.025	4.437
12	0.695	0.873	1.083	1.356	1.782	2.179	2.681	3.055	3.428	3.93	4.318
13	0.694	0.87	1.079	1.35	1.771	2.16	2.65	3.012	3.372	3.852	4.221
14	0.692	0.868	1.076	1.345	1.761	2.145	2.624	2.977	3.326	3.787	4.14
15	0.691	0.866	1.074	1.341	1.753	2.131	2.602	2.947	3.286	3.733	4.073

Table 4   343

TABLE 4.   Percentiles of the t Distribution (*continued*)

One Sided	75%	80%	85%	90%	95%	97.50%	99%	99.50%	99.75%	99.90%	99.95%
Two Sided	50%	60%	70%	80%	90%	95%	98%	99%	99.50%	99.80%	99.90%
df											
16	0.69	0.865	1.071	1.337	1.746	2.12	2.583	2.921	3.252	3.686	4.015
17	0.689	0.863	1.069	1.333	1.74	2.11	2.567	2.898	3.222	3.646	3.965
18	0.688	0.862	1.067	1.33	1.734	2.101	2.552	2.878	3.197	3.61	3.922
19	0.688	0.861	1.066	1.328	1.729	2.093	2.539	2.861	3.174	3.579	3.883
20	0.687	0.86	1.064	1.325	1.725	2.086	2.528	2.845	3.153	3.552	3.85
21	0.686	0.859	1.063	1.323	1.721	2.08	2.518	2.831	3.135	3.527	3.819
22	0.686	0.858	1.061	1.321	1.717	2.074	2.508	2.819	3.119	3.505	3.792
23	0.685	0.858	1.06	1.319	1.714	2.069	2.5	2.807	3.104	3.485	3.767
24	0.685	0.857	1.059	1.318	1.711	2.064	2.492	2.797	3.091	3.467	3.745
25	0.684	0.856	1.058	1.316	1.708	2.06	2.485	2.787	3.078	3.45	3.725
26	0.684	0.856	1.058	1.315	1.706	2.056	2.479	2.779	3.067	3.435	3.707
27	0.684	0.855	1.057	1.314	1.703	2.052	2.473	2.771	3.057	3.421	3.69
28	0.683	0.855	1.056	1.313	1.701	2.048	2.467	2.763	3.047	3.408	3.674
29	0.683	0.854	1.055	1.311	1.699	2.045	2.462	2.756	3.038	3.396	3.659
30	0.683	0.854	1.055	1.31	1.697	2.042	2.457	2.75	3.03	3.385	3.646
40	0.681	0.851	1.05	1.303	1.684	2.021	2.423	2.704	2.971	3.307	3.551
50	0.679	0.849	1.047	1.299	1.676	2.009	2.403	2.678	2.937	3.261	3.496
60	0.679	0.848	1.045	1.296	1.671	2	2.39	2.66	2.915	3.232	3.46
80	0.678	0.846	1.043	1.292	1.664	1.99	2.374	2.639	2.887	3.195	3.416
100	0.677	0.845	1.042	1.29	1.66	1.984	2.364	2.626	2.871	3.174	3.39
120	0.677	0.845	1.041	1.289	1.658	1.98	2.358	2.617	2.86	3.16	3.373
∞	0.674	0.842	1.036	1.282	1.645	1.96	2.326	2.576			

TABLE 5. χ^2 Distribution Values

df	0.995	0.99	0.975	0.95	0.9	0.1	0.05	0.025	0.01	0.005
1	–	–	0.001	0.004	0.016	2.706	3.841	5.024	6.635	7.879
2	0.01	0.02	0.051	0.103	0.211	4.605	5.991	7.378	9.21	10.597
3	0.072	0.115	0.216	0.352	0.584	6.251	7.815	9.348	11.345	12.838
4	0.207	0.297	0.484	0.711	1.064	7.779	9.488	11.143	13.277	14.86
5	0.412	0.554	0.831	1.145	1.61	9.236	11.07	12.833	15.086	16.75
6	0.676	0.872	1.237	1.635	2.204	10.645	12.592	14.449	16.812	18.548
7	0.989	1.239	1.69	2.167	2.833	12.017	14.067	16.013	18.475	20.278
8	1.344	1.646	2.18	2.733	3.49	13.362	15.507	17.535	20.09	21.955
9	1.735	2.088	2.7	3.325	4.168	14.684	16.919	19.023	21.666	23.589
10	2.156	2.558	3.247	3.94	4.865	15.987	18.307	20.483	23.209	25.188
11	2.603	3.053	3.816	4.575	5.578	17.275	19.675	21.92	24.725	26.757
12	3.074	3.571	4.404	5.226	6.304	18.549	21.026	23.337	26.217	28.3
13	3.565	4.107	5.009	5.892	7.042	19.812	22.362	24.736	27.688	29.819
14	4.075	4.66	5.629	6.571	7.79	21.064	23.685	26.119	29.141	31.319
15	4.601	5.229	6.262	7.261	8.547	22.307	24.996	27.488	30.578	32.801
16	5.142	5.812	6.908	7.962	9.312	23.542	26.296	28.845	32	34.267
17	5.697	6.408	7.564	8.672	10.085	24.769	27.587	30.191	33.409	35.718
18	6.265	7.015	8.231	9.39	10.865	25.989	28.869	31.526	34.805	37.156
19	6.844	7.633	8.907	10.117	11.651	27.204	30.144	32.852	36.191	38.582
20	7.434	8.26	9.591	10.851	12.443	28.412	31.41	34.17	37.566	39.997
21	8.034	8.897	10.283	11.591	13.24	29.615	32.671	35.479	38.932	41.401
22	8.643	9.542	10.982	12.338	14.041	30.813	33.924	36.781	40.289	42.796
23	9.26	10.196	11.689	13.091	14.848	32.007	35.172	38.076	41.638	44.181
24	9.886	10.856	12.401	13.848	15.659	33.196	36.415	39.364	42.98	45.559
25	10.52	11.524	13.12	14.611	16.473	34.382	37.652	40.646	44.314	46.928
26	11.16	12.198	13.844	15.379	17.292	35.563	38.885	41.923	45.642	48.29
27	11.808	12.879	14.573	16.151	18.114	36.741	40.113	43.195	46.963	49.645

Table 5   345

TABLE 5. χ^2 **Distribution Values** (*continued*)

df	0.995	0.99	0.975	0.95	0.9	0.1	0.05	0.025	0.01	0.005
28	12.461	13.565	15.308	16.928	18.939	37.916	41.337	44.461	48.278	50.993
29	13.121	14.256	16.047	17.708	19.768	39.087	42.557	45.722	49.588	52.336
30	13.787	14.953	16.791	18.493	20.599	40.256	43.773	46.979	50.892	53.672
40	20.707	22.164	24.433	26.509	29.051	51.805	55.758	59.342	63.691	66.766
50	27.991	29.707	32.357	34.764	37.689	63.167	67.505	71.42	76.154	79.49
60	35.534	37.485	40.482	43.188	46.459	74.397	79.082	83.298	88.379	91.952
70	43.275	45.442	48.758	51.739	55.329	85.527	90.531	95.023	100.425	104.215
80	51.172	53.54	57.153	60.391	64.278	96.578	101.879	106.629	112.329	116.321
90	59.196	61.754	65.647	69.126	73.291	107.565	113.145	118.136	124.116	128.299
100	67.328	70.065	74.222	77.929	82.358	118.498	124.342	129.561	135.807	140.169

TABLE 6.   *F* Distribution Values

F Table for $\alpha = 0.10$

$df_2 = $	$df_1 = 1$	2	3	4	5	6	7	8	12	24	∞
1	39.86346	49.5	53.59324	55.83296	57.24008	58.20442	58.90595	59.43898	60.70521	62.00205	63.32812
2	8.52632	9	9.16179	9.24342	9.29263	9.32553	9.34908	9.36677	9.40813	9.44962	9.49122
3	5.53832	5.46238	5.39077	5.34264	5.30916	5.28473	5.26619	5.25167	5.21562	5.17636	5.1337
4	4.54477	4.32456	4.19086	4.10725	4.05058	4.00975	3.97897	3.95494	3.89553	3.83099	3.76073
5	4.06042	3.77972	3.61948	3.5202	3.45298	3.40451	3.3679	3.33928	3.26824	3.19052	3.105
6	3.77595	3.4633	3.28876	3.18076	3.10751	3.05455	3.01446	2.98304	2.90472	2.81834	2.72216
7	3.58943	3.25744	3.07407	2.96053	2.88334	2.82739	2.78493	2.75158	2.66811	2.57533	2.47079
8	3.45792	3.11312	2.9238	2.80643	2.72645	2.66833	2.62413	2.58935	2.50196	2.4041	2.29257
9	3.3603	3.00645	2.81286	2.69268	2.61061	2.55086	2.50531	2.46941	2.37888	2.27683	2.15923
10	3.28502	2.92447	2.72767	2.60534	2.52164	2.46058	2.41397	2.37715	2.28405	2.17843	2.05542
11	3.2252	2.85951	2.66023	2.53619	2.45118	2.38907	2.34157	2.304	2.20873	2.10001	1.97211
12	3.17655	2.8068	2.60552	2.4801	2.39402	2.33102	2.28278	2.24457	2.14744	2.03599	1.90361
13	3.13621	2.76317	2.56027	2.43371	2.34672	2.28298	2.2341	2.19535	2.09659	1.98272	1.8462
14	3.10221	2.72647	2.52222	2.39469	2.30694	2.24256	2.19313	2.1539	2.05371	1.93766	1.79728
15	3.07319	2.69517	2.48979	2.36143	2.27302	2.20808	2.15818	2.11853	2.01707	1.89904	1.75505
16	3.04811	2.66817	2.46181	2.33274	2.24376	2.17833	2.128	2.08798	1.98539	1.86556	1.71817
17	3.02623	2.64464	2.43743	2.30775	2.21825	2.15239	2.10169	2.06134	1.95772	1.83624	1.68564
18	3.00698	2.62395	2.41601	2.28577	2.19583	2.12958	2.07854	2.03789	1.93334	1.81035	1.65671
19	2.9899	2.60561	2.39702	2.2663	2.17596	2.10936	2.05802	2.0171	1.9117	1.78731	1.63077

Table 6   347

df₂	1	2	3	4	5	6	7	8	12	24	∞
20	2.97465	2.58925	2.38009	2.24893	2.15823	2.09132	2.0397	1.99853	1.89236	1.76667	1.60738
21	2.96096	2.57457	2.36489	2.23334	2.14231	2.07512	2.02325	1.98186	1.87497	1.74807	1.58615
22	2.94858	2.56131	2.35117	2.21927	2.12794	2.0605	2.0084	1.9668	1.85925	1.73122	1.56678
23	2.93736	2.54929	2.33873	2.20651	2.11491	2.04723	1.99492	1.95312	1.84497	1.71588	1.54903
24	2.92712	2.53833	2.32739	2.19488	2.10303	2.03513	1.98263	1.94066	1.83194	1.70185	1.5327
25	2.91774	2.52831	2.31702	2.18424	2.09216	2.02406	1.97138	1.92925	1.82	1.68898	1.5176
26	2.90913	2.5191	2.30749	2.17447	2.08218	2.01389	1.96104	1.91876	1.80902	1.67712	1.5036
27	2.90119	2.51061	2.29871	2.16546	2.07298	2.00452	1.95151	1.90909	1.79889	1.66616	1.49057
28	2.89385	2.50276	2.2906	2.15714	2.06447	1.99585	1.9427	1.90014	1.78951	1.656	1.47841
29	2.88703	2.49548	2.28307	2.14941	2.05658	1.98781	1.93452	1.89184	1.78081	1.64655	1.46704
30	2.88069	2.48872	2.27607	2.14223	2.04925	1.98033	1.92692	1.88412	1.7727	1.63774	1.45636
40	2.83535	2.44037	2.22609	2.09095	1.99682	1.92688	1.87252	1.82886	1.71456	1.57411	1.37691
60	2.79107	2.39325	2.17741	2.04099	1.94571	1.87472	1.81939	1.77483	1.65743	1.51072	1.29146
120	2.74781	2.34734	2.12999	1.9923	1.89587	1.82381	1.76748	1.72196	1.6012	1.44723	1.19256
∞	2.70554	2.30259	2.0838	1.94486	1.84727	1.77411	1.71672	1.6702	1.54578	1.38318	1

F Table for α = 0.05

	$df_1 = 1$	2	3	4	5	6	7	8	12	24	∞
$df_2 = 1$	161.4476	199.5	215.7073	224.5832	230.1619	233.986	236.7684	238.8827	243.906	249.0518	254.3144
2	18.5128	19	19.1643	19.2468	19.2964	19.3295	19.3532	19.371	19.4125	19.4541	19.4957
3	10.128	9.5521	9.2766	9.1172	9.0135	8.9406	8.8867	8.8452	8.7446	8.6385	8.5264
4	7.7086	6.9443	6.5914	6.3882	6.2561	6.1631	6.0942	6.041	5.9117	5.7744	5.6281

(continues)

TABLE 6.   F Distribution Values (continued)

F Table for α = 0.05

df_2	$df_1=1$	2	3	4	5	6	7	8	12	24	∞
5	6.6079	5.7861	5.4095	5.1922	5.0503	4.9503	4.8759	4.8183	4.6777	4.5272	4.365
6	5.9874	5.1433	4.7571	4.5337	4.3874	4.2839	4.2067	4.1468	3.9999	3.8415	3.6689
7	5.5914	4.7374	4.3468	4.1203	3.9715	3.866	3.787	3.7257	3.5747	3.4105	3.2298
8	5.3177	4.459	4.0662	3.8379	3.6875	3.5806	3.5005	3.4381	3.2839	3.1152	2.9276
9	5.1174	4.2565	3.8625	3.6331	3.4817	3.3738	3.2927	3.2296	3.0729	2.9005	2.7067
10	4.9646	4.1028	3.7083	3.478	3.3258	3.2172	3.1355	3.0717	2.913	2.7372	2.5379
11	4.8443	3.9823	3.5874	3.3567	3.2039	3.0946	3.0123	2.948	2.7876	2.609	2.4045
12	4.7472	3.8853	3.4903	3.2592	3.1059	2.9961	2.9134	2.8486	2.6866	2.5055	2.2962
13	4.6672	3.8056	3.4105	3.1791	3.0254	2.9153	2.8321	2.7669	2.6037	2.4202	2.2064
14	4.6001	3.7389	3.3439	3.1122	2.9582	2.8477	2.7642	2.6987	2.5342	2.3487	2.1307
15	4.5431	3.6823	3.2874	3.0556	2.9013	2.7905	2.7066	2.6408	2.4753	2.2878	2.0658
16	4.494	3.6337	3.2389	3.0069	2.8524	2.7413	2.6572	2.5911	2.4247	2.2354	2.0096
17	4.4513	3.5915	3.1968	2.9647	2.81	2.6987	2.6143	2.548	2.3807	2.1898	1.9604
18	4.4139	3.5546	3.1599	2.9277	2.7729	2.6613	2.5767	2.5102	2.3421	2.1497	1.9168
19	4.3807	3.5219	3.1274	2.8951	2.7401	2.6283	2.5435	2.4768	2.308	2.1141	1.878
20	4.3512	3.4928	3.0984	2.8661	2.7109	2.599	2.514	2.4471	2.2776	2.0825	1.8432
21	4.3248	3.4668	3.0725	2.8401	2.6848	2.5727	2.4876	2.4205	2.2504	2.054	1.8117
22	4.3009	3.4434	3.0491	2.8167	2.6613	2.5491	2.4638	2.3965	2.2258	2.0283	1.7831
23	4.2793	3.4221	3.028	2.7955	2.64	2.5277	2.4422	2.3748	2.2036	2.005	1.757
24	4.2597	3.4028	3.0088	2.7763	2.6207	2.5082	2.4226	2.3551	2.1834	1.9838	1.733

Table 6   349

	1	2	3	4	5	6	7	8	12	24	∞
25	4.2417	3.3852	2.9912	2.7587	2.603	2.4904	2.4047	2.3371	2.1649	1.9643	1.711
26	4.2252	3.369	2.9752	2.7426	2.5868	2.4741	2.3883	2.3205	2.1479	1.9464	1.6906
27	4.21	3.3541	2.9604	2.7278	2.5719	2.4591	2.3732	2.3053	2.1323	1.9299	1.6717
28	4.196	3.3404	2.9467	2.7141	2.5581	2.4453	2.3593	2.2913	2.1179	1.9147	1.6541
29	4.183	3.3277	2.934	2.7014	2.5454	2.4324	2.3463	2.2783	2.1045	1.9005	1.6376
30	4.1709	3.3158	2.9223	2.6896	2.5336	2.4205	2.3343	2.2662	2.0921	1.8874	1.6223
40	4.0847	3.2317	2.8387	2.606	2.4495	2.3359	2.249	2.1802	2.0035	1.7929	1.5089
60	4.0012	3.1504	2.7581	2.5252	2.3683	2.2541	2.1665	2.097	1.9174	1.7001	1.3893
120	3.9201	3.0718	2.6802	2.4472	2.2899	2.175	2.0868	2.0164	1.8337	1.6084	1.2539
∞	3.8415	2.9957	2.6049	2.3719	2.2141	2.0986	2.0096	1.9384	1.7522	1.5173	1

F Table for α = 0.25

	$df_1 = 1$	2	3	4	5	6	7	8	12	24	∞
$df_2 = 1$	647.789	799.5	864.163	899.5833	921.8479	937.1111	948.2169	956.6562	976.7079	997.2492	1018.258
2	38.5063	39	39.1655	39.2484	39.2982	39.3315	39.3552	39.373	39.4146	39.4562	39.498
3	17.4434	16.0441	15.4392	15.101	14.8848	14.7347	14.6244	14.5399	14.3366	14.1241	13.902
4	12.21179	10.6491	9.9792	9.6045	9.3645	9.1973	9.0741	8.9796	8.7512	8.5109	8.257
5	10.007	8.4336	7.7636	7.3879	7.1464	6.9777	6.8531	6.7572	6.5245	6.278	6.015
6	8.8131	7.2599	6.5988	6.2272	5.9876	5.8198	5.6955	5.5996	5.3662	5.1172	4.849
7	8.0727	6.5415	5.8898	5.5226	5.2852	5.1186	4.9949	4.8993	4.6658	4.415	4.142
8	7.5709	6.0595	5.416	5.0526	4.8173	4.6517	4.5286	4.4333	4.1997	3.9472	3.67
9	7.2093	5.7147	5.0781	4.7181	4.4844	4.3197	4.197	4.102	3.8682	3.6142	3.333
10	6.9367	5.4564	4.8256	4.4683	4.2361	4.0721	3.9498	3.8549	3.6209	3.3654	3.08

(continues)

TABLE 6. F Distribution Values (*continued*)

F Table for $\alpha = 0.25$

$df_2 = 11$	$df_1 = 1$	2	3	4	5	6	7	8	12	24	∞
11	6.7241	5.2559	4.63	4.2751	4.044	3.8807	3.7586	3.6638	3.4296	3.1725	2.883
12	6.5538	5.0959	4.4742	4.1212	3.8911	3.7283	3.6065	3.5118	3.2773	3.0187	2.725
13	6.4143	4.9653	4.3472	3.9959	3.7667	3.6043	3.4827	3.388	3.1532	2.8932	2.595
14	6.2979	4.8567	4.2417	3.8919	3.6634	3.5014	3.3799	3.2853	3.0502	2.7888	2.487
15	6.1995	4.765	4.1528	3.8043	3.5764	3.4147	3.2934	3.1987	2.9633	2.7006	2.395
16	6.1151	4.6867	4.0768	3.7294	3.5021	3.3406	3.2194	3.1248	2.889	2.6252	2.316
17	6.042	4.6189	4.0112	3.6648	3.4379	3.2767	3.1556	3.061	2.8249	2.5598	2.247
18	5.9781	4.5597	3.9539	3.6083	3.382	3.2209	3.0999	3.0053	2.7689	2.5027	2.187
19	5.9216	4.5075	3.9034	3.5587	3.3327	3.1718	3.0509	2.9563	2.7196	2.4523	2.133
20	5.8715	4.4613	3.8587	3.5147	3.2891	3.1283	3.0074	2.9128	2.6758	2.4076	2.085
21	5.8266	4.4199	3.8188	3.4754	3.2501	3.0895	2.9686	2.874	2.6368	2.3675	2.042
22	5.7863	4.3828	3.7829	3.4401	3.2151	3.0546	2.9338	2.8392	2.6017	2.3315	2.003
23	5.7498	4.3492	3.7505	3.4083	3.1835	3.0232	2.9023	2.8077	2.5699	2.2989	1.968
24	5.7166	4.3187	3.7211	3.3794	3.1548	2.9946	2.8738	2.7791	2.5411	2.2693	1.935
25	5.6864	4.2909	3.6943	3.353	3.1287	2.9685	2.8478	2.7531	2.5149	2.2422	1.906
26	5.6586	4.2655	3.6697	3.3289	3.1048	2.9447	2.824	2.7293	2.4908	2.2174	1.878
27	5.6331	4.2421	3.6472	3.3067	3.0828	2.9228	2.8021	2.7074	2.4688	2.1946	1.853
28	5.6096	4.2205	3.6264	3.2863	3.0626	2.9027	2.782	2.6872	2.4484	2.1735	1.829
29	5.5878	4.2006	3.6072	3.2674	3.0438	2.884	2.7633	2.6686	2.4295	2.154	1.807

Table 6   351

df_2	1	2	3	4	5	6	7	8	12	24	∞
30	5.5675	4.1821	3.5894	3.2499	3.0265	2.8667	2.746	2.6513	2.412	2.1359	1.787
40	5.4239	4.051	3.4633	3.1261	2.9037	2.7444	2.6238	2.5289	2.2882	2.0069	1.637
60	5.2856	3.9253	3.3425	3.0077	2.7863	2.6274	2.5068	2.4117	2.1692	1.8817	1.482
120	5.1523	3.8046	3.2269	2.8943	2.674	2.5154	2.3948	2.2994	2.0548	1.7597	1.31
∞	5.0239	3.6889	3.1161	2.7858	2.5665	2.4082	2.2875	2.1918	1.9447	1.6402	1

F Table for $\alpha = 0.10$

/ $df_1 = 1$	2	3	4	5	6	7	8	12	24	∞
$df_2 = 1$ 4052.181	4999.5	5403.352	5624.583	5763.65	5858.986	5928.356	5981.07	6106.321	6234.631	6365.864
2	98.503	99	99.166	99.249	99.299	99.333	99.356	99.374	99.416	99.458	99.499
3	34.116	30.817	29.457	28.71	28.237	27.911	27.672	27.489	27.052	26.598	26.125
4	21.198	18	16.694	15.977	15.522	15.207	14.976	14.799	14.374	13.929	13.463
5	16.258	13.274	12.06	11.392	10.967	10.672	10.456	10.289	9.888	9.466	9.02
6	13.745	10.925	9.78	9.148	8.746	8.466	8.26	8.102	7.718	7.313	6.88
7	12.246	9.547	8.451	7.847	7.46	7.191	6.993	6.84	6.469	6.074	5.65
8	11.259	8.649	7.591	7.006	6.632	6.371	6.178	6.029	5.667	5.279	4.859
9	10.561	8.022	6.992	6.422	6.057	5.802	5.613	5.467	5.111	4.729	4.311
10	10.044	7.559	6.552	5.994	5.636	5.386	5.2	5.057	4.706	4.327	3.909
11	9.646	7.206	6.217	5.668	5.316	5.069	4.886	4.744	4.397	4.021	3.602
12	9.33	6.927	5.953	5.412	5.064	4.821	4.64	4.499	4.155	3.78	3.361
13	9.074	6.701	5.739	5.205	4.862	4.62	4.441	4.302	3.96	3.587	3.165
14	8.862	6.515	5.564	5.035	4.695	4.456	4.278	4.14	3.8	3.427	3.004
15	8.683	6.359	5.417	4.893	4.556	4.318	4.142	4.004	3.666	3.294	2.868

(continues)

TABLE 6.   F Distribution Values (continued)

F Table for α = 0.10

df_2	$df_1 = 1$	2	3	4	5	6	7	8	12	24	∞
16	8.531	6.226	5.292	4.773	4.437	4.202	4.026	3.89	3.553	3.181	2.753
17	8.4	6.112	5.185	4.669	4.336	4.102	3.927	3.791	3.455	3.084	2.653
18	8.285	6.013	5.092	4.579	4.248	4.015	3.841	3.705	3.371	2.999	2.566
19	8.185	5.926	5.01	4.5	4.171	3.939	3.765	3.631	3.297	2.925	2.489
20	8.096	5.849	4.938	4.431	4.103	3.871	3.699	3.564	3.231	2.859	2.421
21	8.017	5.78	4.874	4.369	4.042	3.812	3.64	3.506	3.173	2.801	2.36
22	7.945	5.719	4.817	4.313	3.988	3.758	3.587	3.453	3.121	2.749	2.305
23	7.881	5.664	4.765	4.264	3.939	3.71	3.539	3.406	3.074	2.702	2.256
24	7.823	5.614	4.718	4.218	3.895	3.667	3.496	3.363	3.032	2.659	2.211
25	7.77	5.568	4.675	4.177	3.855	3.627	3.457	3.324	2.993	2.62	2.169
26	7.721	5.526	4.637	4.14	3.818	3.591	3.421	3.288	2.958	2.585	2.131
27	7.677	5.488	4.601	4.106	3.785	3.558	3.388	3.256	2.926	2.552	2.097
28	7.636	5.453	4.568	4.074	3.754	3.528	3.358	3.226	2.896	2.522	2.064
29	7.598	5.42	4.538	4.045	3.725	3.499	3.33	3.198	2.868	2.495	2.034
30	7.562	5.39	4.51	4.018	3.699	3.473	3.304	3.173	2.843	2.469	2.006
40	7.314	5.179	4.313	3.828	3.514	3.291	3.124	2.993	2.665	2.288	1.805
60	7.077	4.977	4.126	3.649	3.339	3.119	2.953	2.823	2.496	2.115	1.601
120	6.851	4.787	3.949	3.48	3.174	2.956	2.792	2.663	2.336	1.95	1.381
∞	6.635	4.605	3.782	3.319	3.017	2.802	2.639	2.511	2.185	1.791	1

Model Building

In observational data sets, the independent variables are not truly independent because they are usually correlated with each other. If the level of correlation is moderate to high, then the regression coefficients are influenced by the particular set of variables that are in the model. Variable selection methods have been developed to arrive at an optimal subset of variables. However, care is needed when using these methods, as will be discussed.

Stepwise regression involves examining several different regression equations in order to take all possible independent variables and sequentially evaluate them with respect to their statistical significance. This process generates a final set of variables that reflect the best fitting model. Three selection techniques using SAS will be presented here.

1. FORWARD: This technique begins with the best single regressor. The next best variable is added to the model, then the next best, and so on, until no additional variable adds to the significance of the model.
2. BACKWARD: This technique begins with all variables in the model and then drops the most insignificant variable, then the next, until all insignificant variables have been dropped from the model.
3. STEPWISE: This technique is similar to FORWARD, but with an additional step in which all variables in each model are checked again for statistical significance after the new variable has been added.

To illustrate these techniques, let's consider again the data set involving quality-of-life indicators according to voice disorders and voice-related conditions.[1] We are interested in whether emotional well-being, measured on a 100-point scale (with a higher score representing better emotional health), is associated with a history of voice disorders. The emotional well-being variable is based on responses to the SF-36 (short form), developed by the RAND Corporation to assess eight measures of functional health, well being, and psychometrically based physical and mental health.[2] We are also interested in whether age, gender, history of smoking, level of alcohol consumption per day, average number of days of exercise per week, race, marital status, and level of education attained are associated with emotional well-being. The following is the SAS code and partial output for each of the 3 selection techniques.

FORWARD

PROC REG DATA=EXAMPLE;
    MODEL EMOTION = VD GENDER AGE SMOKED DRINK
    EXERCISE RACE MS EDUCATION BMI/SELECTION = FORWARD
    SLE = 0.15;

RUN;

	Summary of Forward Selection						
Step	**Variable entered**	**Number of variables in**	**Partial *r*-square**	**Model *r*-square**	**C(*p*)**	***F* value**	**Pr > *f***
1	Smoked	1	0.0288	0.0288	25.4854	12.14	0.0005
2	VD	2	0.0288	0.0576	14.6642	12.46	0.0005
3	Gender	3	0.0135	0.0711	10.6659	5.9	0.0156
4	Age	4	0.0134	0.0845	6.7115	5.93	0.0153
5	Exercise	5	0.0076	0.0921	5.3054	3.41	0.0655

We generally require the *P* value to be less than 0.05 for the corresponding variable to be significant. However, in exploratory model building, it is common to set an inclusion level of 0.1, 0.15, or even higher.

BACKWARD

PROC REG DATA=EXAMPLE;
    MODEL EMOTION = VD GENDER AGE SMOKED DRINK
    EXERCISE RACE MS EDUCATION BMI/SELECTION = BACKWARD
    SLS = 0.15;

RUN;

Summary of Backward Elimination						
Step	Variable entered	Number of variables in	Partial r-square	Model r-square	C(p)	F value	Pr > f
1	BMI	9	0	0.1018	9.0095	0.01	0.9224
2	MS	8	0	0.1017	7.0225	0.01	0.9093
3	Education	7	0.0019	0.0998	5.8884	0.87	0.3514
4	Drink	6	0.0031	0.0967	5.2696	1.39	0.2394
5	Race	5	0.0046	0.0921	5.3054	2.04	0.1535

The same model was selected using this approach as the forward approach, which is not always the case.

STEPWISE

PROC REG DATA=EXAMPLE;
    MODEL EMOTION = VD GENDER AGE SMOKED DRINK
    EXERCISE RACE MS EDUCATION BMI/SELECTION = STEPWISE
    SLE = 0.15 SLS = 0.15;

RUN;

Summary of Stepwise Selection						
Step	Variable entered	Number of variables in	Partial r-square	Model r-square	C(p)	F value	Pr > f
1	Smoked	1	0.0288	0.0288	25.4854	12.14	0.0005
2	VD	2	0.0288	0.0576	14.6642	12.46	0.0005
3	Gender	3	0.0135	0.0711	10.6659	5.9	0.0156
4	Age	4	0.0134	0.0845	6.7115	5.93	0.0153
5	Exercise	5	0.0076	0.0921	5.3054	3.41	0.0655

The partial r-square value indicates the proportion of variation in emotional well-being that is explained by each variable. The model r-square provides a cumulative indication of the amount of variability in emotional well-being explained by the variables included in the model. Thus, 9.2% of variation in emotional well-being is explained by these five variables.

The final output from the selection techniques is shown in the following table.

Source	Df	Sum of squares	Mean squares	F value	Pr > f
Model	5	8568.93	1713.79	8.22	<0.0001
Error	405	84462	208.55		
Corrected total	410	93031			

Variable	Parameter estimate	Standard error	Type ii ss	F value	Pr > f
Intercept	94.19	6.20	48080.00	230.55	<0.0001
VD	−6.03	1.98	1944.50	9.32	0.00
Gender	3.73	1.44	1400.46	6.72	0.01
Smoked	−6.19	1.61	3068.69	14.71	0.00
Exercise	0.71	0.39	711.54	3.41	0.07
Age	−0.21	0.09	1181.81	5.67	0.02

We see from these results that emotional well-being is significantly lower among individuals with a history of voice disorders, a history of smoking, and older age. Males compared with females have a higher emotional well-being score. There is also some evidence that a higher emotional well-being score may be associated with higher levels of exercise.

REFERENCES

1. Merrill RM, Anderson AE, Sloan A. Quality of life indicators according to voice disorders and voice-related conditions. *Laryngoscope*. 2011;121:2,004–2,011.
2. Ware JE, Gandek B. The SF-36 health survey: development and use in mental health research and the IQOLA project. *Int J Ment Health*. 1994;23(2):49–73.

Answers to Chapter Exercises

CHAPTER 1

1. Because of the interactive nature of these dimensions of health, it is unlikely that you came up with one or more of these six dimensions as being unnecessary. Yet, circumstances at any given time in life may influence the importance placed on any one or a combination of the six dimensions of health.

2. *Assessment* involves monitoring health status to identify and solve community health problems. It also involves diagnosing and investigating health problems and health hazards in the community. *Policy development* involves informing, educating, and empowering people about health issues; mobilizing community partnerships and action to identify and solve health problems; and developing policies and plans that support individual and community health efforts. *Assurance* requires enforcing laws and regulations that protect health and ensure safety; linking people to needed personal health services and providing the provision of health care when it is otherwise unavailable; assuring the availability of competent public and personal healthcare workers; evaluating the effectiveness, accessibility, and quality of personal and population-based health services; and conducting research in order to provide new insights and innovative solutions to health problems.

3. *Monitoring* is a process wherein changes in health status over time or among populations are identified. *Diagnosing* is the act or process of identifying or determining the nature of a case of a disease or distinguishing one disease from another. Monitoring is conducted on a population level, whereas diagnosing is conducted on an individual level. Both are carried out to identify health problems and to assess progress toward health goals or objectives.

4. Health education to influence health behavior change (e.g., nutrition or physical activity); health education and resource allocation to improve immunization levels; regulations to improve housing conditions, sanitation, and water supply; and quarantining to stop the spreading of illness.

5. Epidemiology includes the study of the determinants of health-related states or events, whereas biostatistics does not have a causal focus. In addition, epidemiology is a study involving human populations. Biostatistics is not restricted to the study of just human populations.

6. The study of the distribution and determinants of health-related states or events in human populations can provide useful information for informing public health policy and individual decision making.

7. Epidemiology plays a foundational role because of its central role in carrying out the three core public health functions. Epidemiology offers an approach to assess and monitor the health of populations at risk and identify health problems and priorities, identify risk factors for health problems, and provide a basis for predicting the effects of certain exposures. In turn, epidemiologic information is useful in formulating policies and priorities designed to solve identified health problems and allocating scarce health resources for preventing, protecting, and promoting the public's health.

8. The clinician treats and cares for the patient based on scientific knowledge, experience, and clinical judgment; the epidemiologist explores the source or exposure that caused the adverse health outcome, the number of persons exposed, and the potential for further spread, and applies this information in the development of interventions to prevent additional cases or recurrences.

9. Although a major focus of epidemiology is the study of disease states, it also involves the study of events, behaviors, and conditions associated with health. There are many events that influence health, such as a suicide attempt, a motor vehicle accident, or a workplace injury. Similarly, several lifestyle behaviors can influence health, such as poor diet, a physically inactive lifestyle, or reckless behaviors. Various conditions also play a role in one's health, such as contaminated drinking water or squalid living conditions.

10. A, A, A, A, B, A, C, C, C, C, A, A

11. Confidence in one's ability to take action; emotional.

12. B, A, A

13. Pathogens (organisms or substances such as bacteria, viruses, fungi, and parasites that are capable of producing disease) may be transmitted indirectly from an infected person or animal by a fomite (inanimate object) or a vector (invertebrate animal).

14. Airborne transmission, vector-borne transmission, and vehicle-borne transmission.

15. Direct transmission—rabies, a viral disease of mammals, transmitted from the infected saliva of a rabid animal to an uninfected animal through a bite. Indirect

transmission—rabies transmitted from a rabid animal to an uninfected animal through the air (water droplets or dust particles carrying the infectious agent).

16. The "what" question, which identifies the observed clinical features that distinguish the health-related state or event.
17. A, B, A, B
18. All.
19. Experimental.
20. Descriptive, probability, inferential, and statistical techniques.
21. Knowledge of the fundamentals of epidemiology and biostatistics will make the information in the health and medical literature more accessible. It will also allow you to critically assess the scientific adequacy of the study designs, data collection, and statistical methods employed in the research. In addition, you can assess whether the study conclusions are appropriate and whether chance, bias, or confounding factors may have influenced the results.

CHAPTER 2

1. *Population* refers to a collection of individuals who share one or more observable personal or observational characteristics from which data may be collected and evaluated. Social, economic, family (marriage and divorce), work and labor force, and geographic factors may characterize populations.
2. C, D, B, A
3. A, B, A, B, A
4. Case study.
5. In general, a sample may be studied more quickly and at a lower cost, the entire population may be impossible to access, and sample results may be more accurate than results based on a population.
6.

Number of children	Frequency	Relative frequency	Cumulative frequency	Cumulative relative frequency
0	4	0.2	4	0.2
1	8	0.4	12	0.6
2	4	0.2	16	0.8
3	2	0.1	18	0.9
4+	2	0.1	20	1.0

7. A

8. B

9. D

10. Higher incidence, better survival, and/or poorer recovery for disease A.

11. $Attack\ Rate = \dfrac{34}{63} \times 100 = 54\%$

12. D

13. C, B, A, A

14.

$$Prevalence = \dfrac{90}{9,000} \times 100 = 1\%$$

$$I_e = \dfrac{207}{6,000 - 60} \times 1000 = 34.8\%$$

$$I_0 = \dfrac{61}{3,000 - 30} \times 1000 = 20.5\%$$

$$I_t = \dfrac{268}{9,000 - 90} \times 1000 = 30.1\%$$

15. $Ratio = \dfrac{34.8}{20.5} = 1.70$

16. 120.0 per 100,000; approximately 120 new cases per 100,000 person-years of gonorrhea are reported to the CDC each year.

17. Attack Rate = 7/70 × 100 = 10%; 10% of children attending the child-care facility developed hepatitis A.
Secondary Attack Rate = 5/(32 − 7) × 100 = 20%; 20% of family members of the 7 infected children developed hepatitis A.

18. $Person - time\ rate = \dfrac{350}{5,000 \times 40 + 78 \times 50 + 452 \times 20} \times 1,000 = 1.6$; there were approximately 1.6 injuries per 1,000 hours worked.

19. $Number\ of\ classes = [2 \times 250]^{0.3333} = 7.9 \approx 8$

20. $Approximate\ class\ interval\ (width) = \dfrac{41.9 - 18.5}{8} = 2.9 \approx 3$. Beginning with 18, the boundaries are: 18–<21, 21–<24, 24–<27, 27–<30, 30–<33, 33–<36, 36–<39, 39–<42.

21. Arithmetic mean = 25.53
Median = 25.5
Mode = there is no mode
Variance = 7.05
Standard deviation = 2.65
Standard error = 0.84
Range = 7.1 (22 to 29.1)
Interquartile range = 5.4 (22.8 to 28.2)
Coefficient of variation = 10.40
This information can be obtained using the following statements in SAS:

```
DATA EXERCISE2_21;
INPUT PCTOBESE @@;
DATALINES;
28.2 29.1 26.1 22 22.8 24.5 26.7 24.9 22.3 28.7
;
PROC UNIVARIATE;
RUN;
```

22. $SD = \sqrt{\dfrac{6581.23 - \dfrac{(255.3)^2}{10}}{10-1}} = \sqrt{7.047} = 2.65$

CHAPTER 3

1.

$$Rate_F = \frac{168,086}{18,199,526} \times 100,000 = 923.6$$

$$Rate_U = \frac{14,142}{2,668,925} \times 100,000 = 529.9$$

The ratio of the rate in Florida to the rate in Utah is:

$$Ratio = \frac{923.6}{529.9} = 1.7$$

This result indicates that the mortality rate in Florida is 1.7 times (or 70%) greater than in Utah.

2.

Ages (Years)	Florida, 2007			Utah, 2007		
	# Deaths	Population	Rate per 100,000	# Deaths	Population	Rate per 100,000
0–19	3,181	4,466,929	71.2	531	912,374	58.2
20–39	6,481	4,640,902	139.6	892	843,838	105.7
40–59	24,039	5,009,290	479.9	2,116	583,098	362.9
60–79	57,652	3,085,897	1,868.2	4,390	263,995	1,662.9
80+	76,733	996,508	7,700.2	6,213	65,620	9,468.1
Total	168,086	18,199,526	923.6	14,142	2,668,925	529.9

3.

Age	Ratio	Percent change
0–19	1.224	22.4%
20–39	1.321	32.1%
40–59	1.322	32.2%
60–79	1.123	12.3%
80+	0.813	−18.7%

The mortality rate remains higher in Florida for each age group through age 79, but it is lower in the age group 80 years and older. We also computed the rate ratios for 5-year age intervals and found a similar result (data not shown).

4.

Age	Utah rate		Florida population		Expected number of cases
0–19	0.000582	×	4,466,929	=	2,600
20–39	0.001057	×	4,640,902	=	4,906
40–59	0.003629	×	5,009,290	=	18,179
60–79	0.016629	×	3,085,897	=	51,315
80+	0.094681	×	996,508	=	94,351

The sum of the expected number of cases in Utah if they had the same population as in Florida is 171,351. Dividing this number by the total population in Florida gives the age-adjusted rate, which is:

$$Age - Adjusted\ Rate = \frac{171,351}{18,199,526} = 0.009415$$

The age-adjusted rate is 941.5 per 100,000.

5. The ratio of the rate in Florida to the rate in Utah is:

$$Ratio = \frac{941.5}{951.5} = 0.99$$

Thus, the mortality rate in Florida is 0.99 times (or 1% lower) than that in Utah.

6.

White rate		Black population		Expected number of cases
0.0000078	×	664,888	=	5
0.0000701	×	269,503	=	19
0.0004380	×	94,626	=	41
0.0042820	×	21,862	=	94
Total				159

7. In the previous problem, we computed the expected number of cases for blacks, assuming they had the same rate as whites (i.e., 159). Now, the standardized mortality ratio is:

$$SMR = \frac{129}{159} = 0.81$$

Therefore, the death rate from pneumonia and influenza is 19% lower among blacks than whites, after adjusting for differences in the age distribution.

8. Yes, we would not age-adjust if the age distributions were similar among the groups being compared.

9. Trends in age-specific rates are assumed to be similar.

10. When a rate is age-adjusted, it reflects what the rate would be if the population distribution were the same as some standard. The selection of the standard is somewhat arbitrary. However, the value of the age-adjusted rate is that it allows us to make meaningful comparisons between and among groups with different age distributions, or within a group over time if the age distribution changes. Age-adjustment eliminates the confounding effect of age when there are differences in the age distribution among the comparison groups.

11. If two populations are being compared and one is much larger than the other, we typically use the larger population as the standard. In addition, if rates are being compared over time, we generally choose a standard within the range of years being considered. In addition, if a given standard is used by convention, such as that the 2000 U.S. population is currently the standard for cancer rates in the United States, then, to make comparisons with these rates, we should also use the 2000 U.S. population as our standard.

CHAPTER 4

1.

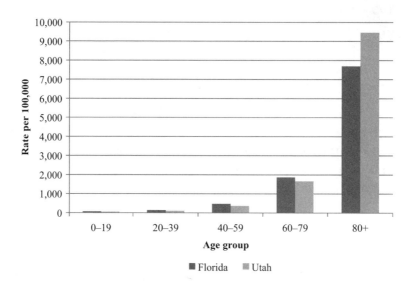

In Excel, highlight the data to be plotted, go to Insert-Chart, and choose the bar graph. To enter the labels on the horizontal axis, go to Design-Select, Data-Edit, and highlight the data for the axis labels, then click OK.

2. A, E; A; A; B, C, D

3.

Stem	Leaf	Stem	Leaf
29	1	25	
28	27	24	59
27		23	
26	17	22	038

The following SAS code can also generate this stem-and-leaf plot:

```
DATA EXERCISE2_21;
INPUT PCTOBESE @@;
DATALINES;
28.2 29.1 26.1 22 22.8 24.5 26.7 24.9 22.3 28.7
;
PROC UNIVARIATE PLOT;
RUN;
```

4. To construct the box plot, you need the following information (left panel): first quartile, second quartile (median), third quartile, minimum, and maximum values. You can plot this by hand, or you can use Excel or SAS to obtain the box plot. The SAS code in the previous problem will generate a box plot.

Average	25.53	Average	25.53
Min	22	25th	22.8
Q1	22.8	50th	2.7
Median	25.5	75th	2.7
Q3	28.2	Min	0.8
Max	29.1	Max	0.9

To construct a box plot in Excel, put the data in the spreadsheet as shown above (right panel). (Note that 2.7 = 25.5 − 22.8; 2.7 = 28.2 − 25.5; 0.8 = 22.8 − 22; and 0.9 = 29.1 − 28.2.) Select the cells 25th and 22.8, go to Insert-Column, and choose the stacked bar chart. Next, copy the cells 50th and 2.7 and paste it on the graph. Then copy the cells 75th and 2.7 and paste it on the graph. Now select the top box and go to Layout-Error, Bars-More Error Bars, Options-Plus-Custom-Specify, Value-Positive, Error Value, choose the cell containing

0.9, and then click OK. Next, select the bottom box and go to Layout-Error, Bars-More Error Bars, Options-Minus-Custom-Specify, Value-Negative, Error Value, choose the cell containing 0.8, and then click OK. Now select the bottom box and go to Format-Shape, Fill, and choose No Fill. Next, highlight the legends on the right and delete. In addition, choose the value on the bottom of the graph and delete. To get rid of the grid lines, go to Layout-Gridlines-Primary Horizontal Gridlines, and click None. Finally, select the boxes and go to Format-Shape, Outline, and choose black. Also, go to Format-Shape, Fill, and select No Fill.

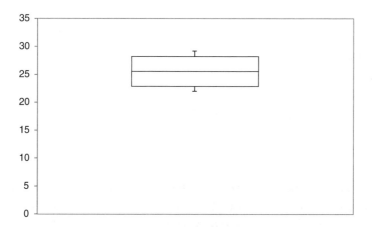

5. Using Excel, the following graph was created. On average, 5-year observed survival is about 6% higher for white males than black males. Survival improved for both black and white male patients over the study period. However, in the most recent 5 years, there is a leveling off around 52% for white males and 44% for black males.

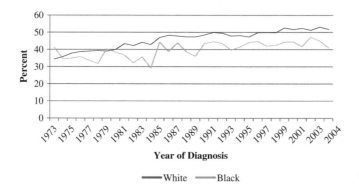

Five-year observed survival for colon cancer in the United States for white and black males.

6. Using Excel, the following graph was created. On average, 5-year observed survival is above 4% higher for white females than black females. Survival improved for both black and white female patients over the study period. However, in the most recent 5 years, there is a leveling off around 51% for white females and 45% for black females.

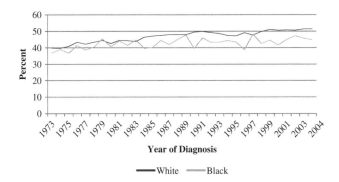

Five-year observed survival for colon cancer in the United States for white and black females.

7. Using Excel, the following graph was created. On average, 5-year observed survival is above 8% higher for whites than blacks across the age span. Survival decreases with age at diagnosis, more so after age 50.

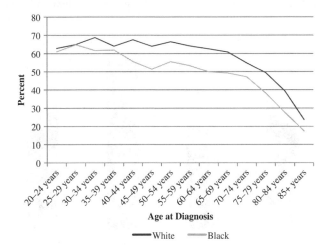

Five-year observed survival for colon cancer in the United States for whites and blacks diagnosed in 2000–2004 by age at diagnosis.

8. Using Excel, the following graph was created. Plotting the data on a logarithmic scale allows us to focus on the rate of change.

The rate of change is nearly constant through about age 50, and then decreases.

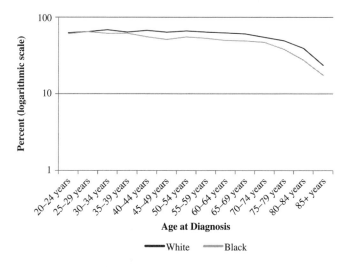

Five-year observed survival for colon cancer in the United States for whites and blacks diagnosed in 2000–2004 by age at diagnosis.

In Excel, the logarithmic scale was obtained by selecting the left axis and going to Format-Format, Selection, and then clicking the box next to Logarithmic Scale.

9.

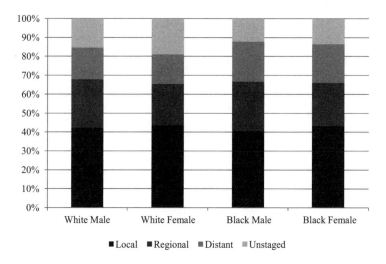

Liver cancer in the United States according to stage, gender, and race.
Source: Surveillance, Epidemiology, and End Results, 2006–2008.

10.

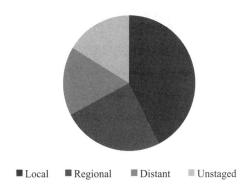

■ Local   ■ Regional   ■ Distant   ■ Unstaged

Liver cancer in the United States according to stage at diagnosis.

11.

$$Approximate\ number\ of\ classes = \lceil 2 \times 30 \rceil^{0.3333} = 3.9 \approx 4$$

$$Approximate\ class\ interval\ (width) = \frac{32 - 0}{4} = 8$$

Number of absences	Number of observations	Number of absences	Number of observations
0–3	8	16–19	3
4–7	5	20–23	3
8–11	5	24–27	1
12–15	4	28–31	1

Using Excel, we obtained the following:

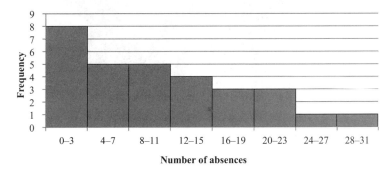

Histogram of absent employees for selected class intervals.

12. Using Excel, the following scatter plot was made.

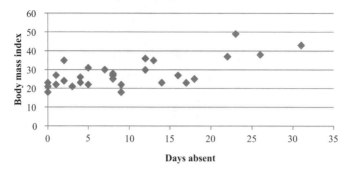

Scatter plot showing the relationship between body mass index and days absent.

There is a positive relationship between days absent and BMI.

13. The site http://www.uvm.edu/~agri99/spring2004/Population_Pyramids_in_Excel.html provides a nice step-by-step example of how to construct a population pyramid in Excel.

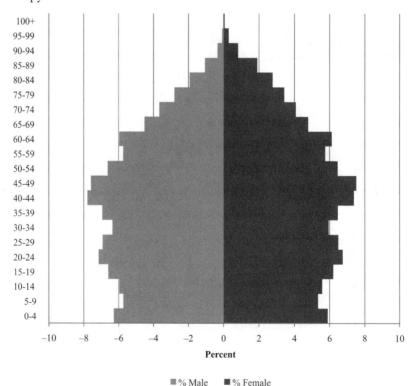

Population pyramid for the United Kingdom, 2010.
Data source: U.S. Census Bureau.

This is a constrictive population pyramid in that there is a lower number or percentage of younger people. The people are generally older, as the country has a long life expectancy and a low death rate, but also a low birth rate. This is a typical pattern of developed countries, probably the result of factors such as easy access and incentive to use birth control, good health care, and few negative environmental factors.

14. To construct this data in Excel, sum the data for the age groups, as follows:

Age	Males	Females	Ratio
0–14	5,555,089	5,283,031	0.95
15–39	10,497,145	10,006,397	0.95
40–69	11,804,941	11,946,711	1.01
70+	3,067,510	4,187,623	1.37

Select the highlighted cells in Excel, go to Insert, and select the 2-D bar option. Select the horizontal axis, then Format and Format Selection. Under Axis Options, Vertical Axis Crosses: choose Axis Value Equal to 1. Click and delete the legend. Finally, select the Layout tab and add a chart title.

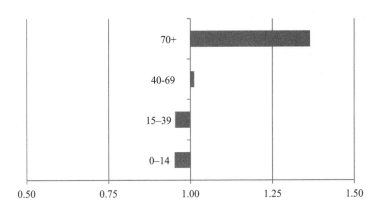

Female-to-male ratio in the United Kingdom.

15. The answer to this question depends on the map you choose to construct.

CHAPTER 5

1.

Age	Probability of dying between ages x to $x + n$ $_nq_x$	Number surviving to age x l_x	Number dying between ages x to $x + n$ $_nd_x$	Person-years lived between ages x to $x + n$ $_nL_x$	Total number of person-years lived about age x T_x	Expectation of life at age x e_x
0–<1	0.006760	100,000	676	99,662	7,792,893	77.9
1–4	0.001140	99,324	113	397,070	7,693,231	77.5
5–9	0.000683	99,211	68	495,884	7,296,161	73.5
10–14	0.000839	99,143	83	495,507	6,800,277	68.5
15–19	0.003089	99,060	306	494,534	6,304,769	63.6
20–24	0.004907	98,754	485	492,558	5,810,235	58.8
25–29	0.004958	98,269	487	490,128	5,317,678	54.1
30–34	0.005524	97,782	540	487,560	4,827,549	49.4
35–39	0.007251	97,242	705	484,447	4,339,990	44.6
40–44	0.011003	96,537	1,062	480,028	3,855,543	39.9
45–49	0.016870	95,475	1,611	473,346	3,375,515	35.4
50–54	0.025217	93,864	2,367	463,402	2,902,168	30.9
55–59	0.035858	91,497	3,281	449,283	2,438,766	26.7
60–64	0.052469	88,216	4,629	429,509	1,989,483	22.6
65–69	0.077793	83,587	6,503	401,681	1,559,975	18.7
70–74	0.119029	77,085	9,175	362,486	1,158,294	15.0
75–79	0.191290	67,910	12,990	307,072	795,807	11.7
80–84	0.297734	54,919	16,351	233,718	488,735	8.9
85–89	0.441765	38,568	17,038	150,244	255,018	6.6
90–94	0.612438	21,530	13,186	74,685	104,773	4.9
95–99	0.778825	8,344	6,499	25,474	30,088	3.6
100+	1.000000	1,846	1,846	4,614	4,614	2.5

2.

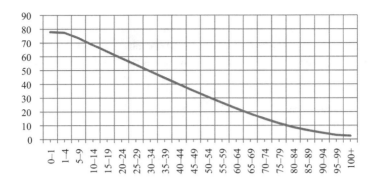

Expected years of life remaining, conditioned on surviving to age *x*.

3.

Age	q_x Population	q_x^1 Malignant cancer	q_x^2 Accidents and adverse effects	q_x^3 Suicide and self-inflicted injury	q_x^4 All other
0–<1	0.00586	0.00002	0.00018	0.00000	0.00567
1–4	0.00107	0.00006	0.00034	0.00000	0.00067
5–9	0.00065	0.00012	0.00023	0.00000	0.00030
10–14	0.00072	0.00011	0.00024	0.00000	0.00037
15–19	0.00191	0.00012	0.00094	0.00015	0.00070
20–24	0.00242	0.00024	0.00109	0.00017	0.00092
25–29	0.00292	0.00023	0.00094	0.00023	0.00152
30–34	0.00345	0.00060	0.00073	0.00025	0.00188
35–39	0.00529	0.00123	0.00087	0.00029	0.00290
40–44	0.00839	0.00234	0.00126	0.00038	0.00441
45–49	0.01317	0.00415	0.00153	0.00041	0.00708
50–54	0.01953	0.00660	0.00143	0.00040	0.01111
55–59	0.02810	0.01070	0.00108	0.00028	0.01604
60–64	0.04346	0.01600	0.00120	0.00031	0.02595
65–69	0.06685	0.02414	0.00130	0.00011	0.04129
70–74	0.10127	0.03168	0.00171	0.00020	0.06768
75–79	0.16141	0.04037	0.00306	0.00021	0.11777
80–84	0.25045	0.04579	0.00599	0.00008	0.19859
85+	1.00000	0.08852	0.02298	0.00026	0.88824

4.

Age	l_x Total	d_x^1 Malignant cancer	d_x^2 Accidents and adverse effects	d_x^3 Suicide and self-inflicted injury	d_x^4 All other
0–<1	1,000,000	20	176	0	5,668
1–4	994,136	62	335	0	665
5–9	993,074	118	224	0	302
10–14	992,430	111	239	0	367
15–19	991,713	117	932	152	692
20–24	989,819	237	1,075	172	908
25–29	987,427	225	928	231	1,502
30–34	984,540	590	715	244	1,848
35–39	981,143	1,206	852	286	2,846
40–44	975,953	2,281	1,228	371	4,308
45–49	967,765	4,017	1,478	399	6,848
50–54	955,024	6,305	1,362	379	10,606
55–59	936,371	10,020	1,015	261	15,016
60–64	910,059	14,560	1,093	286	23,613
65–69	870,508	21,017	1,132	100	35,943
70–74	812,316	25,735	1,392	162	54,975
75–79	730,053	29,469	2,237	153	85,978
80–84	612,216	28,033	3,665	52	121,580
85+	458,885	40,618	10,544	121	407,602

5.

Age	W_x^1 Malignant cancer	W_x^2 Accidents and adverse effects	W_x^3 Suicide and self-inflicted injury	W_x^4 All other
0–<1	184,743	30,622	3,367	781,268
1–4	184,722	30,445	3,367	775,601
5–9	184,661	30,110	3,367	774,936
10–14	184,543	29,886	3,367	774,634
15–19	184,432	29,647	3,367	774,266
20–24	184,315	28,715	3,215	773,575
25–29	184,078	27,640	3,043	772,666
30–34	183,852	26,712	2,812	771,164
35–39	183,262	25,997	2,568	769,316
40–44	182,056	25,145	2,282	766,470
45–49	179,775	23,917	1,911	762,162
50–54	175,758	22,440	1,512	755,313
55–59	169,453	21,077	1,133	744,707
60–64	159,433	20,063	873	729,691
65–69	144,873	18,970	587	706,078
70–74	123,856	17,838	487	670,135
75–79	98,120	16,446	325	615,161
80–84	68,652	14,209	173	529,182
85+	40,618	10,544	121	407,602

6.

Age	F_x^1 Malignant cancer	F_x^2 Accidents and adverse effects	F_x^3 Suicide and self-inflicted injury	F_x^4 All other
0–<1	0.00000	0.00000	0.00000	0.00000
1–4	0.00011	0.00576	0.00000	0.00725
5–9	0.00044	0.01670	0.00000	0.00811
10–14	0.00108	0.02401	0.00000	0.00849
15–19	0.00168	0.03182	0.00000	0.00896
20–24	0.00231	0.06227	0.04528	0.00985
25–29	0.00360	0.09736	0.09641	0.01101
30–34	0.00482	0.12768	0.16492	0.01293
35–39	0.00801	0.15104	0.23750	0.01530
40–44	0.01454	0.17885	0.32237	0.01894
45–49	0.02689	0.21894	0.43242	0.02446
50–54	0.04863	0.26719	0.55088	0.03322
55–59	0.08276	0.31168	0.66338	0.04680
60–64	0.13700	0.34482	0.74081	0.06602
65–69	0.21581	0.38050	0.82579	0.09624
70–74	0.32958	0.41746	0.85545	0.14225
75–79	0.46888	0.46291	0.90343	0.21261
80–84	0.62839	0.53598	0.94874	0.32266
85+	0.78013	0.65568	0.96407	0.47828

7. YPLL: 65,517 for malignant cancers, 53,725 for accidents and adverse effects, and 10,530 for suicide and self-inflicted injury.

Age group	Mid-point (age)	Years to 65	Malignant cancer Deaths	Accidents and adverse effects Deaths	Suicide and Self-Inflicted injury Deaths	Population	Malignant cancer Age-Specific YPLL	Accidents and adverse effects Age-specific YPLL	Suicide and Inflicted Injury Age-Specific YPLL	Malignant cancer Cumulative YPLL	Accidents and adverse effects Cumulative YPLL	Suicide and self-inflicted injury Cumulative YPLL
0	0.5	64.5	4	35	0	197,736	258	2,258	0	65,517	53,725	10,530
1–4	3	62	12	65	0	771,419	744	4,030	0	65,259	51,468	10,530
5–9	7.5	57.5	21	40	0	886,569	1208	2,300	0	64,515	47,438	10,530
10–14	12.5	52.5	19	41	0	850,680	998	2,153	0	63,308	45,138	10,530
15–19	17.5	47.5	20	159	26	844,815	950	7,553	1,235	62,310	42,985	10,530
20–24	22.5	42.5	40	181	29	832,569	1,700	7,693	1,233	61,360	35,433	9,295
25–29	27.5	37.5	40	165	41	876,216	1,500	6,188	1,538	59,660	27,740	8,063
30–34	32.5	32.5	99	120	41	824,416	3,218	3,900	1,333	58,160	21,553	6,525
35–39	37.5	27.5	211	149	50	856,043	5,803	4,098	1,375	54,943	17,653	5,193
40–44	42.5	22.5	394	212	64	839,219	8,865	4,770	1,440	49,140	13,555	3,818
45–49	47.5	17.5	715	263	71	855,627	1,2513	4,603	1,243	40,275	8,785	2,378
50–54	52.5	12.5	1,032	223	62	773,939	1,2900	2,788	775	27,763	4,183	1,135
55–59	57.5	7.5	1,422	144	37	655,083	10,665	1,080	278	14,863	1,395	360
60–64	62.5	2.5	1,679	126	33	513,329	4,198	315	83	4,198	315	83
65–69	67.5		1,894	102	9	379,124						
70–74	72.5		2,071	112	13	310,299						
75–79	77.5		2,318	176	12	263,955						
80–84	82.5		2,172	284	4	207,471						
85+			2,350	610	7	214,904						

8. Ages 50–54 for malignant cancers, ages 20–24 for accidents and adverse effects, and ages 25–29 for suicide and self-inflicted injury.
9. 619 per 100,000 for malignant cancer, 508 per 100,000 for accidents and adverse effects, and 100 per 100,000 for suicide and self-inflicted injury.
10. This value is often used because it is the retirement age and is thus seen from a strictly economic point of view. However, we may wish to consider social aspects as well, such that average life expectancy may be a more appropriate endpoint.

CHAPTER 6

1. If an experiment is repeated n times under the same conditions, and if the event A occurs m times, then as n grows larger, the ratio m/n approaches a fixed limit that is the probability of A. $P(A) = P(A) = \dfrac{m}{n}$.
2. Intersection, union, and complement. Refer to Figure 6.1.
3. Mutually exclusive events involve two or more events for which the occurrence of one event precludes the occurrence of the other(s). Independent events are events whose occurrence or outcome has no effect on the probability of the other. There is a link between mutually exclusive events in that they cannot both happen at once. However, there is no link between independent events.
4. When the events are mutually exclusive.
5. $P(A \cup B) = P(A) + P(B) - P(A \cap B)$
6. $P(A \cup B) = P(A) + P(B) = 0.15 + 0.10 = 0.25$
7. When events are independent. $P(A \cap B) = P(A)P(B)$
8. $P(A \cap B) = P(A)P(B|A)$
9.

$$P(Man|No) = \frac{P(Man \ and \ No)}{P(No)} = \frac{189/461}{384/461} = \frac{189}{384} = 0.492$$

$$P(Man) = \frac{219}{461} = 0.475$$

Because, $P(Man|No) \neq P(No)$, the events Man and No Voice Disorder are not independent.

10. We know $P(G_1)$ equals ½. We also know that $P(G_2)$ equals ½. Because this is an independent process, $P(G_2|G_1) = P(G_2) = ½$. Thus, $P(G_1, G_2) = P(G_2|G_1) \times P(G_1) = P(G_2) \times P(G_1) = (½)(½) = ¼$.

11. $P(Unmarried) = \dfrac{1,693,848}{4,131,019 + 1,693,848} = 0.291$

12. $P(Unmarried | < 15) = \dfrac{P(Unmarried\ and\ < 15)}{P(< 15)} = \dfrac{4,980/5,824,867}{10,010/5,824,867} = \dfrac{4,980}{10,010} = 0.498$

13. No, because $P(Unmarried) \neq P(Unmarried | < 15)$.

14. $1 - (0.198 + 0.097 + 0.24) = 1 - 0.319 = 0.681$

15. $P(< 20 | < 30) = \dfrac{0.133}{0.681} = 0.1953$

16. $P(married\ and\ 20 - 29) = 0.6808 \times 0.5480 = 0.373$

17. $P(Married) = 1 - P(Unmarried) = 1 - 0.291 = 0.709$

18. Bayes' Theorem relates the probability of the occurrence of an event to the presence or nonpresence of an associated event; that is, it shows that if we know the conditional probability of B given A, we can identify the conditional probability of A given B.

19. $Sensitivity = \dfrac{285}{285 + 15} = 0.95;\ Specificity = \dfrac{8,730}{970 + 8,730} = 0.90$. Therefore, of those who are abused, 95% are identified through the physical exam. Of those who are not abused, 90% are determined to not be physically abused through the physical exam.

20. PV+ = 0.227, meaning of those who have a positive physical exam, 22.7% are abused. PV– = 0.998, meaning of those who have a negative physical exam, 99.8% are not abused.

21. Cluster sampling.

22. Stratified random sample.

23. When a cyclic repetition is inherent in the sampling frame. For example, systematic sampling should not involve months of the year if we are evaluating skiing injuries or automobile accidents because these events are more common in cold-weather months.

24. If the convenience sample sufficiently represents the target population.

25. Once the spreadsheet is open, put the curser in any given cell. Then type =RANDBETWEEN(1, 500) and press the Enter key. This will give a random number, somewhere from the bottom to the top number specified. Then, copy this formula and paste it down the next 99 cells.

CHAPTER 7

1. A variable is any characteristic that can be measured or categorized. If any particular outcome of a variable is determined by chance, it is a random variable.

2. Every random variable has a corresponding probability distribution. A probability distribution describes the behavior of the random variable.

3. A parameter is a measure from a population, whereas a statistic is a measure from a sample. We denote population parameters using Greek letters (e.g., σ, β, μ, ρ) and sample statistics using Roman letters (e.g., s, b, $\overline{X}$, r).

4. (1) There is a fixed number of trials n of an experiment with only two possible outcomes for each trial ("success" and "failure"). (2) The probability of a success on any given trial, designated as π, remains constant from trial to trial. Therefore, the probability of a failure is $1 - \pi$. (3) The trials are independent of one another in that the probability associated with the outcome in one trial is not influenced by the outcome in another trial.

5. (1) Sampling is conducted over an interval on some continuous medium, such as area, distance, or time. (2) Events occur independently from one interval of the medium to another. (3) Probability of the occurrence of an event increases if the interval increases. (4) The probability of more than one event occurring in a very small interval is negligible.

6. When the number of trials (n) is large, and the chance of success (f) for each trial is small, then the binomial probability is approximately equal to the Poisson probability.

7. Forms a symmetric bell-shaped curve; 50% of the scores lie above and 50% below the midpoint of the distribution; the curve is asymptotic to the x-axis; and the mean, median, and mode are located at the midpoint of the x-axis.

8. By converting normally distributed variables to the standard normal distribution, probabilities can be obtained from the standard normal distribution table. This saves us having to apply integral calculus each time we want to estimate probabilities for normally distributed variables.

9.

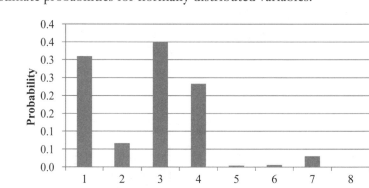

Probability distribution for eight combinations of services for cancer patients.

10. 0.310
11. 0.349
12. 0.387
13. 0.88, 2.06, 1.5
14. 0.896, 1.279, 1.129
15. 0.167, 0.302, 0.276
16. 0.180
17. 0.967
18. 0.380
19. 0.368
20. 0.252
21. A statistical rule stating that for any normal distribution, 68.2% of the data lie within ±1 standard deviation of the mean, 95.4% of the data lie within ±2 standard deviations of the mean, and 99.8% of the data lie within ±3 standard deviations of the mean. It applies when the sample size is sufficiently large such that the central limit theorem holds for smaller sample sizes that are normally distributed.
22. Chebyshev's inequality is appropriate to summarize a distribution of values when the standard deviation does not express the range clearly because of skewed data or outliers. It is a more conservative estimate for spread.
23. (1) The mean of the sampling distribution of $\overline{X}$ equals the mean of the population μ from which the sample is taken. (2) The standard deviation in the sampling distribution of $\overline{X}$ equals the standard deviation of the sampled population divided by the square root of the sample size. That is, $\dfrac{\sigma}{\sqrt{n}}$ is called the standard error of the mean. (3) If the distribution in the population is normal, then the sampling distribution of the mean is also normal. However, regardless of the shape of the original population distribution, if the sample size is sufficiently large, the sampling distribution of the mean is approximately normally distributed. A rule of thumb is that 30 is sufficient for any distribution.
24. $Z = \dfrac{X - 4.35}{4.64}$, so the mean of 4.35 is transformed to $Z = \dfrac{4.35 - 4.35}{4.64}$ and the standard deviation for the standard normal curve is 1.
25. 0.0228, 0.1587
26. 0.6826
27. 2.03

28.

$$\mu = 1{,}000 \times 0.674 = 674$$

$$\sigma^2 = 1{,}000 \times 0.674 \times 0.326 = 219.724$$

$$\sigma = \sqrt{219.724} = 14.823$$

The standardization formula is:

$$Z = \frac{X - 674}{14.823}$$

Hence,

$$P(X > 700) = P\left(\frac{X - 674}{14.823} > \frac{700 - 674}{14.823}\right) \approx P(Z > 1.75)$$

$$= 0.0401$$

Thus, there is approximately a 4.0% chance of there being at least 70% that have had a flu shot within the last year.

29. 0.0427, or 4.3%.

30. $P(Z < 4) = P\left(Z < \dfrac{\overline{X} - 4.35}{4.64/\sqrt{75}}\right) = P\left(Z < \dfrac{4 - 4.35}{4.64/\sqrt{75}}\right) = P(Z < -0.65) = 0.2578$

31. $P\left(Z \geq \dfrac{30 - 35}{12/\sqrt{30}}\right) = P\left(Z \geq \dfrac{30 - 35}{12/\sqrt{30}}\right) = P(-2.28) = 0.9887$

32.

$$3.2 \pm 2 \times 1.9 \rightarrow -0.6 \text{ to } 7$$

$$3.2 \pm 3 \times 1.9 \rightarrow -2.5 \text{ to } 8.9$$

Thus, these intervals encompass 75% and 88.9% of the number of children, respectively. However, because having fewer than 0 children is meaningless, we can say 0 to 7 encompasses 75% of the number of children, and 0 to 8.9 encompasses 88.9% of the number of children.

CHAPTER 8

1. An estimator is a statistic that is a measure from a sample. For instance, the sample mean $\overline{X}$ is a point estimator of the population mean μ. Confidence intervals define an upper limit and a lower limit with an associated probability.

The ends of the confidence interval are called the confidence limits. An interval estimate is called a confidence interval.

2. If we were to take 100 different samples from the same population and calculate the confidence limits for each, then we would expect that 95 out of these 100 intervals would contain the true value of μ, and 5 would not contain the true value of μ. Because we usually only have one sample, and hence one confidence interval, we do not know whether our interval is one of the 95 or one of the 5. In that sense, we are 95% confident.

3. Sample size, standard deviation, and the confidence coefficient. As the sample size goes up, the confidence interval gets smaller; as the standard deviation goes up, the confidence interval gets bigger; and as the confidence coefficient goes up, the confidence interval gets bigger.

4. Like the Z distribution, the t distribution is symmetric, bell-shaped, and has mean 0. It is unlike the Z distribution in that there is more area in the tails and it is not as high in the middle. The thicker tails in the t distribution result because s will vary more from sample to sample for small samples. However, s remains constant for large samples. The variability in the sampling distribution of t depends on the sample size n. As the sample size increases to 30 or more, the t distribution approximates the Z distribution.

5. A conjecture about the nature of a population.

6. A statistical hypothesis test begins with a statement about the value of the population parameter. This is called the null hypothesis, or H_0. We then make a statement that contradicts H_0, which is called the alternative (research) hypothesis, or H_a.

7. When a statistical test is used to draw a conclusion about a population, a corresponding P value is obtained. This is a measure of the probability that our result is due to chance.

8. The P value is inversely associated with sample size, so as the sample size goes up, the P value goes down. The P value is only relevant when a sample from a population is involved. The P value reflects the role of chance. Because statistical significance is directly related to sample size, it is possible for an association to be of practical significance although it is not of statistical significance (small sample size). An association may not be of practical significance, but it may be statistically significant (large sample size).

9. If the study design is used to test a specific predetermined hypothesis, then it is an analytic study.

10. Power is the probability that a statistical test will reject the null hypothesis when H_0 is false. Power is related to $\beta = P(type\ II\ error)$, where a *type II error* means to accept H_0 when H_0 is false, as follows:

$$Power = 1 - \beta = 1 - P\left(Accepting\ H_0 | H_0\ is\ false\right)$$
$$= P\left(Reject\ H_0 | H_0\ is\ false\right)$$

11.

   1. $H_0: \mu = 65\%$
   2. $H_a: \mu > 65\%$
   3. $\alpha = 0.05$, $n = 200$
   4. t statistic and $(200 - 1) = 199$ degrees of freedom
   5. $t = \dfrac{69.7 - 65}{32.5/\sqrt{200}} = 2.05$
   6. On the basis of the alternative hypothesis, we see that the rejection region is in the upper tail of the t distribution. Referring to Table 4 in Appendix B, the critical value is 1.645. Because the calculated value is in the rejection region, we reject H_0 and accept that the percentage of adults in the United States who visited the dentist within the past year is significant.

12. The 95% confidence interval is 65.2 – 74.2. Thus, we are 95% confident that the population percentage of adults who visited the dentist within the past year is between 65.2 and 74.2.

13.

   1. $H_0: \delta = 0$
   2. $H_a: \delta \neq 0$
   3. $\alpha = 0.05$, $n = 348$
   4. t statistic and $(348 - 1) = 347$ degrees of freedom
   5. $t = \dfrac{-1.53 - 0}{3.38/\sqrt{348}} = -8.44$
   6. On the basis of the alternative hypothesis, we see that the rejection region is in the lower and upper tail of the t distribution. Referring to Table 4 in Appendix B, the critical values are −1.96 and 1.96. Because the calculated value is in the rejection region, we reject H_0 and accept that the mean Beck Depression Inventory score significantly decreased.

14. −1.89 to −1.17. Thus, we are 95% confident that the mean change in the Beck Depression Inventory score over 6 weeks is between −1.89 and −1.17. Given that

the mean change is significant based on the test statistic, we also know that the confidence interval would not overlap zero, which also indicates significance.

15.

DATA EX8_15;
INPUT CHANGE @@;
DATALINES;
-8 -2 -1 1 -5 0 -5 0 -3 0

;
PROC UNIVARIATE DATA=EX8_15 PLOT;
RUN;

Results from this SAS code gave:
Signed Rank S = −12.5, with P=0.0469
Because the *P* value is less than 0.05, we reject the null hypothesis of no change and conclude otherwise.

16.

1. H_0: $\pi \geq .80$
2. H_a: $\pi < .80$
3. $\alpha = 0.05$, $n = 50$
4. Z statistic
5. $Z = \dfrac{0.75 - 0.80}{\sqrt{\dfrac{0.80(1 - 0.80)}{50}}} = -0.88$
6. The critical value is −1.645. Because our calculated value is not less than the critical value, we fail to reject the null hypothesis.

17.

1. H_0: $\pi_B - \pi_A = 0$
2. H_a: $\pi_B - \pi_A \neq 0$
3. $\alpha = 0.05$, $n = 348$
4. McNemar test, degrees of freedom = $(r - 1)(c - 1) = (2 - 1)(2 - 1) = 1$
5. $McNemar = \dfrac{(|33 - 9|)^2}{33 + 9} = 13.71$
6. To obtain the rejection region for the McNemar test, refer to Table 5 in Appendix B, which gives a critical value of 5.02. Because our calculated value is greater than the critical value, we reject the hull hypothesis and conclude that a significant decrease in depression did occur.

18. To simplify my life, I typed the following code into SAS and let the computer generate Cohen's kappa.

DATA EX8_18;
INPUT S1 S2 COUNT;
DATALINES;

1 1 22
1 2 3
2 1 8
2 2 27
;
PROC FREQ DATA=EX8_18;
TABLE S1*S2/AGREE;
WEIGHT COUNT;
RUN;
The result is Kappa = 0.6333, which reflects fair agreement.

19. $H_0: \sigma_1^2 = \sigma_2^2$ $H_a: \sigma_1^2 \neq \sigma_2^2$. $F = \dfrac{13.032}{7.453} = 1.75$. $F_{.05,173,173} \approx 1$, so reject H_0.

20.

1. $H_0: \mu_1 = \mu_2$
2. $H_a: \mu_1 \neq \mu_2$
3. $\alpha = 0.05, n = 348$

4. t $statistic$ and $v = \dfrac{\left(\left[\dfrac{13.03}{174}\right] + \left[\dfrac{7.45}{174}\right]\right)^2}{\left(\left[\dfrac{13.03}{174}\right]^2 \Big/ (174-1) + \left[\dfrac{7.45}{174}\right]^2 \Big/ (174-1)\right)} = 322.107$

5. $t_{322} = \dfrac{(-2.62 - [-0.44]) - 0}{\sqrt{\left(\dfrac{13.03}{174} + \dfrac{7.45}{174}\right)}} = -6.35$

6. Referring to Table 4 in Appendix B, the critical values are −1.96 and 1.96. Because the calculated value is in the rejection region, we reject H_0 and conclude that a decrease in depression is significantly greater for those in the intervention group.

21. $-2.18 \pm 1.96 \sqrt{\left(\dfrac{13.03}{174} + \dfrac{7.45}{174}\right)} \rightarrow -2.84$ to -1.51

22.

1. $H_0: \pi_I \geq \pi_C$
2. $H_a: \pi_I < \pi_C$

3. $\alpha = 0.05, n = 348$
4. From our sample:

$$n_1 = 174, \ f_1 = 0.1839$$

$$n_C = 174, \ f_C = 0.3046$$

$$f_{pooled} = \frac{32+53}{174+174} = 0.2443$$

5.

$$Z = \frac{0.1839 - 0.3046}{\sqrt{0.2443(1-0.2443)\left[\dfrac{1}{174} + \dfrac{1}{174}\right]}} = -2.62$$

6. Referring to Table 3 in Appendix B, the critical value is −1.645. Because the calculated value is in the rejection region, we reject H_0 and conclude that those in the intervention group compared with the control group have significantly lower levels of restless sleep after 6 weeks.

23. $(0.1839 - 0.3046) \pm 1.96 \sqrt{0.2443(1-0.2443)\left[\dfrac{1}{174} + \dfrac{1}{174}\right]} \rightarrow 0.211 \ to - 0.030$

24.

1. $H_0: \pi_I \geq \pi_C$
2. $H_a: \pi_I < \pi_C$
3. $\alpha = 0.05, n = 348$
4. Chi-square (χ^2) test with 1 degree of freedom
5.

$$\chi^2 = \frac{(32-42.5)^2}{42.5} + \frac{(53-42.5)^2}{42.5} + \frac{(142-131.5)^2}{131.5} + \frac{(121-131.5)^2}{131.5} = 6.865$$

6. Referring to Table 3 in Appendix B, the critical value is 3.84. Because the calculated value is in the rejection region, we reject H_0 and conclude that those in the intervention group compared with the control group have significantly lower levels of restless sleep after 6 weeks.

25. $H_0: \mu_1 = \mu_2 = \mu_3; \ H_a: Otherwise$
26. $F, v_1 = 3 - 1 = 2, v_2 = 348 - 3 = 345$

27. First calculate SS_W

$$SS_W = 7469.526 - 366.895 = 7102.631$$

$$MS_A = 183.447$$

$$MS_W = 20.587$$

$$F = \frac{183.447}{20.587} = 8.91$$

28. Referring to Table 6 in Appendix B, we see that the critical value that corresponds with the degrees of freedom and $\alpha = 0.05$ is approximately 3. Because our calculated F statistic is greater than this value, we reject H_0 and conclude that there is a difference in mean Beck Depression Inventory for the three weight classifications.

29. A post-hoc test would be appropriate, such as the Student-Newman-Keuls (SNK) procedure. We used the following SAS code to evaluate further:
PROC ANOVA;
CLASS BMI_CATEGORY;
MODEL BDI= BMI_CATEGORY;
MEANS BMI_CATEGORY/SNK;
RUN;

A partial output is shown here.

SNK Grouping Mean N BMI_CATEGORY

A	5.3222	180	4
B	3.5743	101	3
B	2.9254	67	2

This indicates that at baseline, there is not a significant difference in BDI between normal and overweight groups, but that obese individuals had significantly higher BDI than either the normal or the overweight group.

30. A one-way ANOVA was performed because means in the dependent variable were assessed according to the levels of a single independent variable.

CHAPTER 9

1. Applying the steps of sample size calculation gives:
   1. H_0: $\mu = 4$
   2. H_a: $\mu \neq 4$
   3. 1 or more
   4. From a prior study, we found $s = 4.6$

5. $\alpha = 0.05, \beta = 0.20$

6. $n = \left[\dfrac{(1.96 - [-0.84])4.6}{1} \right]^2 = 67.8$. Thus, to conclude that mean Beck Depression Inventory of ≤ 3 or ≥ 5 is a significant departure from the assumed BDI of 4 (with standard deviation of 4.6), we need a sample of 68.

2.

1. $H_0: \pi \leq 0.20$
2. $H_a: \pi > 0.20$
3. Assumed truth is 0.30
4. The proportion itself determines the estimated standard deviation: $\pi(1 - \pi)$
5. $\alpha = 0.05, \beta = 0.20$

6. $n = \left[\dfrac{1.645\sqrt{0.20(1-0.20)} - (-0.84)\sqrt{0.30(1-0.30)}}{0.30 - 0.20} \right]^2 = 108.8$

Rounding up to a sample size of 109 is required.

3.

1. $H_0: \mu_1 = \mu_2$
2. $H_a: \mu_1 \neq \mu_2$
3. Effect size: 0.3 (20% $\times$ 1.5)
4. 1
5. $\alpha = 0.05, \beta = 0.20$

6. $n = 2\left[\dfrac{(1.96 - [-0.84])1}{0.3} \right]^2 = 348.4$ Thus, the required sample size is 175 per group.

4.

1. $H_0: \pi_1 = \pi_2$
2. $H_a: \pi_1 \neq \pi_2$
3. 15% to 25%
4. The null hypothesis assumes the proportions are equal, and the proportion itself determines the estimated standard deviation: $\pi(1 - \pi)$
5. $\alpha = 0.05, \beta = 0.10$

6. $n = \dfrac{\left[\begin{array}{c} 1.96\sqrt{0.2(1-0.2)(1/0.5 + 1/0.5)} \\ -[-1.282]\sqrt{0.15(1-0.15)(1/0.5) + 0.25(1-0.25)(1/0.5)} \end{array} \right]^2}{(0.15 - 0.25)^2} = 668.5$

A sample size of 335 per group is required.

5. $\dfrac{1}{1 - 0.1} = 1.111$. Thus, 373 per group.

6. $\mu_1 - \mu_2 = \dfrac{2(1.96 - [-0.84])4}{\sqrt{100}} = 2.24$. In other words, 50 in each group will be able to detect a difference of 2.24 between the two groups.

7. $n' = \dfrac{3+1}{2 \times 3} \times 30 = 20$ cases; $c = 3$; 20 cases and 60 controls.

8. This requires a smaller sample size because the standardized effect size is always larger due to the fact that taking two measurements removes the between-subject part of the variability.

9.

    1. A confidence level of 95%, $\dfrac{Z_{0.05}}{2} = 1.96$

    2. Width of the confidence interval of 10

    3. The standard deviation equal to 20

$$n = \frac{4 \times 1.96 \times 20^2}{10^2} = 31.36$$

Rounding up a sample size of $n = 32$ will give us an interval that allows us to estimate the population mean of cholesterol to within 5 points with 95% confidence. A larger sample size is required if dropouts are expected.

10. The sample size formula for estimating the mean when σ is not known is:

$$n = \frac{4 \times \left(t_{\alpha/2, n-1}\right)^2 s^2}{\text{width}^2}$$

To estimate s, we take an initial sample, on a small scale. Then, once we've estimated n, the second stage of sampling occurs, which is the sample size required, minus the initial sample size.

11. From the statement of the problem, we know the following:

    1. A confidence level of 99%, $Z_{0.01/2} = 2.576$

    2. Width of the confidence interval of 0.1

    3. The standard deviation equal to $(0.80)(1 - 0.80) = 0.16$

$$n = \frac{4 \times 2.576^2 \times 0.16}{(0.1)^2} = 424.7$$

Thus, the researcher needs to test $425 - 10 = 415$ more patients.

12. Using the conservative approach where $f = 0.5$ gives:

$$n = \frac{4 \times 2.576^2 \times 0.5(0.5)}{(0.1)^2} = 663.6 \approx 664$$

CHAPTER 10 _____

1. Cross-sectional.
2. Case-study design (i.e., case report, case series).
3. Ecologic.
4. A, A, C, B, A, C, C, C, C, B
5. In observational analytic studies, researchers observe relationships between variables. In analytic experimental studies, a subset of the study participants is assigned the intervention. Alternatively, the participants are grouped according to their receipt of different levels of the intervention.
6. Prospective cohort study.
7. In the context of the cohort study design, the terms *prospective* and *retrospective* have to do with when the investigator comes on the scene to evaluate the data. If the investigator participates in classifying the cohort according to exposure status and then follows the cohort into the future to evaluate health outcome status, it is referred to as a prospective cohort study. On the other hand, if data on exposure and outcome variables are available for a cohort of people, and the investigator evaluates existing exposure and outcome data for the given cohort, it is a retrospective cohort study. Be careful not to confuse a retrospective cohort study design with a case-control study design. Although a case-control study is also considered retrospective, the word *retrospective* is used in a different sense in the context of a case-control study from its use in the context of a cohort study.
8.
   1. Enroll a group with disease ("cases") and an appropriate group without disease ("controls") and compare their patterns of previous exposure.
   2. Generally used to explore rare diseases.
   3. Useful for exploring several risk factors for a given outcome.
   4. Retrospective.
   5. The number of cases to controls may be up to 1:4. The larger number of controls to cases typically occurs to increase power in studies where only a small number of cases are available.
9.
   1. Categorize subjects on the basis of exposure and then follow up to see if they develop the health condition of interest.
   2. After some time, compare the disease rate for the exposed with that of the unexposed.
   3. The period of follow-up varies from a few days for acute diseases to several decades for chronic diseases (e.g., cancer, heart disease).

4. Generally used when the exposure is rare.
5. Useful when there are several outcomes related to a given exposure.
6. Generally prospective, although may be retrospective.

10. In a standard cohort study, the cohort is classified according to exposure status. The cohort may reflect an entire population or a representative sample from the population. In a double-cohort study, two distinct populations or samples of individuals are obtained. One sample may represent exposure to a potential risk factor, and the second sample may be taken from a group of individuals with no exposure or with a lower level of exposure.

11.

1. It is useful for deriving incidence and for describing the natural history of disease and health-related events.
2. It allows us to establish the temporal sequence of events from an exposure to an adverse health outcome.
3. It is an appropriate design to study certain rapidly fatal diseases.
4. It allows us to study multiple potential adverse health outcomes related to a given exposure, such as selected health outcomes related to smoking. The longer a cohort is followed, the more potential health outcomes can be assessed.

12. (1) Less prone to recall bias than a case-control study; (2) smaller sample size required than in a cohort study.

13. A, C, A, D, B

14. Selection bias occurs when the way participants are selected into a study causes the association between exposure and outcome variables to differ from the relationship in the population of interest.

15. Recruit from all individuals in the population.

16. Systematic error that arises from inaccurate measurements or misclassification of subjects according to exposure and outcome status (also called measurement bias). For example, in a case-control study, observation bias results from differential accuracy of recall between cases and controls (recall bias), or because of differential accuracy of exposure information because an interviewer probes cases differently than controls (interviewer bias).

17. If workers represent the exposed group and a sample from the general population represents the unexposed group, bias occurs if the workers are healthier on average than the general population.

18. Selection bias results in the estimated association between exposure and outcome variables if the extent of loss to follow-up is associated with both the exposure and the outcome.

19. Excluding those not likely to remain in the study; having periodic contact with participants; and providing incentives for continued participation.
20. A; A, B; C

CHAPTER 11

1. C, D, A, B
2. The scatter plot shows whether there is a linear relationship between the variables. Outliers can be readily seen using a scatter plot. Many of the statistical measures of association for measuring the relationship between numerical variables assume a linear relationship.
3. Spearman's rank correlation.
4. We will use the t ratio with 441 degrees of freedom. Then:

$$t = \frac{0.394\sqrt{443-2}}{\sqrt{1-0.394^2}} = 9.00$$

which corresponds with $P < 0.0001$. So we reject H_0 and conclude there is a positive relationship between these variables. (A negative t value would have indicated a negative relationship.)
5. $r^2 = 0.155$; 15.5% of the variation in emotional health is explained by general health.
6. If the scatter plot had indicated outlying values. Because the data associating general health and emotional health were fairly linear, Spearman's rank correlation (i.e., 0.394) is similar in value to the Pearson correlation coefficient (i.e., 0.378).
7. a.

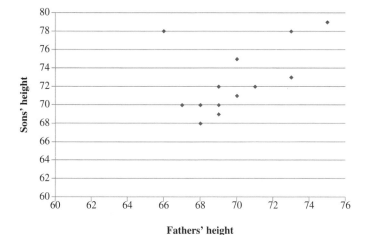

Fathers' height

b.   There is one outliers.

c. $r = 0.522$

d. $t = 2.12$. Because this value is less than the critical value of 2.179, we fail to reject H_0.

e. $r_s = 0.535$

f.   The Spearman rank correlation coefficient is smaller than the Pearson correlation coefficient.

g. $t = 2.19$. We reject H_0 and conclude that there is a positive association between the heights of the fathers and of the sons.

8.   Consider transforming the data.

9.   The correlation coefficient ranges from –1 to 1 and indicates the strength of the linear relationship between variables. The slope coefficient of simple regression also assumes a linear relationship but indicates the amount of variation in the dependent variable explained by a unit change in the independent variable.

10.   This method assumes that (1) for each value of X, Y is normally distributed; (2) that the standard deviation of the outcomes Y do not change over X; (3) that the outcomes Y are independent; and (4) that a linear relationship exists between X and Y.

11.   Often the results no longer make sense as we obtain unrealistic estimates.

12.   It can indicate whether the model assumptions hold (see response to question 9).

13.

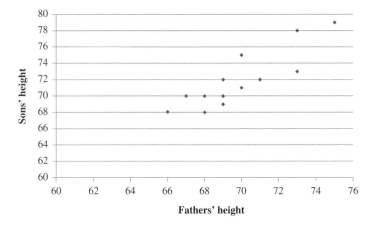

Each of the assumptions is satisfied. Note that for a simple linear regression model, we can evaluate a scatter plot to evaluate the assumptions. In a multiple regression model, a residual plot is needed.

14. $r^2 = 0.867$. The amount of variability in the son's height explained by the father's height is 86.7%.

15. *Slope* = 1.15. For each inch increase in the father's height, the son's height increases by 1.15 inches, on average.

16. $t = \dfrac{1.15}{0.190} = 6.05$. At the 0.05 level of significance, the critical value is 2.179 for a two-tailed test or 1.782 for a one-tailed test. In either case, we reject H_0 and conclude that there is a positive association between the heights of the fathers and sons.

17. Normality, constant variance, independence, and linearity.

18. First, the model explains 14.3% of the variation in emotional health. Second,

   1. $H_0: \beta_1 = 0$

   2. $H_a: \beta_1 \neq 0$

   3. $\alpha = 0.05$, $n = 443$

   4. t statistic with $n - 2 = 441$ degrees of freedom

   5. $t = \dfrac{0.366}{0.043} = 8.51$

   6. At the 0.05 level of significance, the critical value is 1.96 for a two-tailed test, so we reject H_0 and conclude that there is a positive association between general health and emotional health.

19. The assumptions appear to be satisfied.

20. $0.366 \pm 1.96 \times 0.043 \rightarrow 0.282$ to 0.450

21. The t value for general health is 8.21 ($P < 0.0001$), for age is -1.77 ($P = 0.0773$), and for gender is 2.59 ($P = 0.0100$). Hence, age is marginally insignificant and gender is significant at the 0.05 level. General health remains statistically significant after adjusting for both age and gender. Finally, including age and gender in the model increased the coefficient of determination to 16.0%. General health and gender are positively associated with emotional health, and age is negatively associated with general health (albeit marginally insignificant). (Note that in a multiple regression model, the adjusted r^2 should be used.)

22. The dependent variable does not follow a normal distribution.

23. An alternative to using PROC GENMOD is PROC LOGISTIC. The SAS code for this problem is as follows:

DATA EXERCISE11_23;

INPUT DISTANCE CASE $ COUNT;

DATALINES;

1 YES 40

```
1 NO 100
2 YES 35
2 NO 100
3 YES 30
3 NO 100
4 YES 15
4 NO 100
5 YES 12
5 NO 100
;
```
PROC LOGISTIC DATA=EXERCISE11_23 DESC;
MODEL CASE = DISTANCE;
WEIGHT COUNT;
RUN;

The output indicates that the model is significant (likelihood ratio $P < 0.0005$). $OR = 0.737$; 95% CI: 0.638–0.852. Thus, there is a significant negative relationship between the putative site and farther distance away from the site. We are 95% confident that the true OR is between 0.638 and 0.852.

24.

Odds Ratio $= exp(-0.3045) = 0.737$

95% $CI : exp(-0.3045 \pm 1.96 \times 0.0739) \rightarrow 0.638 - 0.852$

25.

1. $H_0: \beta_1 = 0$
2. $H_a: \beta_1 \neq 0$
3. $\alpha = 0.05$, $n = 366$
4. Chi-square (χ^2), 1 degree of freedom
5. Using PROC GENMOD in SAS to compute a Poisson regression for this data resulted in the following:

    $\ln(rate) = -7.142 + 1.121 \times type\ 2\ diabetes$

    $e^{1.121} = 3.069$

6. The chi-square is 60.47, with $P < 0.0001$. Hence, we reject H_0 and conclude that type 2 diabetes is positively associated with POAG.

26. 95% CI: $2.313 - 4.071$. Because this does not overlap 1, it also indicates statistical significance at the 0.05 level.

27. The rate ratio is 1.431 and the 95% *CI*: 1.160–1.766. Thus, those who smoke are 1.431 times (or 43.1%) more likely to develop coronary heart disease.
PROC GENMOD;
CLASS SMOKE AGE/DESC;
MODEL DEATH=SMOKE AGE/DIST=POISSON LINK=LOG
OFFSET=LPYEARS;
ESTIMATE 'SMOKER' SMOKE **1-1**/EXP;
RUN;

28. Odds Ratio = 1.43, 95% *CI*: 1.13 – 1.80. Because the confidence interval does not overlap 1, we reject H_0 and conclude a positive relationship between proximity to residence by a hazardous dump site and low birth weight.
DATA EXERCISE11_28;
INPUT X Y COUNT;
DATALINES;
1 1 181
1 2 4268
2 1 126
2 2 4236
;
PROC FREQ DATA=EXERCISE11_28;
TABLE X*Y/CMH;
WEIGHT COUNT;
RUN;

29.

$$Odds\ Ratio = 2.33$$

$$X^2_{df=1} = \frac{(|35-15|-1)^2}{(35+15)} = 7.22$$

$$95\%CI(1.75) = exp\left[\ln(2.33) \pm 1.96 \times \sqrt{\frac{1}{35} + \frac{1}{15}}\right]$$

$$\rightarrow 1.27 - 4.27$$

Referring to Table 5 in Appendix B, the critical value is 3.84, so we reject H_0 and conclude a positive relationship between teaching in secondary grades and a history of voice disorders.

30.

1. H_0: $OR = 1$
2. H_a: $OR \neq 1$

3. $\alpha = 0.05$, $n = 4,156$
4. Chi-square (χ^2) test with 1 degree of freedom
5. $\chi_1^2 = 0.985$; OR = 0.99; 95% CI: 0.847 – 1.146.
6. Because the 95% confidence interval overlaps 1, we conclude that there is not a statistical association between oral contraceptive use and breast cancer.

31. *Risk Ratio* $= \dfrac{0.389}{0.306} = 1.27$, with 95% CI: 1.14 – 1.43, and $\chi^2 = 17.55$. The association is statistically significant. Therefore, white men diagnosed with stage IV prostate cancer in the age range 70–79 years are 1.27 times (or 27%) more likely to survive 5 years after diagnosis than black men.

32. $RR_{MH} = 1.29$, with 95% CI: 1.15 – 1.44, and $\chi^2_{MH} = 19.11$. There remains a significant association between race and survival among prostate cancer after adjusting for age.

33. Daughters of mothers with a postsecondary education compared with a secondary education are 1.94 times (or 94%) more likely to have an eating disorder, with 95% CI: 1.07 – 3.54. $\chi^2 = 4.75$, $P = 0.0293$. The confidence interval and chi-square both indicate statistical significance.

```
DATA EXERCISE11_33;
INPUT EXPOSED $ CASES PYEARS;
LPYEARS = LOG(PYEARS);
DATALINES;
1 21 80468
2 22 43358
;

PROC GENMOD DATA=EXERCISE11_33;
CLASS EXPOSED;
MODEL CASES = EXPOSED/DIST = POISSON
LINK=LOG OFFSET = LPYEARS;
ESTIMATE 'MOTHER_EDU' EXPOSED -1 1/EXP;
RUN;
```

34.

1. H_0: *Prevalence Ratio* $= 1$
2. H_a: *Prevalence Ratio* $\neq 1$
3. $\alpha = 0.05$, $n = 453$
4. Chi-square with 1 degree of freedom
5. *Prevalence Ratio* $= 2.25$, $\chi^2_{df=1} = 14.84$

6. Referring to Table 5 in Appendix B, the calculated chi-square corresponds with $P < 0.001$, so we reject H_0 and conclude that there is a positive association between respiratory allergies and voice disorders.

35. 95% *CI*: 1.50 – 3.39

36. The odds ratio approximates the risk ratio when the outcome of interest is rare, affecting less than 10% of the population.

37. $AR = 24.6$ per 100,000; the excess risk of having an eating disorder among mothers with a postsecondary education attributed to the higher education is 24.6 per 100,000.

$AR\% = 48.6\%$; among daughters with an eating disorder whose mothers had a postsecondary education, 48.6% of those cases are attributed to the higher education of their mothers.

$PAR = 8.6$ per 100,000; the excess risk of daughters with eating disorders in the population attributed to the higher education of their mothers is 8.6 per 100,000.

$PAR\% = 24.8\%$; 24.8% of daughters with eating disorders can be attributed to the higher education of their mothers.

Each of these statements assumes that a causal relationship exists between the risk of eating disorder and education.

38. Herd immunity is a characteristic of a population or group of people wherein the population or group is mostly protected from a disease by immunity, making the chance of a major epidemic very unlikely. Herd immunity thresholds for vaccine-preventable diseases are generally 80 to 90%. Jonas Salk, who helped develop the polio vaccine, suggested that a herd immunity threshold of 85% was adequate to prevent a polio epidemic.

39.

1. $H_0: \rho \leq 0$
2. $H_a: \rho > 0$
3. The anticipated effect size $(r) = 0.25$
4. Variability is a function of r and is included in the formula
5. α (one-tailed) $= 0.05$ and $\beta = 0.2$

$$C = 0.5 \times \ln\left(\frac{[1 + 0.25]}{[1 - 0.25]}\right) = 0.255$$

$$n = ([1.645 + 0.84] \div 0.255)^2 + 3 = 97.7$$

Thus, a sample size of 98 is required.

CHAPTER 12 _____

1. The strongest methodological design is a between-group design in which the outcome of interest is compared between one group receiving the intervention of interest and another group receiving no active treatment (preferably a placebo) or a currently accepted treatment. A within-group design (also called a time-series design) may also be used, but the outcome of interest is compared before and after an intervention. The between-group design is more prone to individual type confounding factors (e.g., gender, race, genetic susceptibility). The within-group design is more susceptible to confounding from time-related factors (e.g., learning effects where participants do better on follow-up cognitive tests because they learned from the baseline test, influences from the media, or other external factors).

2. A placebo is an inactive substance or treatment (i.e., containing no pharmacological activity) given to satisfy a patient's expectation of treatment. Placebos are commonly used in drug trials. For example, one group is given a real medication and another group is given a placebo that looks just like the real medication to determine whether differences between treated and control groups are from the medication or from the power of suggestion.

3. Randomization eliminates the source of bias in treatment assignment, assuming the sample size is sufficiently large; randomization facilitates blinding the type of treatment to participants, investigators, and evaluators; and randomization permits the use of probability theory to express the level of chance in explaining the difference between outcomes.

4. Blinding is used to control for bias. The cast of characters in a clinical trial are the treating physicians, patients, and assessing investigators. A problem may arise if patients try to get well in order to please their physicians. A placebo effect is a response to medical intervention that results from the intervention itself, not from the specific mechanism of action of the intervention. In a drug study, a placebo is a pill of the same size, color, and shape as the treatment. However, in nondrug studies, it may be impossible or unethical to use a placebo. Even in drug studies, one treatment may have characteristic side effects known to the patient, making blinding ineffective (e.g., flushing and headache with nitrites). More subjective outcomes call for a more serious consideration of placebo. Placebos also improve comparability of treatment groups in terms of compliance and follow-up. Treating physicians and outcome-assessing investigators are often the same people. Most investigators are honest, but believe strongly in their work. Unconscious bias in assessing an outcome is

difficult to rule out in such cases. The most effective way to rule out unconscious bias is to blind.

5. A, B, C, C, A, A
6. Intent-to-treat analysis compares outcomes between intervention and control groups, with each participant analyzed according to his or her random group assignment, regardless of whether he or she adhered to the assigned intervention. Although this approach may underestimate the treatment effect, it also minimizes bias.
7. A, B, E, D, C
8. This is an efficient design that allows us to test two hypotheses for the price of one.
9. Run-in design.
10. Randomized matched-paired design.
11. Ensure the accumulation of an adequate number of cases that will develop the outcome.

CHAPTER 13

1. Survival analysis involves modeling time to failure or time to event. The outcome variable is dichotomous (binary). Survival analysis is able to account for censoring, compare survival between two or more groups, and assess the relationship between covariates and survival time.
2. Censoring is when we do know the exact survival time. Censoring generally occurs because an individual does not experience the event before the end of the study, is lost to follow-up, or withdraws from the study.
3. A survival function $S(t)$ characterizes a distribution of survival times. It is the probability that an individual survives beyond some specified time t. When T is a continuous random variable, then $S(t) = P(T > t)$.
4. The life table method groups survival times into intervals, whereas the product limit method uses exact survival times.
5.

Time since beginning of follow-up (months)	Number at beginning l_t	Deaths d_t	Probability of dying during the time interval $q_t = \dfrac{d_t}{l'}$	Probability of surviving the time interval $p_t = 1 - q_t$	Cumulative survival $\hat{S}(t)$
0	17	0	0.0000	1.0000	1.0000

(continues)

Time since beginning of follow-up (months)	Number at beginning I_t	Deaths d_t	Probability of dying during the time interval $q_t = \dfrac{d_t}{I'}$	Probability of surviving the time interval $p_t = 1 - q_t$	Cumulative survival $\hat{S}(t)$
1	17	5	0.2941	0.7059	0.7059
2	12	4	0.3333	0.6667	0.4706
3	8	1	0.1250	0.8750	0.4118
4	7	0	0.0000	1.0000	0.4118
5	7	1	0.1429	0.8571	0.3529
6	6	1	0.1667	0.8333	0.2941
7	5	0	0.0000	1.0000	0.2941
8	5	0	0.0000	1.0000	0.2941
9	5	0	0.0000	1.0000	0.2941
10	5	1	0.2000	0.8000	0.2353
11	4	0	0.0000	1.0000	0.2353
12	4	0	0.0000	1.0000	0.2353
13	4	0	0.0000	1.0000	0.2353
14	4	0	0.0000	1.0000	0.2353
15	4	0	0.0000	1.0000	0.2353
16	4	0	0.0000	1.0000	0.2353
17	4	1	0.2500	0.7500	0.1765

Time since beginning of follow-up (months)	Number at beginning l_t	Deaths d_t	Probability of dying during the time interval $q_t = \dfrac{d_t}{l'}$	Probability of surviving the time interval $p_t = 1 - q_t$	Cumulative survival $\hat{S}(t)$
18	3	1	0.3333	0.6667	0.1176
19	2	1	0.5000	0.5000	0.0588
20	1	0	0.0000	1.0000	0.0588
21	1	0	0.0000	1.0000	0.0588
22	1	0	0.0000	1.0000	0.0588
23	1	0	0.0000	1.0000	0.0588
24	1	0	0.0000	1.0000	0.0588
25	1	0	0.0000	1.0000	0.0588
26	1	0	0.0000	1.0000	0.0588
27	1	0	0.0000	1.0000	0.0588
28	1	0	0.0000	1.0000	0.0588
29	1	0	0.0000	1.0000	0.0588
30	1	0	0.0000	1.0000	0.0588
31	1	0	0.0000	1.0000	0.0588
32	1	0	0.0000	1.0000	0.0588
33	1	0	0.0000	1.0000	0.0588
34	1	1	1.0000	0.0000	0.0000

6.

Months	q_t	p_t	$\hat{S}(t)$
0	0.0000	1.0000	1.0000
1	0.2941	0.7059	0.7059
2	0.3333	0.6667	0.4706
3	0.1250	0.8750	0.4118
5	0.1429	0.8571	0.3529
6	0.1667	0.8333	0.2941
10	0.2000	0.8000	0.2353
17	0.2500	0.7500	0.1765
18	0.3333	0.6667	0.1176
19	0.5000	0.5000	0.0588
34	1.0000	0.0000	0.0000

DATA EXERCISE13_7_8_9;
INPUT PN TIME CENSOR;
DATALINES;

```
1    1    1
2    1    1
3    1    1
4    1    1
5    1    1
6    2    1
7    2    1
8    2    1
9    2    1
10   3    1
11   5    1
12   6    1
13   10   1
14   17   1
15   18   1
16   19   1
17   34   1
;
```

PROC LIFETEST DATA=EXERCISE13_7_8_9 PLOTS=(S);
TIME TIME*CENSOR(**0**);
RUN;

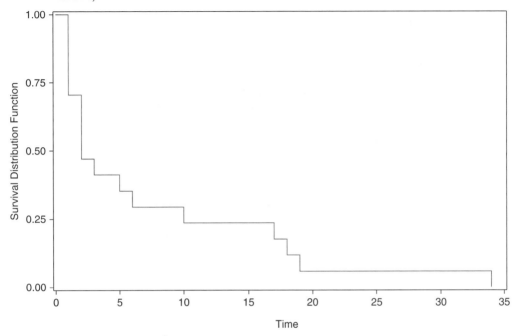

7. 2
8. 7.35
9.

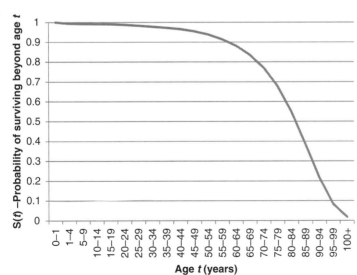

10.

1. H_0: *No difference in survival curves*
2. H_a: *Difference in survival curves*
3. $\alpha = 0.05$, $n = 38$
4. Log-rank test with 1 degree of freedom
5. Using the PROC LIFETEST in SAS gives the following:

Test of Equality over Strata			
Test	Chi-square	DF	Pr > Chi-square
Log-rank	6.1753	1	0.0130
Wilcoxon	7.0629	1	0.0079

6. Because the *P* value is less than 0.05, we reject H_0 and conclude that the survival among the ovarian cancer cases is different between the two age groups.

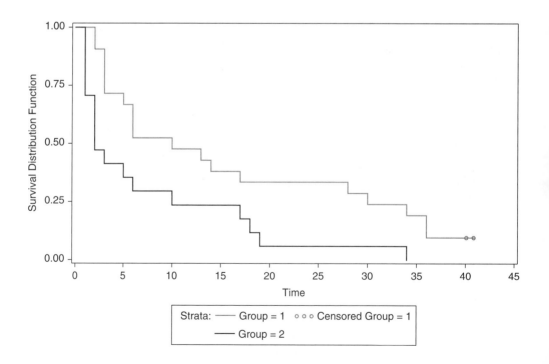

CHAPTER 14 _____

1. Causal inference involves making conclusions about associations based on lists of criteria or conditions applied to the results of scientific studies. Causal inference considers the totality of evidence in making a "judgment" about causality.

2. Statistical inference involves drawing a conclusion about a population based on information from a sample, using probability to indicate the level of reliability of the conclusion. A sufficiently large random selection of individuals assures representation. After the sample data are evaluated using appropriate statistical methods, conclusions about the prevalence and association of variables are inferred.

3. A cause produces an effect, result, or consequence in a health-related state or event. It is an event, condition, or characteristic that precedes the outcome. A change in the causal factor results in a change in the health-related state or event. If a factor is required for the outcome to occur, the causative factor is "necessary." If the outcome always occurs because of the factor, the causative factor is "sufficient."

4. Etiology is the study of causation; that is, etiology is the study of why and how things occur.

5. A risk factor is a condition or behavior that is associated with an increased risk of developing a health problem. (It may also be thought of as a component cause.) For example, risk factors for food poisoning from *Salmonella* include risk behaviors that may bring you in closer contact with *Salmonella* bacteria. Typically, a single risk factor (e.g., high blood pressure, high cholesterol, physical inactivity, obesity) is not a "sufficient cause." In other words, it often takes a combination of risk factors before conditions are sufficient to cause a health problem. For example, you may know of someone who was a chronic smoker most of his or her life, but lived to an old age and died of a disease not associated with tobacco smoking. Yet, if that person had familial adenomatous polyposis, the combination of this inherited condition and smoking may have been sufficient for death from colon cancer to occur prior to death from another cause.

6. B, A, C

7. B, A, A, D, C

8. Establishing a temporal sequence of events is fundamental to there being a causal association.

9. The prospective cohort study design. Note that an experimental study design is a special type of cohort design that is also effective at establishing a temporal sequence of events.

10. The outcome variable is usually easier to measure, because the exposure variable often occurred in the distant past and may not be directly measureable. We often must rely on indirect measures of exposure (e.g., distance lived from a waste treatment plant, or amount of water consumed). Insights into causality may still be made with indirect measures of exposure.

11. Consistency occurs when associations are replicated by different investigators in different settings and populations, using different methods. If similar associations are consistently replicated, it is unlikely that the results could be due to chance, bias, or confounding.

12. Specificity of association means that an exposure is associated with only one health outcome or that the health outcome is associated with only one exposure. Although this condition may support a causal hypothesis, failure to satisfy this criterion cannot rule out causality if more than one exposure is related to a given health outcome or if more than one health outcome is related to a given exposure.

13. If an association is causal, we would expect an increasing gradient of risk associated with greater exposure; however, it is possible that a biological gradient may be entirely explained by confounding, such as was the case between birth order and Down syndrome, where maternal age confounded this relationship.

14. Biological plausibility is the association between an exposure and disease outcome supported in terms of basic human biology. Biological evidence often requires controlled laboratory experiments. This is a vague and subjective criterion that may be difficult or impossible to apply.

15. A causal association should be consistent with known epidemiologic patterns of health-related states or events. This is a vague criterion that is difficult to distinguish from consistency or biological plausibility.

16. The ideal study design for providing information about causality is the randomized, blinded experimental control trial. This is because randomization balances the effect of confounding factors between and among groups, blinding helps minimize bias, and the comparison group allows us to evaluate the strength of statistical association. Furthermore, a temporal sequence of events and a dose-response relationship between exposure and health outcome can be effectively assessed. The next best study design for supporting causality is the cohort study, followed by the case-control study. The cohort study is better than the case-control study for supporting causal associations, because temporality and risk can be determined. All analytic epidemiologic study designs are better able to determine temporality and to control for confounding and bias than descriptive epidemiologic study designs. However,

ethics and feasibility greatly limit application of this criterion in human populations.

17. 8, 6, 7, 5, 3, 4, 1, 2

18. The agent is a causative factor, such as a pathogen or chemical; the host is an organism and is usually a human, which may be expanded to groups or populations and their characteristics; environmental factors are extrinsic factors that affect the agent and the opportunity for exposure. The agent, host, and environment interact in complex ways to produce adverse health-related states or events in humans. When we look for causes of disease, we must consider all three components. In addition, each component has time-related issues (e.g., duration of exposure, time the pathologic changes occur prior to clinical symptoms, and time in which a vector is capable of spreading an infectious agent).

19. Webs are graphic, pictorial, or paradigmatic representations of complex sets of events or conditions caused by an array of activities. The final outcome is the disease or condition. Webs can have many arms, branches, sources, inputs, and causes that are somehow interconnected or interrelated to the outcome. Webs can also have a chain of events in which some events must occur before others can take place.

20. First, a complete understanding of the causal factors and mechanisms is not required or necessary for the development of effective prevention and control measures. Second, it is possible to interrupt the production of a health problem by cutting the link(s) of occurrences of the various factors at strategic points that will stop the chain of events in the causation of the health problem.

INDEX

Figures and tables are represented by an italic *f* or *t* following the page number.